Nuclear Endocrinology

Doina Piciu

Nuclear Endocrinology

Second Edition

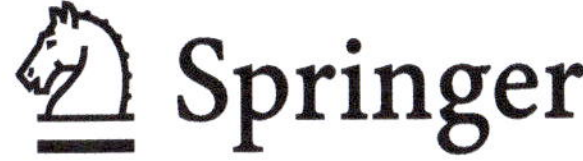

Doina Piciu
Institute of Oncology "Prof. Ion Chiricuță"
Nuclear Medicine & Endocrine Tumors
Cluj-Napoca
Romania

ISBN 978-3-319-85949-1 ISBN 978-3-319-56582-8 (eBook)
DOI 10.1007/978-3-319-56582-8

Printed on acid-free paper

This Springer imprint is published by Springer Nature
The registered company is Springer International Publishing AG
The registered company address is: Gewerbestrasse 11, 6330 Cham, Switzerland

Preface

Nothing in life is to be feared; it is only to be understood

Marie Curie

The main purpose of this book was to help educate new experts in the field of nuclear endocrinology and help clinicians to better integrate nuclear medicine methods of diagnosis and therapy into their practice. I was trying to create a brief, didactic, easy-to-use guide, dedicated to the daily activities of the endocrinologists. Even if the first major contribution of radionuclide therapy in 1940 was the application of radioactive iodine in therapy of Graves' disease, after more than 75 years, nowadays, a special clinical interest of nuclear medicine continues to be devoted to endocrinology. Spectacular achievements continue to be developed in this specialty, every day. A multidisciplinary team of endocrinologists, nuclear medicine physicians, endocrine surgeons, oncologists, etc. devoted their lives and their research to many of the issues related to both topics, endocrinology and nuclear medicine; their work inspired me and gave me the courage to put them together in this book: *Nuclear Endocrinology*.

There have been several significant advances in nuclear medicine since the publication of the first edition of *Nuclear Endocrinology*. Hybrid PET imaging, mainly PET/CT, has become a milestone of many clinical settings, including endocrinology. Nuclear and molecular medicine is a rapidly changing field, maybe with the most impressive and challenging development in the last decade. The concept of functional imaging, molecular and targeted nuclear diagnostic, and treatment of diseases is sometimes difficult to be assimilated by other medical specialties, so a dedicated update would be firstly in the benefit of patient care improvement. The purpose of the book was to give the endocrinologist a nuclear medicine physician point of view. This book is designed to ensure an update, to be an easy-to-use tool in clinical practice of endocrinologists, and to provide the most relevant information about nuclear medicine applicable to endocrine pathology.

The experience from the first edition showed that the book was equally of great interest for nuclear medicine physicians, so the detailed description of techniques was highly appreciated by these specialists; all necessary information was summarized and updated and easily accessible by those with specific interest in this topic. The book is divided into two sections: the first part of general nuclear medicine covers also general principles of nuclear physics; the second part consists of nuclear endocrinology used in diagnosis and therapy, organized by organ and by pathology. The last chapter is exclusively dedicated to hybrid imaging, mainly PET/CT in the pathologies of endocrine glands.

This book expresses my work during the past 25 years in an important nuclear medicine and endocrine tumor department, as nuclear medicine physician and endocrinologist, with thousands of patients being diagnosed and more than 10,000 patients being treated by nuclear medicine procedures. All the interesting clinical cases presented in this book are some of my patients. Behind the words and images are destinies and memories; I want to address my gratitude to all of them for being steps in further knowledge for the readers of this book.

Often, in the endocrine pathologies the success of treatment is ensured only if there is teamwork, if there is excellent collaboration between many specialists: endocrinologists, nuclear medicine physicians, surgeons, oncologists, radiologists, pathologists, geneticists, etc. To all my colleagues who honored me as part of the team, I address special thanks and deep consideration.

It is not possible to end this foreword without mentioning Mss. Ute Heilmann, Wilma McHugh, and Anna-Lena Buchholz from Springer, names that during our exceptional collaboration became friends. Only because of their confidence and their proficiency my experience, my words, and my voice are ready to be shared and heard.

I want to thank my husband Radu, for his continuous support of my profession, and my daughter Andra, who became the proudest part of my life.

Cluj-Napoca, Romania — Doina Piciu, M.D., Ph.D.

Note

All cases presented in this book are from the personal database collection, from the Institute of Oncology "Prof. Dr. Ion Chiricuță" Cluj-Napoca.

Contents

Contributors

Patriciu Achimaş-Cadariu, M.D., Ph.D. Department of Oncological and Gynecological Surgery, University of Medicine and Pharmacy "Iuliu Haţieganu", Cluj-Napoca, Romania

Călin Căinap, M.D., Ph.D. Department of Medical Oncology, University of Medicine and Pharmacy "Iuliu Haţieganu", Cluj-Napoca, Romania

Alexandru Irimie, M.D., Ph.D. Department of Oncological and Gynecological Surgery, University of Medicine and Pharmacy "Iuliu Haţieganu", Cluj-Napoca, Romania

Andra Piciu, M.D. Department of Medical Oncology, University of Medicine and Pharmacy "Iuliu Haţieganu", Cluj-Napoca, Romania

Introduction

Endocrinology is one of the "youngest" and dynamic medical specialties and had celebrated in 2005 its centenary as a recognized science and branch of medicine, with very impressive recent discoveries of hormones, new molecules, peptides, and pathways of action.

In endocrinology, nuclear medicine has a major contribution both in imagistic procedures and in therapeutic approaches.

Nuclear medicine is a part of medicine that uses radioisotopes for diagnostic and treatment of different diseases. As a continuously growing medical specialty, nuclear medicine has a history directly related with the discovery of different radioactive substances with potential role in diagnostic and treatment.

The spectacular development of technology and medical instruments gave the opportunity of newly nuclear medicine procedures to lead to the improvement of patient's medical care. The areas that have been particularly affected are hybrid imaging with both PET/CT and SPECT/CT, as well as radionuclide therapy. The ability to fuse physiologic and anatomic information with hybrid imaging has greatly enhanced the information available for patient management. The addition of newer therapeutic interventions has provided additional choices for managing several medical areas, such as oncology, endocrinology, and cardiology, as well as other fields.

Even if the first successful radioisotope treatment in human happened between 1939 and 1941, when phosphorus-32 was used for the treatment of polycythemia vera (Lawrence 1941), the first major achievement was in endocrinology and came at the beginning of the 1940s. A. Hertz and A. Roberts published in 1942 the results of the first application of radioactive iodine in therapy of Graves' disease; in 1946, a dose of iodine-131 halted the growth of thyroid cancer and was found to be a useful tool in diagnosing and treating thyroid diseases. This new method of organ imaging was invaluable and marked the beginning of a new era in medical history.

Today, there are over 100 procedures involving radioisotopes for both diagnosis and treatment of many diseases; the major clinical interest continues to be devoted to endocrinology and oncology.

The present work intends to offer the support of a brief, synthetic, and easy way for integrated nuclear medicine in the daily practice of endocrinologists.

Realizing that nuclear medicine is a rapidly changing field, the author tried to emphasize principles and specific details; introduction of new technologies results in new training requirements, both for nuclear medicine physicians and for endocrinologists. Endocrinologists need to be familiar with the concept of functional imaging, molecular and targeted nuclear diagnostic, and treatment of endocrine disorders, generally named "nuclear endocrinology."

Further Reading

Erf LA, Lawrence JH (1941) Clinical studies with the aid of radiophosphorus III. The absorption and distribution of radiophosphorus in the blood, its excretion by and its therapeutic effect on patients with polycythemia. Ann Intern Med 15:276

Erf LA, Jones HW (1943) Radiophosphorus – an agent for the satisfactory treatment of polycythemia and its associated manifestations. Ann Intern Med 19:587

Hertz S, Roberts A, Salter WT (1942) Radioactive iodine as an indicator in thyroid physiology. IV. The metabolism of iodine in Graves' disease. J Clin Invest 21(1):25–29

Seidlin SM, Marinelli LD, Oshry E (1946) Radioactive iodine therapy; effect on functioning metastases of adenocarcinoma of the thyroid. J Am Med Assoc 132(14):838–847

Part I

General Nuclear Medicine

1 Principles of Nuclear Medicine

Look deep into nature, and then you will understand everything better.

Albert Einstein

1.1 Principles and History of Nuclear Medicine

Nuclear medicine is a medical specialty involving the application of radioactive substances in the diagnostic and therapy of diseases. The most important characteristic of nuclear medicine methods is the ability of the substances used as tracers to reflect the function of different organs; these methods can reveal also structure and anatomy.

Nuclear medicine procedures and images show function, physiology, and metabolism and have the capacity to determinate the cause, nature, or manifestations of a disease or condition. This may include monitoring the progression or regression of the disease or injury in response to therapy.

The collaboration between Professor Karl T. Compton, President of the Massachusetts Institute of Technology, and Saul Hertz, the Director of the Thyroid Clinic of Massachusetts General Hospital, Boston, was part of the early history of nuclear medicine. In the letter wrote by Saul Hertz in December 23, 1936, he underlined the fact that if the radioiodine artificially obtained by the team of Professor Compton is selectively taken up by the thyroid gland, this will be a useful method of therapy in cases of overactivity of the thyroid gland. Doctor Saul Hertz was one of the scientists whose pioneering work played an important part in the foundation of nuclear medicine. In 1937 he used radioiodine in studying thyroid physiology, and he was the first who used the "atomic cocktail" (iodine-131) for thyroid treatment, in 1941. Another pioneer scientist that suggested the use of radionuclides to label compounds in biology and medicine was the Hungarian chemist G. Hevesy, awarded with the Nobel Prize in 1943.

Comparing to standard radiography, nuclear medicine images (scans or scintigraphies) always require the administration of radioactive tracers. These radiolabeled drugs, named radiopharmaceuticals, usually reflect the blood flow, the capillary permeability, the specific tissue extraction, or the specific pathways of metabolism and pathophysiologic processes.

One of the most well-known examples regarding the fundamental differences between nuclear scans and standard radiology is the evaluation of brain activity, for example, a computer tomography (CT) performed in a situation of a corpse or a patient being in cerebral death can reveal a normal brain structure, while a nuclear scan confirms the lack of neurological activity and death.

Comparing to X-ray methods, nuclear medicine has specific patterns of activity. A radiograph results when an external beam passes through the patient and is recorded on the other side. This principle is equally true for a simple classic radiography or a computed tomography (CT). Nuclear scans result when a radioactive tracer administered inside the patient allows the

D. Piciu, *Nuclear Endocrinology*, DOI 10.1007/978-3-319-56582-8_1

external record of the radiation activity. This difference explains the need for specific instruments and equipment in nuclear medicine, comparing to radiology.

All nuclear medicine methods are using radioactive tracers called radiopharmaceuticals. Most of them consist of two parts: a radioactive compound that provides the signal, which will be detected in the exterior, and a ligand that determines the tracer's distribution in the body.

Most of the nuclear imaging procedures are "in vivo" and involve the administration to the patient of relatively short-lived radionuclides and the use of some specific instruments called gamma cameras or other specialized instrumentation to form the images; these images will be either planar or tomographic ones.

The planar images are static or dynamic, and they are obtained as if the distribution of the radiopharmaceutical within the patient's body was from a single "plan."

Tomographic images are those that have been composed and constructed from linear projection data, acquired by placing the radiation detectors 360° around the patient. The tomographic images in nuclear medicine are single-photon emission tomography (SPECT), when the camera rotates around the patient, and positron emission tomography (PET), when the radiation detectors are located in a ring around the patient and their use leads to detection. The idea to combine PET with CT was made in the early 1990s by Townsend, Nutt, and co-workers, and it was to be 7 years before the first prototype combined PET/CT scanner was completed and installed in the University of Pittsburgh Medical Center, USA.

The clinical importance of hybrid imaging has rapidly increased. The images obtained are fused, providing anatomical information from CT or MRI and the functional information from PET. Each system performs a different type of tomography: transmission for CT and emission for PET. Due to this, the detection and acquisition systems of the two modalities are different and highly specialized for the specific requirements of each modality.

1.2 Basics of Nuclear Physics

1.2.1 Atomic Structure

The atom is the basic unit of matter; originally, the sense of the word atom denoted a particle that cannot be divided into smaller particles, but in modern scientific usage, the atom is composed of various subatomic particles. The constituting particles of an atom are the electrons, the protons, and the neutrons. Even if the atomic models described in the last several decades (the quantum models) are more complex, the structure of the three particles is one of the simplest being the first model discovered by E. Rutherford and by the Nobel Prize-awarded Danish physicist Niels Bohr; this model is sufficient to explain the basic physical concepts necessary in nuclear medicine.

Atoms consist of small and very dense nucleus composed of neutrons and protons, surrounded by electrons. The number of electrons in one atom is equal to the number of protons from the nucleus. The number of protons from the nucleus represents the *Z* number, and it is named *atomic number.*

The atoms having the same atomic number form a chemical element.

As the heavy particles, protons and neutrons, are gathered in the nucleus, the atomic mass is concentrated within it.

The atomic number *Z* is typically subscripted preceding the element symbol ($_{Z}X$).

Another characteristic element of the atom is the *atomic mass*. The atomic mass is measured in atomic mass unit, where 1 AMU = 1/12 mass of carbon measured in grams. The atomic mass number is equal to the number of protons plus neutrons and provides the average weight of all isotopes of any given element.

The protons (p or p^+) weigh 1 atomic mass unit (AMU) and carry a positive electric charge. Neutrons (n or n^0) are minimally heavier and have no electric charge, while electrons (e or e^-) have a mass of only 0.000548 AMU and carry a negative charge.

The atomic mass is usually represented as superscript preceding the element symbol (^{A}X).

The chemical symbol of an element is represented as follows:

$$^{A}_{Z}X$$

Atoms with the same atomic number, but different atomic mass numbers, are called isotopes. The isotopes of an element have the same chemical properties. The electron's configuration of an atom determines its chemical properties and reactivity.

A nuclide is a nuclear configuration that contains a specific number of neutrons and protons. Some nuclides are inherently stable, while others are not. Unstable nuclides are called radionuclides. The radionuclides trend to move to stable configuration through the process of radioactive decay. There is a large spectrum in the degree of radioactivity among different nuclides. Some are extremely unstable and decay within microseconds, and others decay over billions of years. The time required for one-half of the original radioactive sample to decay is the physical half-life ($T_{1/2}$) of the nuclide. Size is one of the main determinants of nuclear stability; therefore, heavy nuclides, which have large atomic diameters, are less stable than the light- or medium-weight nuclides.

Elements can be grouped into families:

- Isotopes: Nuclides having the same atomic number, Z
- Isobars: Nuclides with the same mass number, A
- Isotones: Nuclides with the same neutron number, N

All isotopes of the elements having the mass numbers above bismuth-209 (atomic number $Z = 83$) are radioactive. The heaviest stable (non-radioactive) element in the nature is bismuth-209, at least according to nowadays knowledges; in 2003 the researchers from the Institut d'Astrophysique Spatiale were able to calculate the half-life of bismuth-209 as 1.9×10^{19} years, which is about a billion (10^9) times the age of the universe. If a nuclide does not contain the stable neutron/proton ratio between 1 and 1.5, it is probably radioactive.

The type of decay is largely determined by whether there is neutron excess or a neutron deficiency relative to a stable configuration. Radioactive species often contain nuclei that are in an excited state, and thus, they carry excess of energy. As the nucleus decays to the ground state, it emits the excess of energy. The entire process of relaxation and energy emission usually occurs within 10^{-12} s.

A few radioactive species remain in excited state longer periods ranging from nanoseconds to days. These longer-lived nuclides are called *metastable*. By far, the best-known example in nuclear medicine is technetium-99m (Tc-99m).

1.2.2 Radioactivity

Another component of the atom are the photons, which have no mass. These units have energy and are the basic units of electromagnetic radiation, originated from changes in either orbital electrons or the nucleus. Nuclear medicine images result from recording the photons that arise from radioactive decay.

Excitation results when an incident photon imparts some of its energy, raising the energy level of an orbital electron. Ionization takes place when the photon interacts with a target atom and dislodges one or more of its orbital electrons.

Ionizing radiation is a general term for high-energy electromagnetic radiation. Photons arising either from deflection of electrons or from orbital electron rearrangements are called *X-rays*. From the nuclear decay results energetic radiation called *gamma rays*.

Gamma rays and X-rays have the energy measured in kiloelectron volts, *keV*. One electron volt is the amount of energy needed to move one electron through an electric potential difference of 1 V.

In 1903, H. Becquerel and Pierre and Marie Curie were awarded with the Nobel Prize in physics for the discovery of radioactivity. Almost all of radioactive decays occur with the emission of some combination of alpha (α), beta (β), or gamma (γ) rays. Beta particles may be positively or negatively charged.

1.2.2.1 Radioactive Decay: Alpha Decay (Eq. 1.1)

$$\text{Source : Nucleus}$$

$$\text{Primary emission :}{}^{4}_{2}\text{He, helium}-4$$

$$\text{Nuclide transformation scheme :}$$

$$^{A}_{Z}X \Rightarrow {}^{(A-4)}_{(Z-2)}Y + {}^{4}_{2}He \quad (1.1)$$

Alpha decay is a type of radioactive decay, in which an alpha particle (α-particle) is emitted from the nucleus of an atom. The alpha particle is made of a pair of protons and a pair of neutrons, which implies the existence of a helium-4 nucleus. The ejection of the alpha particle from a nucleus will decrease its atomic number by 2 and its mass by 4. Alpha decay is a possible decay scheme for a number of different radionuclides, having the *Z* atomic number greater than 82. In this case, an unstable nucleus reaches a point where it can no longer remain intact, and an alpha particle is ejected from the nucleus. The nucleus can then "rearrange" itself and decide whether or not the new arrangement is convenient. In case it is still unstable, a new radioactive decay will take place. These particles are positively charged.

There are a few numbers of different radioisotopes that undergo this decay process, and one example is radon-222. Radon-222 decays by alpha emission, into polonium-218.

The following equation (Eq. 1.2) describes the decay process:

$$^{222}_{86}Rn \Rightarrow {}^{4}_{2}He + {}^{218}_{84}Po \quad (1.2)$$

Note that all subscript and superscript numbers on each side of the equation are balanced. In this case, 86 = 2 + 84, and 222 = 4 + 218. In alpha decay, one element has changed into another. Elements and isotopes that release alpha particles are called alpha emitters.

Considering how far the particles can go, the alpha particle is quite heavy, so it will only travel a few centimeters in the air, and it will not penetrate the skin or clothing, posing little health risk if it remains outside the body. If alpha-emitting elements enter the body through cuts or by inhaling, the risks can be quite high. Actually, people who smoke inhale into their lungs the radioactive isotope polonium-210, a naturally occurring alpha emitter found in tobacco, highly increasing the risk of lung cancer.

1.2.2.2 Radioactive Decay: Beta Decay (Eq. 1.3)

$$\text{Source : Nucleus}$$

$$\text{Primary emission : } b^{+}, b^{-}$$

$$\text{Nuclide transformation scheme :}$$

$$^{A}_{Z}X \Rightarrow {}^{A}_{(Z-1)}Y + {}^{0}_{+1}e + n$$
$$^{A}_{Z}X \Rightarrow {}^{A}_{(Z+1)}Y + {}^{0}_{-1}e + n \quad (1.3)$$

Beta particles are a form of ionizing radiation made of high-energy, fast-moving, electrically charged subatomic particles. The production of beta particles is therefore named "beta decay."

As it turns out, there are two types of beta particles:

$$\beta^{+} \text{and } \beta^{-}$$

The symbol may be notated also in Latin alphabet as b^+ and b^-.

Beta minus decay occurs when one neutron contained in the nucleus of an unstable atom is converted into a proton. During this conversion, an electron and an antineutrino are ejected from the nucleus. This type of beta decay is also known as electron emission.

Beta minus decay (β^-) is synthetized as follows:

$$\text{Neutron} \Rightarrow \text{proton} + \beta^{-} + \text{antineutrino}$$

An example of beta minus decay is the first step of radioiodine I-131 decay (Eq. 1.4):

$$^{131}_{53}I \Rightarrow {}^{131}_{54}Xe^{*} + e^{-} + \nu \quad (1.4)$$

e^- is the beta minus particle.

ν is the antineutrino.

$^{131}_{54}Xe^{*}$ is the unstable xenon.

The neutrinos are particles that have neither mass nor charge; there are neutrino and antineutrino, particles with opposite spin directions. These particles were postulated to balance the energy and spin considerations of nuclear decay equations and were later discovered experimentally.

Beta plus decay, also known as positron emission, is the opposite situation. Beta plus decay occurs when a proton in the nucleus of an unstable atom is converted into a neutron. Typically, when beta decay occurs, a small amount of gamma radiation is also emitted.

Beta plus decay (β^+) is presented in the following reaction:

$$\text{Proton} \Rightarrow \text{neutron} + \beta^+ + \text{neutrino}$$

An example of beta plus decay is presented in the following equation (Eq. 1.5):

$$^{15}_{8}\text{O} \Rightarrow ^{15}_{7}\text{N} + e^+ + \nu \quad (1.5)$$

e^+ is the beta plus particle.
ν is the neutrino.

Beta particles can travel a few meters through the air and can be stopped by a thin sheet of aluminum or a piece of wood a few centimeters thick. However, they do travel fast enough to penetrate clothing and do pose a health risk, especially if, like alpha particles, they are inhaled or ingested.

Radioactive isotopes that release beta particles are called beta (β) emitters. Beta emitters exist in our environment from both natural and man-made sources. Some beta emitters such as carbon-14 and potassium-40 exist naturally in our body.

1.2.2.3 Radioactive Decay: Gamma Decay (Eq. 1.6)

$$\text{Source : Nucleus}$$
$$\text{Primary emission : } \gamma \text{ rays}$$
$$\text{Nuclide transformation scheme: } ^{A}_{Z}\text{X} \Rightarrow ^{A}_{Z}\text{Y} \quad (1.6)$$

Gamma decay produces only photons of ionizing radiation. A nucleus in excited state emits its excess of energy producing one or more gamma rays. Fundamental from X-rays, the gamma rays have the same energy if these rays are arising from the same specific transition. This transition is also called isomeric transition.

Some emitted photons encounter an orbital electron and may transfer all their energy to the electron and eject it from the atom; unstable, the void will be immediately completed with another electron from other levels, with emission of an X-ray photon. These X-ray photons result from rearrangements of electrons on the orbital levels, while gamma rays originate from the nucleus. This process is also called internal conversion.

Each radionuclide that decays by isomeric transition has also a specific ratio of conversion, ratio that suggests the possibility of an internal conversion. A low conversion ratio has more benefit for the diagnostic purpose, due to the lower radiation exposure of the patient.

1.2.2.4 Electron Capture

Electrons fill the energy levels outside the nucleus of an atom. The electrons are spread out in space somehow—they can be found even in the space "occupied" by the nucleus. Under certain circumstances, a nucleus will absorb one electron by changing a proton into a neutron and emitting a neutrino. This process is known as electron capture.

The process produces a different nucleus from the initial one: the new nucleus will have a Z of 1 less than the parent because one proton has been released, but its mass number A will be the same because the neutron is also a nucleon with almost the same mass as the proton.

Because of the rearrangement of the electrons, there is an X-ray emission, as in the case of internal conversion.

Electron capture and positron emission cause the same end effect by increasing the ratio of neutrons/protons. As a general rule, light nuclides with neutron deficiency usually decay by positron emission, while heavy nuclides decay by capture of electrons.

Several radionuclides that decay by electron capture are routinely used in clinical practice, as iodine-125, indium-111, etc.

1.2.2.5 Decay Equations

The probability of a radioactive atom decaying in 1 s is called the transformation constant, λ.

If there are N radioactive atoms, the number of atoms decaying every second will be $N\lambda$. In a period of time Δt, the number decaying ΔN is presented in Eq. 1.7:

$$\Delta N = -N\lambda \times \Delta t$$
$$N = N_0 \times e^{-\lambda t} \quad (1.7)$$

N_0 is the original number of atoms at $t = 0$.

The term *half-life* is defined as the time it takes for one-half of the atoms of a radioactive material to disintegrate.

The *half-life* can be related to the decay constant as is presented in the Eq. 1.8:

$$\frac{N_0}{2} = N_0 \times e^{-\lambda t_{1/2}}$$
$$\frac{1}{2} = e^{-\lambda t_{1/2}}$$
$$t_{1/2} = \frac{0.693}{\lambda} \quad (1.8)$$

1.2.3 Interaction of Radiation with Matter

The most important effects of radiation interactions with the matter, having definite importance in nuclear medicine, are the photoelectric effect and the Compton effect.

1.2.3.1 Photoelectric Effect

The photoelectric effect appears when the atom absorbs the whole energy of an incident photon and releases an electron. The energy of the electron is equal with the difference between the photon energy and the energy needed for the liaison of the electron in the atom. The probability of attenuation by photoelectric interaction is more likely when a low-energy photon strikes a substance with a high atomic number Z.

1.2.3.2 Compton Effect

The Compton effect consists of the partial absorption of the energy of an incident photon by an electron. The electron and the photon will be deviated under an angle depending on the energy of the incident photon; the resulting photon has energy, lower than the initial one. This effect is important for elements with a low atomic number Z and high photon energy.

Further Reading

Beck NR (1976) Some essential characteristics of radioactive materials. In: Diagnostic nuclear medicine. Waverly Press, Baltimore

Bohr N (1913) On the constitution of atoms and molecules. Philos Mag 26:1–25

Cook ND (2010) Atomic and nuclear physics. In: Models of the atomic nucleus, 2nd edn. Springer, Berlin

Cutnell JD, Kenneth WJ (1998) Physics, 4th edn. Wiley, New York, pp 910–930

Emsley J (2001) Nature's building blocks: an A-Z guide to the elements. Oxford University Press, New York, pp 422–425

Hevesy G (2011) The Nobel prize in chemistry 1943. Nobelprize.org. http://www.nobelprize.org/nobel_prizes/chemistry/laureates/1943/

IAEA (2006) Advances in medical radiation imaging for cancer diagnosis and treatment. Nucl Technol Rev 110–127. August, Annex VI

Muggli ME, Ebbert JO, Robertson C et al (2008) Waking a sleeping giant: the tobacco industry's response to the polonium-210 issue. Am J Public Health 98:1643–1650

Palmer EL, Scott JA, Strauss HW (1992) Radiation and radionuclides. In: Practical nuclear medicine. WB Saunders Company, Harcourt Brace Jovanovich, Philadelphia, pp 1–26

2 Specific Measurements, Units, and Terms

The beginning of wisdom is to call things by their right names.

– Chinese proverb –

- *Radioactivity*—The rate at which nuclear transformations occur; the International System of Units (SI) unit is becquerel (Bq) = 1 transformation/s.
- *Becquerel (Bq)*—Unit of radioactivity, corresponding to one radioactive disintegration per second.
  - 1 Bq = 1 disintegration/s
  - 1 MBq (megabecquerel) = 10^6 Bq
  - 1 GBq (gigabecquerel) = 10^9 Bq
- *Curie (Ci)*—Former unit of radioactivity, corresponding to 3.7×10^{10} radioactive disintegrations per second. Now replaced by the becquerel.
  - 1 Ci = 3.7×10^{10} disintegrations/s
  - 1 Ci = 3.7×10^{10} Bq = 37×10^9 Bq = 37 GBq
- *Absorbed dose*—The amount of energy imparted by ionizing radiation to mass unit. The absorbed dose is measured in a unit called gray (Gy). A dose of 1 Gy is equivalent to a unit of energy J (joule) deposited in 1 kg of substance.
  - 1 Gy = 1 J/kg
- *Gray (Gy)*—The name for the unit of absorbed dose, in the SI. The previous, old, unit of absorbed dose, rad, has been replaced by the gray.
  - 1 Gy = 100 rad
- *Rad*—The former unit of absorbed dose, equivalent to an absorption energy of 10^{-2} J/kg; one rad is equal approximately to the absorbed dose delivered when soft tissue is exposed to one roentgen of medium-voltage radiation.
  - 1 rad = 0.01 Gy
- *Equivalent dose*—The absorbed doses in the tissue or organ due to radiation. The radiation weighting factor W_R measures the relative harmfulness of different radiations; the SI unit is sievert (Sv).
- *Effective dose*—The sum of the weighted equivalent doses in all tissues or organs of the body. It is also called the biological dose, used in radioprotection, as it determines how dangerous an individual's exposure to radiations can be; the SI unit is sievert (Sv).
- *Sievert (Sv)*—Unit of the equivalent dose or effective dose in the SI system. Sv replaces the classical radiation unit: the rem. Submultiples of sievert (symbol Sv) used in practice include millisievert (mSv) and microsievert (μSv).
  - 1 Sv = 100 rem
  - 1 mSv = 100 mrem = 0.1 rem
- *Rem*—Former unit of equivalent and effective dose. It is the product of absorbed dose (in rads) and the radiation weighting factor.
  - 1 rem = 1×10^{-2} Sv = 0.01 Sv = 10 mSv
  - 1 mrem = 0.01 mSv
  - 1 mrem = 0.01×10^3 μSv = 10 μSv
- *Collective effective dose equivalent*—The sum of individual effective doses in a population used to assess collective risks, unit person-Sv (man-Sv).
- *Roentgen (R)*—A unit of exposure to ionizing radiation. It is the amount of γ- or X-rays

D. Piciu, *Nuclear Endocrinology*, DOI 10.1007/978-3-319-56582-8_2

required to produce ions carrying one electrostatic unit of the electric charge (either positive or negative) in 1 cm^3 of dry air under standard conditions of pressure and temperature.

- A coulomb (C) per kilogram (C/kg) is the derived SI unit of ionizing radiation exposure. It is a measure of the amount of radiation required to create 1 C of charge of each polarity in 1 kg of matter.
- 1 C/kg = 3876 R
- 1 R = 2.58 × 10^{-4} C/kg

- *X-ray*—A penetrating form of electromagnetic radiation admitted either if the inner orbital electrons of an excited atom return to their normal state (these are characteristic X-rays) or if a metal target is bombarded with high-speed electrons. X-rays are always nonnuclear in origin.
- *Gamma rays* (γ)—High-energy, short-wavelength electromagnetic radiation. γ-radiation frequently accompanies α- and β-emissions and always accompanies fission. γ-Rays are very penetrating. Dense materials such are lead or depleted uranium stop the γ-rays. The γ-rays originate inside the nucleus, while X-rays originate from the outside.
- *Beta particle* (β)—An elementary particle emitted from a nucleus during radioactive decay, with a single electric charge and a mass equal to 1/1837 part of a proton. A negatively charged β-particle is identical to an electron. A positively charged β-particle is called a positron. β-radiation may cause skin burns, and β-emitters are harmful if they enter the body. A thin sheet of metal, however, stops β-particles, easily.
- *Alpha particle* (α)—A positively charged particle emitted by radioactive materials. It consists of two neutrons and two protons bound together; hence, it is identical with the nucleus of a helium atom. It is the least penetrating of the common types of radiation—alpha, beta, and gamma—since a single sheet of paper could stop it.
- *Half-life* ($T_{1/2}$), *physical* (T_p)—The time taken for the activity of a radionuclide to decay to half of its initial value. Thus after one half-life, 50% of the initial activity remains. After two half-lives, only 25% of the initial activity remains, etc.
- *Half-life, biological* (T_b)—The time required for a biological system, such as a human or an animal, to eliminate by natural processes half of the amount of a substance, such as a radioactive material, which has entered the system.
- *Half-life, effective* (T_{eff})—The effective half-life is defined as is presented in Eq. 2.1:

$$T_{eff} = \frac{T_b \times T_p}{T_b + T_p} \tag{2.1}$$

T_{eff} is effective half-life of the radionuclide.
T_b is biological half-life of the radionuclide.
T_p is physical half-life of the radionuclide.

A schematic presentation of the specific doses useful for the daily practice of endocrinologists goes as follows:

Absorbed dose (Gy)
The energy of radiation in *one* kilogram of a substance

Equivalent dose (Sv)
Absorbed dose weighted *for* the degree of the effect of different radiations

Effective dose (Sv)
Equivalent dose measured according *to* susceptibility of different tissues *to* the effect

Table 2.1 Metric system

Prefix	Yotta	Zetta	Exa	Peta	Tera	Giga	Mega	Kilo	Hecto	Deca
Symbol	Y	Z	E	P	T	G	M	K	H	Da
10^n	10^{24}	10^{21}	10^{18}	10^{15}	10^{12}	10^9	10^6	10^3	10^2	10^1
Unit 1										
Prefix	Deci	Centi	Mili	Micro	Nano	Pico	Femto	Atto	Zepto	Yocto
Symbol	d	c	m	μ	n	p	f	a	z	y
10^{-n}	10^{-1}	10^{-2}	10^{-3}	10^{-6}	10^{-9}	10^{-12}	10^{-15}	10^{-18}	10^{-21}	10^{-24}

Regarding the doses and the units of measurements in nuclear medicine, endocrinologists should be familiar with some of the multiples or submultiples of these units. The most frequent amounts of radioactive substances used in the diagnosis and treatment of endocrinology diseases are submultiples of 10^{-3} (μCi) or multiples of 10^3 (MBq) and 10^6 (GBq).

The metric system introduced in 1975 is presented in Table 2.1.

The most frequent nuclear units' transformations are presented below:

100 μCi = 0.1 mCi
1000 μCi = 1 mCi
1000 mCi = 1 Ci
1 mCi = 37 MBq
100 MBq = 0.1 GBq
1000 MBq = 1 GBq
100 mCi = 3.7 GBq

Further Reading

[SI Brochure] International Bureau of Weights and Measures (2006) The international system of units (SI), 8th edn. International Bureau of Weights and Measures, Sèvres, ISBN:92-822-2213-6

Cook ND (2010) Atomic and nuclear physics. In: Models of the atomic nucleus, 2nd edn. Springer, Berlin

Cutnell JD, Kenneth WJ (1998) Physics, 4th edn. Wiley, New York, pp 910–930

ICRP (2007) The 2007 recommendations of the international commission on radiological protection. ICRP publication 103. Ann ICRP 37(2–4):1–332

ICRP (2008). Radiation dose to patients from radiopharmaceuticals—addendum 3 to ICRP publication 53. ICRP publication 106. Ann ICRP 38(1–2):1–197

ICRP (2009) Education and training in radiological protection for diagnostic and interventional procedures. ICRP publication 113. Ann ICRP 39(5):1–68

International Commission on Radiological Protection (1977) Recommendations of the international commission on radiological protection. ICRP publication 26. Pergamon, Oxford

Palmer EL, Scott JA, Strauss HW (1992) Radiation and radionuclides. In: Practical nuclear medicine. WB Saunders Company, Harcourt Brace Jovanovich, Philadelphia, pp 1–26

Sorenson JA, Phelps ME (1987) Physics in nuclear medicine, 2nd edn. Grune & Stratton, Orlando

3 Dosimetry

"Multum in parvo"
– Much in little –

Latin proverb

According to our knowledge so far, the dosimetric approach in nuclear medicine is less extensive than in external beam radiotherapy. The strategy of fixed doses of radiopharmaceuticals is almost a routine in diagnosis and also in many nuclear therapeutic procedures.

During the last decade, many studies were performed on this topic, especially concerning the treatments of neuroendocrine tumors, limiting the side effects and toxicity of radiopharmaceuticals, and, in thyroid carcinoma, trying to improve the management of some radioiodine resistant forms of the disease. The most relevant issues regarding the strict calculation of doses refer to:

- Decay of radionuclide and dose activity calculation for the administration
- Dose rates for radiation protection
- Dose rates to the target organ (the tested or treated organ) and critical organ (the most susceptible to irradiation during the diagnosis test or treatment)

Most up-to-date publications on radiation dosage of radiopharmaceuticals used to patients, during the nuclear medicine procedures, appear in the International Commission on Radiological Protection (ICRP) Publication 106, addendum 3 to ICRP Publication 53, and ICRP Publication 133. The most important dosage rates of labeled radionuclides used in human studies are listed in these publications. It is important for the clinical practice to underline that all radiopharmaceuticals used in nuclear medicine suffer decays, with half-times varying from seconds to years. The clinician should organize the activity and the testing or treating procedures, taking into account the following special feature: the estimated dosage to be administrated may decrease until its total disappearance.

The decays of the most important radiopharmaceuticals used in nuclear endocrinology will be presented in this section of the book; these data are very important in daily practice, in order to calculate the activities and to decide which radiopharmaceutical will be used for each patient and the type of diagnostic test or therapy to be used.

Key Point

- In nuclear medicine, it is mandatory to respect the physic characteristics of the radiopharmaceuticals used, and further, the time schedules of any nuclear medicine procedure became essential.

D. Piciu, *Nuclear Endocrinology*, DOI 10.1007/978-3-319-56582-8_3

3.1 Decays of Radionuclides and Doses Calculation

The doses that need to be administered are calculated according to the purpose of the diagnosis or the therapeutic test, to the decay of the radionuclide, and to the patient's body weight and age.

The pediatric doses are adjusted using two different methods, presented in Eqs. 3.1 and 3.2:

$$\text{By body weight: pediatric activity} = \frac{\text{Patient weight (kg)}}{70\,(\text{kg})} \times \text{Adult activity} \quad (3.1)$$

$$\text{Webster's rule (not useful for infants): pediatric activity} = \frac{\text{Age}+1}{\text{Age}+7} \times \text{Adult activity} \quad (3.2)$$

Some of the radioisotopes are nuclear reactor products, and others are cyclotron radioisotopes. Carbon C-11, nitrogen N-13, oxygen O-15, and fluorine F-18, these are cyclotron products and are positron emitters used in positron emission tomography (PET); they are used for studying brain physiology and pathology, in particular in dementia, psychiatry, and neuropharmacology studies. They also have a significant role in cardiology. F-18 in FDG has become essential in detection of cancers and the monitoring of progress in their treatment, using PET. In the following pages, the characteristics of the most frequently used radioisotopes in endocrinology, in practical clinic, are presented.

3.1.1 Fluorine F-18

Radiation:

- Gamma: 511 keV (194% abundance), positron annihilation radiation
- Beta: 249 keV (97% abundance)

Half-life ($T_{1/2}$):

- Physical $T_{1/2}$: 109.8 min
- Biological $T_{1/2}$: 6 h
- Effective $T_{1/2}$: 1.4 h

Critical organ: lung, stomach

Exposure routes: ingestion, inhalation, puncture, skin contamination absorption

Radiological hazard: external and internal exposure, contamination

3.1.2 Gallium Ga-68 and Gallium Ga-67

Ga-68:

Radiation:

- Gamma and X-rays: 511 keV (178% abundance), 1077 keV (3%)
- Beta: 1899 keV (88% abundance), 822 keV (1%)

Half-life ($T_{1/2}$):

- Physical $T_{1/2}$: 78 h
- Biological $T_{1/2}$: 12 years (gallium citrate)
- Effective $T_{1/2}$: 3.3 days

Critical organ: lung, gastrointestinal tract

Exposure routes: ingestion, inhalation, puncture, skin contamination (absorption)

Radiological hazard: external and internal exposure, contamination

Ga-67:

Radiation:

- There are in principal three gamma emissions at 93, 185, and 300 keV.

Half-life ($T_{1/2}$):

- Physical $T_{1/2}$: 1.13 h
- Biological $T_{1/2}$: 12 years (gallium citrate)
- Effective $T_{1/2}$: 1 h

Critical organ: bone marrow, gastrointestinal tract (the lower bowel)

Exposure routes: ingestion, inhalation, puncture, wound, skin contamination (absorption)

3.1.3 Radioiodine I-123

Radiation:

- Gamma and X-rays: 159 keV (83% abundance), others
- Electrons: 3 keV (94% abundance), 24 keV, 127 keV (others)

Half-life ($T_{1/2}$):

- Physical $T_{1/2}$: 13.22 h
- Biological $T_{1/2}$: 120–138 days
- Effective $T_{1/2}$: 12 h

Critical organ: thyroid gland

Exposure routes: ingestion, inhalation, puncture, skin contamination absorption

Radiological hazard: external and internal exposure, contamination

Table 3.1 presents the decays for radioiodine I-123 useful for the diagnosis in endocrinology

3.1.4 Radioiodine I-124

Radiation:

- Gamma and X-ray: 511 keV (46%), 603 keV (61%), 1691 keV (11%), others
- Beta: 1532 keV (11%), 2135 keV (11%)

Half-life ($T_{1/2}$):

- Physical $T_{1/2}$: 4.18 days
- Biological $T_{1/2}$: 120–138 days (unbound iodine)
- Effective $T_{1/2}$: 4 days (unbound iodine)

Critical organ: thyroid gland

Exposure routes: ingestion, inhalation, puncture, skin contamination absorption

Radiological hazard: external and internal exposure, contamination

3.1.5 Radioiodine I-125

Radiation:

- Gamma and X-rays: 35.5 keV (7% abundance), 27 keV (113% abundance), others

Half-life ($T_{1/2}$):

- Physical $T_{1/2}$: 59.4 days
- Biological $T_{1/2}$: 120–138 days
- Effective $T_{1/2}$: 42 days

Critical organ: thyroid gland

Exposure routes: ingestion, inhalation, puncture, skin contamination absorption

Radiological hazard: external and internal exposure, contamination

Table 3.2 presents the decays of I-125.

The calculation formula for the activity is presented in Eq. 3.3:

$$A = A_0 e^{-\lambda t} \tag{3.3}$$

A is the final activity after the time t.
A_0 is the initial activity.
λ is the disintegration (decay) constant.
t is the time.
$\lambda = 0.0693/T_{1/2}$.

Table 3.1 Decays of radioiodine I-123

Hours	0	1	2	3	4	5	13	15	18	20	24
The decay factor	1	0.948	0.900	0.854	0.810	0.769	0.505	0.454	0.388	0.349	0.283

Table 3.2 Decays of radioiodine I-125

Days	0	10	20	30	40	50	60	70	80	100	110
The decay factor	1	0.889	0.791	0.704	0.627	0.558	0.496	0.441	0.393	0.349	0.3

3.1.6 Radioiodine I-131

Radiation:

- Gamma and X-rays: 364 keV (81% abundance), others 723 keV
- Beta emission: 606 keV (89% abundance), 248–807 keV (others)

Half-life ($T_{1/2}$):

- Physical $T_{1/2}$: 8.04 days
- Biological $T_{1/2}$: 120–138 days
- Effective $T_{1/2}$: 7.6 days

Critical organ: thyroid gland

Exposure routes: ingestion, inhalation, puncture, skin contamination absorption

Radiological hazard: external and internal exposure, contamination

The most commonly used radionuclide for therapy in endocrinology is I-131. The main decay data are presented in Table 3.3.

As an example, the calculation of a therapeutic dose of I-131 of 370 MBq (10 mCi) at the calibration moment and at 24 h and 8 days is presented in Table 3.4.

3.1.7 Indium In-111

Radiation:

- Gamma: 245 keV (94% abundance), 171 keV (90% abundance), others

Half-life ($T_{1/2}$):

- Physical $T_{1/2}$: 2.84 days
- Biological $T_{1/2}$: 120–138 days
- Effective $T_{1/2}$: 42 days

Critical organ: depends on the linked substances

Exposure routes: ingestion, inhalation, puncture, skin contamination absorption

Radiological hazard: external and internal exposure, contamination

Indium (In-111) is a radionuclide used in endocrinology as tracer for neuroendocrine tumors, linked to somatostatin analogues. In-111 decays by electron capture to cadmium Cd-111 (stable). The decays are presented in Table 3.5.

3.1.8 Lutetium Lu-177

Radiation:

- Gamma and X-rays: 113 keV (3% abundance), 210 keV (11% abundance), others
- Beta: 490 keV

Half-life ($T_{1/2}$):

- Physical $T_{1/2}$: 6.73 days
- Biological $T_{1/2}$: 120–138 days
- Effective $T_{1/2}$: 6.65 days

Critical organ: gastrointestinal tract, lungs

Table 3.3 Decay factors for I-131

Days	0	1	2	3	4	5	6	7	8	10	12	18	24
Decay factors	1	0.918	0.841	0.772	0.708	0.649	0.595	0.546	0.50	0.421	0.355	0.211	0.106

Table 3.4 Activities of a given dose of I-131 after 24 h and after 8 days

First day, calibration time	At 24 h	At 8 days
370 MBq (10 mCi)	370 × 0.918 = 339.66 MBq	370 × 0.50 = 185 MBq
	339.66 MBq (9.18 mCi)	185 MBq (5 mCi)

Table 3.5 Decays factors for In-111

Hours	0	1	6	12	24	36	48	72
The decay factor	1	0.988	0.940	0.885	0.781	0.690	0.610	0.477

Exposure routes: ingestion, inhalation, puncture, skin contamination absorption

Radiological hazard: external and internal exposure, contamination

3.1.9 Techentium-99m (Tc-99m)

Obtained from generator elution, the comparison between the theoretical and the practical yield should not differ more than 10%. In the generator eluate, the parent radionuclide Mo-99 should not be more than 0.1%.

Radiation:

- Gamma: 141 keV (89% abundance)
- X-rays: 18 keV (6% abundance), 21 keV (1.2% abundance)
- Gamma constant: 0.77 R/h at 1 cm from an unshielded 1 mCi point source

Half-life ($T_{1/2}$):

- Physical $T_{1/2}$: 6 h
- Biological $T_{1/2}$: 1 day
- Effective $T_{1/2}$: 4.8 h

Critical organ: thyroid gland, upper gastrointestinal tract

Exposure routes: ingestion, inhalation, puncture, skin contamination absorption

Radiological hazard: external and internal exposure, contamination

Table 3.6 presents the decays for Tc-99m.

It is essential for the clinician to know the main energy of the radiation and the halftime, in order to assess correctly the necessary activity that will be used for the diagnostic or therapy tests.

As an example:

The dose of Tc-99m pertechnetate necessary for a thyroid scan test is of 370 MBq (10 mCi). If the dose is administrated exactly at the moment of the elution and preparation, the measured activity will be the one calculated and indicated by the physician. In case the injection is made after 6 h, at noon, or after 9 h during the afternoon, the activities decrease as follows (Table 3.7):

3.1.10 Thallium Tl-201

Radiation:

- Gamma: 71 keV (47%), 135 keV (3%), 167 keV (10%)

Half-life ($T_{1/2}$):

- Physical $T_{1/2}$: 3.04 days
- Biological $T_{1/2}$: 10 days
- Effective $T_{1/2}$: 2.3 days

Critical organ: lungs, upper gastrointestinal tract

Exposure routes: ingestion, inhalation, puncture, skin contamination absorption

Radiological hazard: external and internal exposure, contamination

3.1.11 Yttrium Y-90

Radiation:

- There are no gamma rays, so the isotope is not useful for diagnostic.
- Maximum beta: 2.28 MeV.

Table 3.6 Decays factors for Tc-99m

Hours	0	1	2	3	4	5	6	7	8	9	10	11	12
Decay factor	1	0.891	0.794	0.707	0.630	0.562	0.500	0.446	0.397	0.354	0.315	0.281	0.250

Table 3.7 Calculation of different doses of Tc-99m

Morning 8:00 a.m.	Noon at 2:00 p.m.	Afternoon 5:00 p.m.
370 MBq (10 mCi)	370 MBq × 0.5 = 185 MBq 185 MBq (5 mCi)	370 MBq × 0.354 = 130.9 MBq 130.9 MBq (3.5 mCi)

Half-life ($T_{1/2}$):

- Physical $T_{1/2}$: 64.1 h

Critical organ: kidneys
Exposure routes: ingestion, puncture, skin contamination absorption, urinary contamination
Radiological hazard: external exposure, contamination

3.2 Dose Rates to Target and Critical Organ

The organ to be tested or treated is the targeted organ, but not always this one is also the critical organ, defined as the most susceptible to irradiation.

Radiation dose estimates for an adult of 70 Kg and for the most used therapy radionuclide in endocrinology, I-131 sodium iodide, is presented in Table 3.8. The doses are different for adults and children, underlining the necessity of dose adjustment according to age. In case of radioiodine I-131 sodium iodide, the targeted organ and the critical organ is the thyroid gland.

Note that these rate doses are especially important for the establishment of radiotherapy, in case of associate diseases. These rate doses are determined for the most of radiotracers and are listed in specific documents.

The critical organs for Tc-99m are the heart wall, lungs, and urinary bladder.

For thallium-201, the effective dose equivalent resulting from an administrated activity of 78 MBq is 18 mSv (per a 70 kg individual), the typical radiation dose to the target organ (myocardium) is 18 mGy, and to the critical organs, kidneys and descending colon are 42 mGy and 28 mGy, respectively.

Table 3.8 Radiation dose estimates for I-131

Estimated radiation dose (mGy/MBq)		
Organ	mGy/MBq	rad/mCi
Adrenals	3.9E – 02	1.4E – 01
Brain	1.1E – 01	4.1E – 01
Breasts	4.2E – 02	1.6E – 01
Gallbladder	4.5E – 02	1.7E – 01
Intestine	2.4E – 01	8.8E – 01
Stomach	3.6E – 01	1.3E + 00
Heart wall	5.7E – 02	2.1E – 01
Kidneys	3.6E – 02	1.3E – 01
Liver	1.1E – 01	3.9E – 01
Lungs	7.9E – 02	2.9E – 01
Muscle	1.0E – 01	3.7E – 01
Ovaries	4.7E – 02	1.8E – 01
Pancreas	5.2E – 02	1.9E – 01
Red marrow	8.3E – 02	3.1E – 01
Bone	1.0E – 01	3.7E – 01
Skin	5.1E – 02	1.9E – 01
Spleen	4.1E – 02	1.5E – 01
Testes	2.8E – 02	1.0E – 01
Thymus	1.2E – 01	4.4E – 01
Thyroid	3.4E + 02	1.3E + 03
Bladder	6.2E – 01	2.3E + 00
Uterus	5.9E – 02	2.2E – 01
Effective dose equivalent	1.1E + 01 mSv/MBq	3.9E + 01 rem/mCi

Further Reading

Gelfand MJ, Treves ST, Parisi MT (2009) Survey of radiopharmaceutical administered activities used for tumour and whole body imaging in children. Pediatr Radiol 39(Suppl 2):S281–S282

ICRP (1996) Radiological protection and safety in medicine. ICRP publication 73. Ann ICRP 26(2)

ICRP (2000) Prevention of accidental exposures to patients undergoing radiation therapy. ICRP publication 86. Ann ICRP 30(3)

ICRP (2004) Release of patients after therapy with unsealed radionuclides. ICRP publication 94. Ann ICRP 34(2)

ICRP (2007a) The 2007 recommendations of the international commission on radiological protection. ICRP publication 103. Ann ICRP 37(2–4)

ICRP (2007b) Radiological protection in medicine. ICRP publication 105. Ann ICRP 37(6)

ICRP (2008a) Nuclear decay data for dosimetric calculations. ICRP publication 107. Ann ICRP 38(3)

ICRP (2008b) Radiation dose to patients from radiopharmaceuticals—addendum 3 to ICRP publication 53. ICRP publication 106. Ann ICRP 38(1–2)

ICRP (2009) Education and training in radiological protection for diagnostic and interventional procedures. ICRP publication 113. Ann ICRP 39(5)

ICRP (2016) The ICRP computational framework for internal dose assessment for reference adults: specific absorbed fractions. ICRP publication 133. Ann ICRP 45(2)

Krenning EP, Kwekkenboom DJ, Bakker WH et al (1993) Somatostatin receptor scintigraphy with In-111-DTPA-D-Phe1-and[I-123-tyr3]-octreotide: the Rotterdam experience with more than 1000 patients. Eur J Nucl Med 20:716–731

Lassmann M, Biassoni L, Monsieurs M et al (2007) The new EANM pediatric dosage card. Eur J Nucl Med Mol Imaging 34:796–798. Additional notes and erratum found in Eur J Nucl Med Mol Imaging (2008) 35:1666–1668 and Eur J Nucl Med Mol Imaging 35:2141

Treves ST, Davis RT, Fahey FH (2008) Administered radiopharmaceutical doses in children; a survey of 13 pediatric hospitals in North America. J Nucl Med 49:1024–1027

4 The Radiation Protection

Salus populi suprema lex esto.
—Health of the people should be the supreme law—Marcus Tullius Cicero

4.1 Basic Factors in Radiation Protection

One delicate issue in nuclear endocrinology is radiation protection. There are a multitude of documents, legislations and rules, recommendations, and approvals that endocrinologists should obtain from the national authorities before starting to work with nuclear products and to treat patients with radiopharmaceuticals.

Depending on the national legislation, there are different restrictions in the usage of radiopharmaceuticals. There are countries or states where the use of radiopharmaceuticals is allowed only for inpatients, while other countries permit treatments of the outpatients, restricted only by an established national dose limit.

In any of these conditions, endocrinologists should know the basic requirements of safety both for medical staff and for patient and his family. In this section of the book, there are provided several general rules available in direct relation with the basic principles of radiation protection, recognized worldwide.

All medical activities using ionizing radiation must be held under strict regulation respecting the legal requirements: the International Commission on Radiological Protection (ICRP) recommendations; European Union directives regarding medical exposure and basic safety standards; National Council on Radiation Protection and Measurements, legislation, and national codes of practice; and local hospital radiation protection arrangements, reporting, and record-keeping regulations.

The issues related to radiation protection are strictly dependent on the type of radiation; different rays need various modalities of protection to be efficient in relation with humans.

Radiation effects are deterministic and stochastic, also being influenced by the sensitivity of different types of cells to radiation.

Schematic Fig. 4.1 presents three different materials in relation with radiation protection.

Considering the above example, we conclude that the attenuation of the radiation through a given medium might be summarized as follows: the thicker the absorbing material is, the greater is the attenuation, and the greater the atomic number of the material is, the greater is the attenuation. An important characteristic for attenuation is the half-value layer (HVL). HVL can be defined as the thickness of an absorbing material that reduces the radiation beam intensity to half of its original value.

The main factors affecting radiation doses in nuclear medicine are:

1. The radionuclide used (the dose depends on the energy, type, and number of emissions). Gamma emitters provide imaging information but give local and long-range dose to other organs. Beta emitters do not give imaging information and give much higher local doses.

D. Piciu, *Nuclear Endocrinology*, DOI 10.1007/978-3-319-56582-8_4

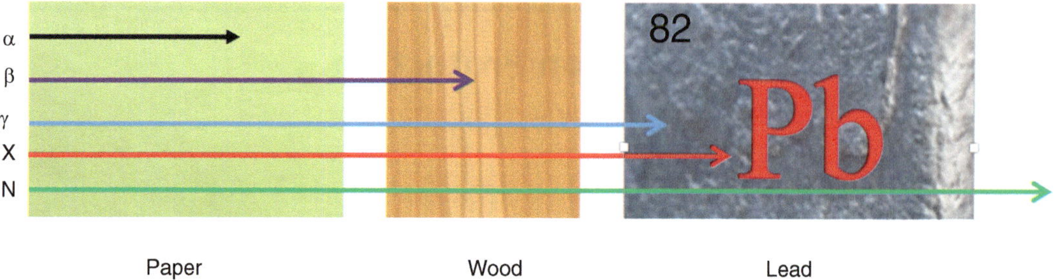

Fig. 4.1 Different materials in relation with radiation protection and ionizing radiations. α—alpha rays are stopped by a piece of paper of 2 mm; β—beta rays pass the paper, but are stopped by wood; γ—gamma rays pass through paper and wood, but are stopped by lead; X-rays pass the paper, wood and are stopped by lead; N-neutrons need special precaution

2. The physical half-life of the radionuclide (the dose increases when half-life increases). The half-life should be long enough to complete the study but short enough for the radiation to effectively disappear after the study.
3. The administered activity for the procedures (the dose increases when the activity increases). The activity should be kept to a minimum level but high enough to obtain the required diagnosis information.
4. The target and critical organs. Although usually one organ is targeted, other organs also receive a radiation dose.
5. Physiological factors. For example, in case of investigations involving isotopes of iodine, the radiation dose targeted to the thyroid may be decreased, by blocking it with stable iodine. In general, the radiation dose will be reduced, if there is fast excretion.

There are three basic requirements in daily medical practice with ionizing radiation:

1. No practice shall be adopted unless its introduction produces a positive relevant benefit (*justification*).
2. All exposures shall be kept as low as reasonable achievable—ALARA principle (*optimization*).
3. The patient doses should not exceed those prescribed by the International Commission on Radiological Protection (*ICRP dose limits*).

All over the world, the national authorities have published and implemented regulations, which represent the basic legal patterns in order to be able to work with radiation. In Europe, the European Atomic Energy Community (EURATOM) has specific legislation regarding the basic safety standards for the health protection of the general public and workers against the dangers of ionizing radiation. This standard, 96/29/EURATOM, was implemented on May 13, 1996, and renewed by 2013/59/EURATOM.

The directive applies to all practices, which involve a risk from ionizing radiation, either from an artificial source or from a natural source, where natural radionuclides are processed because of their radioactive, fissile, or fertile properties. Prior authorization is required for the disposal, recycling, or reuse of radioactive substances or materials containing radioactive substances resulting from any practice, which is compulsory, reported, or authorized, unless the clearance levels established by the competent national authorities are complied with.

Before they are adopted or approved for the first time, member states must ensure that all new classes or types of practices involving exposure to ionizing radiation are justified regarding their economic, social, or other benefits outweighing any adverse effects they may have on health. Persons under the age of 18 may not be assigned to any work, which would make them exposed workers.

The effective dose for exposed workers is limited to 100 mSv during a period of 5 consecutive years and must not exceed 50 mSv/year.

As soon as a pregnant woman or nursing mother informs an undertaking of her situation, she may not be assigned to work involving a significant risk of bodily radioactive contamination.

Regarding the medical exposure directive, EURATOM has established the effective dose limits, which must be complied with by the authorized personnel (occupational dose limits) and by the general public (public dose limits).

The effective dose limit for the occupational personnel (workers with ionizing radiation) is 20 mSv/year/averaged during defined periods of 5 years (Table 4.1).

Areas where there is a risk of exposure must be designated as controlled or supervised areas; designation depends on the extent of likely exposure.

Controlled and supervised areas must include: monitoring and recording of the activities, doses and dose rates, lay down working instructions, indication of area types, nature of the sources, and correct signs for hazardous risks.

Controlled areas must be delineated and must have controlled access.

The effective dose limit for the general public is 1 mSv in a year (Table 4.2).

Justification and optimization of the ionizing medical procedures underline that the ionizing radiation exams must outweigh radiation risk. The results may be sufficiently consistent to improve the management of the patient. Any errors should be avoided in any part of the procedure starting from patient selection to the interpretation of final results. The misadministration leads to an increased radiation dose not only to the patient but also to the staff.

Table 4.1 The effective dose limits for authorized personnel

The annual dose limits (mSv)	
Whole body	20
Lens	150
Skin (cm^2)	500
Hands and feet	500

Table 4.2 The effective dose limits for general public

Annual dose limits (mSv)	
Whole body	1
Lens	15
Skin (cm^2)	50
Hands and feet	50

4.2 Staff Protection in Nuclear Medicine Units

For staff protection, there are several rules that must be respected: adequate dose monitoring, continuous education and training, implementation of local hospital rules, informing the supervisor as soon as a pregnancy is confirmed, employer must undertake risk assessment, reassignment of staff if required, restriction of tasks if required (e.g., injection), remember principles of time and distance and shielding, and escort staff for nuclear medicine patients must not be pregnant.

Radiation protection measures for handling radiopharmaceuticals:

- Wear dedicated single-use coat.
- Remove coat when leaving the area.
- Wear gloves when handling radioactive materials or containers that may have been contaminated.
- Wash and monitor hands frequently.
- Do not eat, drink, or smoke in an area where radioactive materials are used.
- Remove gloves when leaving the area.
- Work in a suitable contained workstation.
- Use different gloves to touch instrument switches.
- Prepare all materials required before starting to handle radioactive materials so that there is no need to open recipients, etc.
- Routine quality control of equipment.

Practical information for pregnant and breastfeeding staff:

- Unborn child should be protected as a member of the public.
- Radiation dose should be limited to 1 mSv after declaration of pregnancy.
- Breastfeeding staff: in case of breastfeeding, work must not involve significant risk of bodily contamination (e.g., iodine therapy).

4.3 General Measures to Reduce the Irradiation of Patient

- Examination must be clinically justified.
- Refer to previous results.
- Choose the most appropriate technique.
- Consider the usage of alternative techniques.
- Choose the radiopharmaceuticals appropriately.
- Prepare the patient adequately, e.g., instructions on diet, drug, etc.
- Administered activity should be minimum consistent with obtaining required diagnostic information.
- Ensure about the accuracy of the injected doses.
- Consider a layout of the waiting area.
- Increased fluid intake and frequent voiding.
- For children, pregnant women, and breast-feeding mothers, take additional measures.
- Use of appropriate equipment.
- Continuous training of the staff.
- Particular attention to justification and optimization for children examinations.
- When I-123, I-125, and I-131 are administered as iodine or iodine-labeled compounds such as albumin or fibrinogen, a substantial part of the effective dose equivalent stems from thyroid gland irradiation. Use thyroid's blocking protocol to reduce dose for non-thyroid imaging studies, e.g., I-123 MIBG studies.

  Blocking protocol:

- Blocking typically begins 1–2 days before the test and continues for 7 days afterward.
- Oral dose of 100 mg KI (or 140 mg KIO_3) or Lugol's solution reduces uptake to less than 1%.
- The most important side effect may be hyperthyroidism (particular problem in elderly or those with cardiovascular disease). The clinician should take additional specific measures.

4.4 Physical Factors in Radiation Protection

In nuclear medicine, radiation protection uses three fundamental principles of physical factors:

4.4.1 Time

Due to the particularities of radiopharmaceuticals used in nuclear endocrinology, for patients submitted to diagnostic or treatment procedures with radionuclides, the principle of time is one of the simplest and most important to reduce the radiation exposure both for the medical staff, patient, and for the patient's family.

Keeping in mind that the less time is spent with the patient after the dose is administrated, the less is the exposure; therefore, all procedures, treatments, examinations, information, and discussion should be carried out *before* the administration of the radioactive dose. The contact with the patient, especially in the first several hours after the dose administration, must be limited as much as possible to strict situations or emergency events.

- Minimize the time spent close to the radioactive sources.
- The examination of the patient and the discussion with the patient should take place before the radiopharmaceutical is injected or orally administrated.
- Remove contaminated items to a safe, shielded place as soon as possible.

Key Point
Time (t) and exposure (absorbed dose—Gy) are directly proportional:

$$\uparrow t \rightarrow \uparrow Gy$$

The time that may be spent near a source of radiation (including the patient who has been treated or injected with radiopharmaceuticals) is calculated according to the following formula (Eq. 4.1):

$$\text{Stay time}(\text{h}) = \frac{\text{Dose limit}(mSv)}{\text{Dose rate}(mSv/\text{h})} \quad (4.1)$$

4.4.2 Distance

The next important factor that influences the dose rates in radiation protection is distance.

- Makes use of the inverse square law, by maximizing distance away from sources. For example, by doubling the distance from a point source, one reduces the dose rate by a factor of 4.
- Use handling tools to lift sources thereby to minimize the dose.
- Because of this particularity of inverse proportionality, the distance is even more important than the time in radiation protection.
- At an appropriate distance, the time spent with the patient may be increased significantly, by a factor of 4.

Key Point
Distance (D) and exposure (absorbed dose—Gy) are inverse square proportional:

$$\uparrow D \rightarrow \downarrow Gy^2$$

Example:
After the treatment with 33 mCi (1.2 GBq) of I-131 of a patient with thyroid carcinoma, the radiation exposure at 1 m (D_1) is 0.07 mSv/h (7 mrem/h)—E_1.
If the distance is increased at 2 m (D_2), the final dose rate (E_2) is inexistent, being almost 0 (Eqs. 4.2 and 4.3):
D_1—1 m
E_1—0.07 mSv/h
D_2—2 m
E_2—?

$$\text{Dose rate}(E_2) = \frac{\text{Dose rate}(E_1) \times \text{Distance}(D_1)}{\text{Distance}(D_2)^2}$$

(4.2)

$$E_2 = \frac{0.07 \frac{mSv}{\text{h}} \times 1\text{ m}}{(2)^2\text{ m}} = 0.0175\ mSv/\text{h} \sim 0.$$

(4.3)

4.4.3 Shielding

If reducing the time or increasing the distance may not be possible, one can choose shielding materials to reduce the external radiation hazard. The proper material to be used depends on the type of radiation and its energy.

The half-value layer (HVL) is the thickness of the shielding material required to reduce the intensity (I) to one-half of its original intensity (I_0) and can be calculated from Eqs. 4.4 and 4.5:

$$\frac{I}{I_0} = e^{-\mu x^{1/2}} = 0.5 \quad (4.4)$$

μ is the linear attenuation coefficient.
$x^{1/2}$ is the half-value layer (HVL).

$$x^{1/2} = \text{HVL} = \frac{0.693}{\mu} \quad (4.5)$$

- Use quick release syringe shields at all stages when handling radiopharmaceuticals.
- Locate generators, sharps containers, etc., behind or within shields.
- Use enclosed vial shields for radiopharmaceuticals, liquid isotopes, and elution vials.
- Cover vial shields when they are not used.
- When working in the radiopharmacy, work behind protective shielding, contained workstation.

4.5 Special Recommendations for Patients Undergoing Nuclear Medicine Procedures

- Instruction sheet detailing activity administered and duration of restrictions required should accompany the patient.
- Nursing and clinical staff, in contact with the patient, should be informed that the patient is radioactive.
- Pregnant visitors or small children should not be allowed to visit the patient during the period of restrictions.

4.5.1 For Female Patients of Childbearing Age and Breastfeeding

Prescriber and practitioner should inquire whether she is pregnant or breastfeeding. In the case of a female breastfeeding in nuclear medicine, special attention must be accorded to justification and optimization of the exposure for mother and child; there are two standard rules that are used worldwide for application.

10 Days Rule

Examinations involving ionizing radiation are only carried out in the first 10 days of the menstrual cycle.

28 Days Rule

Women of childbearing age could undergo medical exposures during the first 4 weeks following last menstrual period (LMP). Practical implementation of LMP rule varies nationally.

Assess if patient is pregnant:

- A pregnancy test or the serological determination of beta HCG (human chorionic gonadotropin), as an early marker of pregnancy, might be used.
- If pregnancy cannot be ruled out, treat patient as pregnant.
- If pregnant, review justification for exam, and consider alternative techniques or deferring exam.
- If exam to proceed, optimize with respect to radiation protection of unborn child.
- Assess fetal dose before and after exam.

After radioisotope scan:

- If breastfeeding to be continued after procedure, express milk before scan and store for use in period immediately after scan.
- Express and discard milk immediately after scan.
- Period of interruption of breastfeeding may be required for certain radiopharmaceuticals; the time is dependent to the isotope. For example, for Tc-99m pertechnetate used for a thyroid scan, a maximum period of 24 h may be recommended.
- Minimize time holding child.
- For most diagnostic procedures, avoidance of pregnancy is not indicated.

In case of therapies with radioiodine:

- Patients should be advised in advance that pregnancy is a contraindication to I-131 therapy, and they should take measures to prevent pregnancy once treatment is planned. Pregnant women should never be treated; the therapy is postponed after delivery.

- Check of pregnancy:
  - Pregnancy tests within 72 h prior to treatment
  - Historical evidence of hysterectomy
  - No menses for a minimum of 2 years and >48 years old
  - Other incontrovertible evidence for absence of pregnancy
- Pregnancy should be delayed for at least 6 months after radioiodine therapy; a delay is based on the need to normalize thyroid levels for a successful pregnancy and healthy infant development and to ensure that additional radiation treatment is not imminent.
- There may be some treated patients who later discover that they were pregnant; such cases should be handled on a case-by-case basis, and a qualified medical physicist should estimate the absorbed radiation dose to the fetus. If a pregnant woman is treated, data must be provided to her obstetrician, and the patient must be counseled on possible pregnancy outcomes and treatment options.
- In meta-analysis study (Sawka et al. 2008a), no evidence was found that I-131 treatments impaired fertility. The latest 2017 American Thyroid Association guideline (Alexander et al. 2017) referring to the diagnosis and management of thyroid disease during pregnancy and the postpartum underlines that there are no relations between the I-131 therapy for ablation in thyroid cancer and any of the following conditions: an increased risk of infertility, pregnancy loss, stillbirths, neonatal mortality, congenital malformations, preterm births, low birth weight, death during the first year of life, or cancers in offspring.
- Radioiodine therapy for thyroid cancer in young men has been associated with transient testicular dysfunction; men should be advised to wait a period of at least 3 months (Sawka et al. 2008b).

Breastfeeding after radioiodine therapies:

- Women who are lactating or have recently stopped breastfeeding should not be treated with I-131.
- Breastfeeding must be stopped at least 6 weeks before administration of I-131 therapy, and a delay of 3 months will more reliably ensure that lactation-associated increase in breast sodium iodide symporter activity has returned to normal.
- If the I-131 treatment is urgent or there is concern regarding residual breast uptake, an I-123 scan will detect whether breast concentrations of radioactivity greater than normal (substantially above background) impose a delay in therapy.

4.5.2 Procedures in Case of Nuclear Events

During the preparation and administration of radiopharmaceuticals, or because of an unexpected intolerance in the patient's body, nuclear events, mainly incidents, may appear.

According to the International Atomic Energy Agency (IAEA), the events related to nuclear materials are divided in nuclear accidents and nuclear incidents. These events are classified on a scale of seven levels and are defined in direct relation with their impact on the safety of general population (INES, International Nuclear and Radiological Event Scale).

- Major accident—level 7
- Major release of radioactive material, with widespread health and environmental effects, requiring the implementation of planned and extended countermeasures.
- Serious accident—level 6
- Significant release of radioactive material likely to require implementation of planned countermeasures.
- Accident with wider consequences—level 5
- Limited release of radioactive material; requires implementation of some planned countermeasures; several deaths from radiation may occur.
- Accident with local consequences—level 4
- Minor release of radioactive material unlikely to result in implementation of planned countermeasures other than local food controls; at least one death from radiation occurs.

- Serious incident—level 3
- Exposure in excess of ten times the statutory annual limit for workers.
- Leads to nonlethal deterministic health effects (e.g., burns) from radiation.
- Severe contamination in an area not expected by design, with a low probability of significant public exposure.
- Incident—level 2
- Exposure of a member of the public exceeds 10 mSv.
- A worker is exposed in excess comparing with the statutory annual limits.
- Radiation level in an operating area exceeds 50 mSv/h.
- A significant contamination into an area not expected by design, to be affected.
- Anomaly—level 1
- Overexposure of a member of the public, in excess comparing to the statutory annual limit, occurs.
- Low activity lost or stolen radioactive source, device, or transport package.
- Levels 1, 2, and 3 are defined as nuclear incidents and may occur as possible events in the daily nuclear endocrinology practice.
- In this situation, it is mandatory to ensure the safety of individuals and to avoid the spread of radioactivity.

There are two categories of actions: decontamination of persons and decontamination of rooms.

4.5.2.1 Actions for Person Decontamination

- Urgent notification of the responsible with radiation protection.
- Avoid external contamination entering the body through damaged skin or ingestion.
- Remove contaminated clothing as soon as possible, taking care not to spread the contamination.
- Store contaminated clothing until contamination is reduced to an acceptable level.
- Clean affected areas; wash contaminated areas repeatedly with large quantities of soap and running water. Avoid contamination of the mouth or eyes. Irrigate eyes with sterile 0.9% saline solution.
- If the skin is broken or cut in the area of contamination, open the wound and irrigate immediately with tap water.

4.5.2.2 Actions for Room Decontamination

In case of a nuclear incident occurring in the department of nuclear medicine or in the clinical department of endocrinology, the following measures should be taken:

- *For minor spills*, put on gloves, cover the spill with paper towels to soak up the liquid, mark the area of contamination, then work inward from the marked boundary, and scrub the area with detergent; avoid spreading the contamination; label and store all contaminated cleaning equipment. Monitor the area and continue to clean until the activity is within acceptable limits. Monitor all the personnel involved in the cleaning process.
- *For major spills*, vacate the room, post signs, decontaminate the personnel, and then assemble cleaning equipment; put on overshoes, gloves, and plastic apron. Proceed as for minor spills but use forceps to handle cleaning equipment; enclose monitor in protective cover; when contamination is short-lived, consider covering the affected area and restricting access until activity is within acceptable limits. For long-lived contamination, try to remove the paint and to use organic solvents for plastics and steel for woodwork. Wear facemask during treatment and ensure adequate ventilation. If all measures fail, take the area out of service.

Further Reading

Azizi F, Smyth P (2009) Breastfeeding and maternal and infant iodine nutrition. Clin Endocrinol (Oxf) 70:803–809

Brzozowska M, Roach PJ (2006) Timing and potential role of diagnostic I-123 scintigraphy in assessing radioiodine breast uptake before ablation in

postpartum women with thyroid cancer. Clin Nucl Med 31:683–687
Council Directive 96/29/Euratom of 13 May 1996 laying down basic safety standards for the protection of the health of workers and the general public against the dangers arising from ionizing radiation. 1–114
Germain JS, Silberstein EB, Vetter RJ et al (2007) National Council on Radiation Protection and Measurements (NCRP) Report no. 155 management of radionuclide therapy patients
Greenlee C, Burmeister LA, Butler RS et al (2011) Current safety practices relating to I-131 administered for diseases of the thyroid: a survey of physicians and allied practitioners. Thyroid 21:151–160
Grigsby PW, Siegel BA, Baker S, Eichling JO (2000) Radiation exposure from outpatient radioactive iodine (I-131) therapy for thyroid carcinoma. JAMA 283:2272–2274
ICRP (1996) Radiological protection and safety in medicine. ICRP publication 73. Ann ICRP 26(2)
ICRP (1997) General principles for the radiation protection of workers. ICRP publication 75. Ann ICRP 27(1)
ICRP (2000) Prevention of accidental exposures to patients undergoing radiation therapy. ICRP publication 86. Ann ICRP 30(3)
ICRP (2004a) Doses to infants from ingestion of radionuclides in mothers' milk. ICRP publication 95. Ann ICRP 34(3–4)
ICRP (2004b) Release of patients after therapy with unsealed radionuclides. ICRP publication 94. Ann ICRP 34(2)
ICRP (2006) The optimisation of radiological protection—broadening the process. ICRP publication 101b. Ann ICRP 36(3)
ICRP (2007a) The 2007 recommendations of the international commission on radiological protection. ICRP publication 103. Ann ICRP 37(2–4)
ICRP (2007b) Radiological protection in medicine. ICRP publication 105. Ann ICRP 37(6).
ICRP (2008a) Nuclear decay data for dosimetric calculations. ICRP publication 107. Ann ICRP 38(3)
ICRP (2008b) Radiation dose to patients from radiopharmaceuticals—addendum 3 to ICRP publication 53. ICRP publication 106. Ann ICRP 38(1–2)
ICRP (2009) Education and training in radiological protection for diagnostic and interventional procedures. ICRP publication 113. Ann ICRP 39(5)
Pearce A et al (2017) Guidelines of the American Thyroid Association for the diagnosis and management of thyroid disease during pregnancy and the postpartum. Thyroid. doi:10.1089/thy.2016.0457
Sawka AM, Lakra DC, Lea J et al (2008a) A systemic review examining the effects of therapeutic radioactive iodine on ovarian function and future pregnancies in female cancer survivors. Clin Endocrinol (Oxf) 69:479–490
Sawka AM, Lea J, Alsheri B et al (2008b) A systemic review of the gonadal effects of therapeutic radioactive iodine in male thyroid cancer survivors. Clin Endocrinol (Oxf) 68:610–617
The American Thyroid Association Taskforce on Radioiodine Safety (2011) Radiation safety in the treatment of patients with thyroid diseases by radioiodine I-131: practice recommendations of the American Thyroid Association. Thyroid 21(4):335–346

5 Equipments in Nuclear Medicine

Nature is the source of all true knowledge. She has her own logic, her own laws, she has no effect without cause nor invention without necessity.

Leonardo Da Vinci

5.1 Gamma Camera

The revolutionary metabolic image provided by nuclear medicine has in its background a tremendous effort for the improvement of instruments and equipments.

Especially during the last two decades, the spectacular development of positron emission tomography and of fusion/hybrid images was possible due to the new and astonishing equipment and software, able to give us the best functional and structural information of the human body.

With respect to pathology occurring in endocrinology, the most frequent instruments used are gamma cameras, also called gamma scanners; nevertheless, in the last years, it significantly increased the use of hybrid equipments, as PET/CT or SPECT/CT.

The principle of these procedures consists of radiopharmaceutical administration into patient's body, mainly intravenously; after a period of time, the emitted gamma rays from patient's organs are registered by gamma camera alone or fused with CT, and an image is obtained in the final software station.

The order of the procedures is presented in the next schema in Figs. 5.1, 5.2, and 5.3.

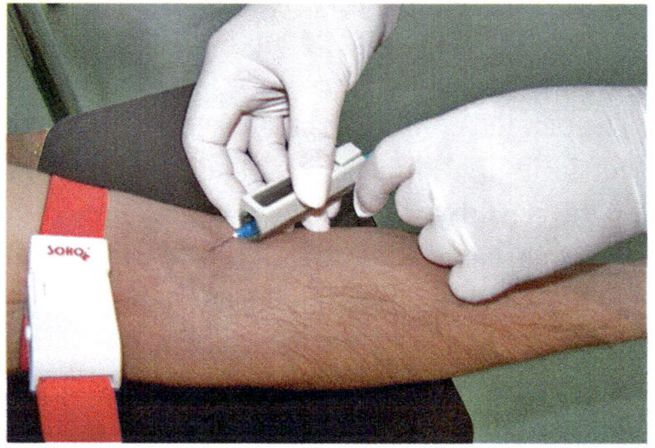

Fig. 5.1 Intravenous administration of radiopharmaceutical, protection holder of the syringe

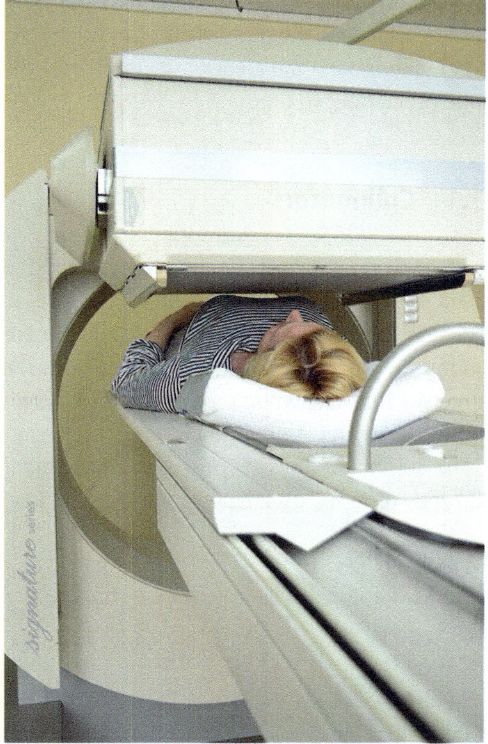

Fig. 5.2 Patient examined by gamma camera (Model Siemens e.cam Signature)

D. Piciu, *Nuclear Endocrinology*, DOI 10.1007/978-3-319-56582-8_5

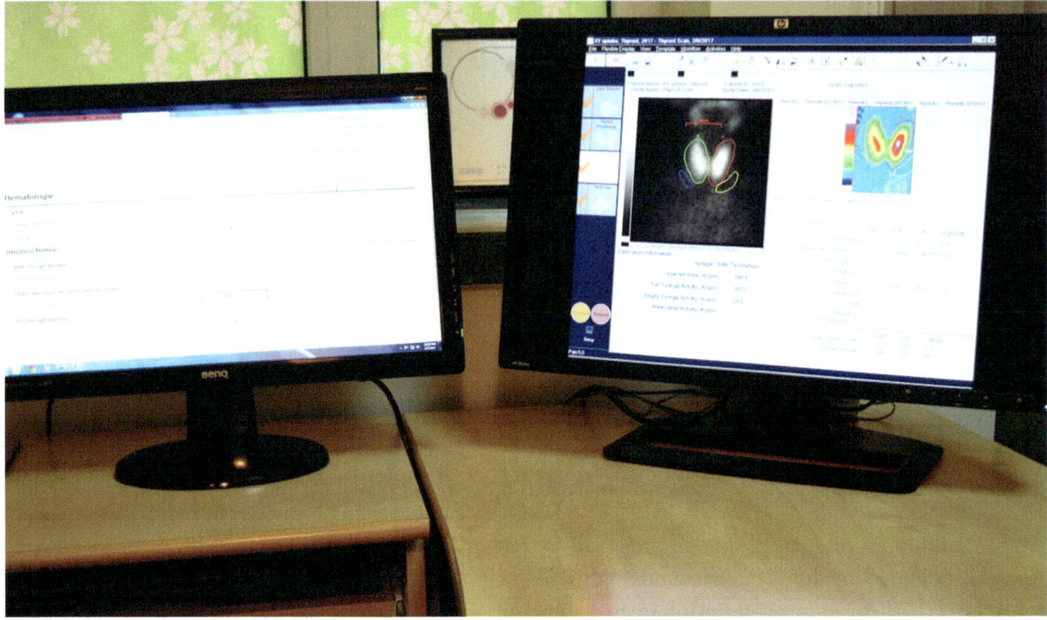

Fig. 5.3 Image processing by gamma camera's software station (Model Siemens e.cam Signature)

The main parts of gamma camera are the crystal, the collimator, the photomultiplier tubes, the lead shielding, and the electronic circuit and the image processing station.

5.1.1 Collimators

Gamma rays take random directions from the patient's body. The collimator has the role to block the emitted rays that are not suitable for creating the image. It restricts the rays from the source so that each point in the image corresponds to a unique point in the source.

The collimator consists of a different number and types of holes distributed in a piece of lead (Fig. 5.4).

The holes may be:

- Hexagonal
- Circular
- Square
- Triangular

Manufacturers have different preferences in order to maintain the best resolution and sensitivity at low costs and ease of manufacture. The difference in spacing creates differences in the thickness of the walls or of the septa. The collimator septa must be accurately aligned to avoid any distortion or artifacts.

Collimators are specially designed for:

- Different energies of radionuclides
- Different resolution
- Different sensitivity
- Different image, size, or shape

All these characteristics are reflected in different types of collimators: parallel, divergent, converging, and pinhole.

The parallel collimator creates an image of the object in its real dimensions. The design of the hole, the sensitivity, and the spatial resolution of the gamma camera are changing. The field of view (FOV) of this does not change with the distance between the object (the organ in the human body) and the collimator (Fig. 5.5).

(a) Divergent collimator: The size of the object in the image from gamma camera's crystal is smaller than the original object (Fig. 5.6).

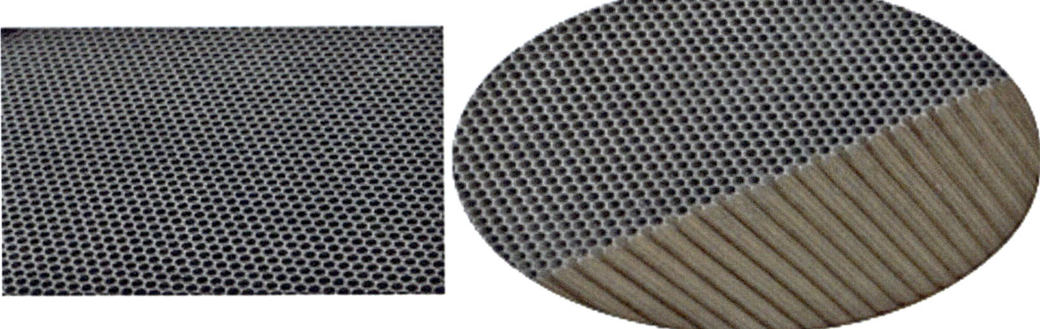

Fig. 5.4 The core of a collimator with hexagonal holes

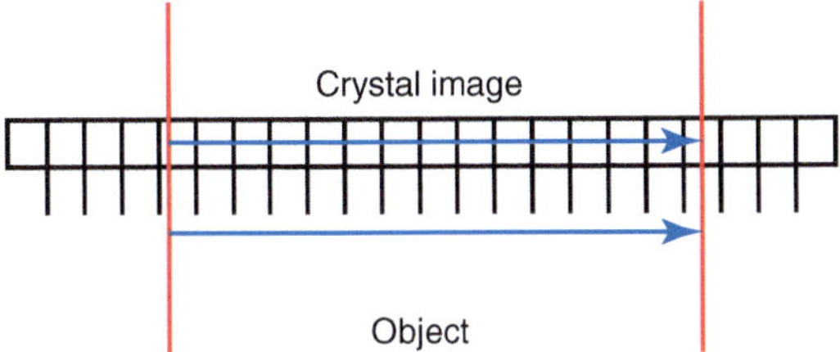

Fig. 5.5 Collimator with parallel holes

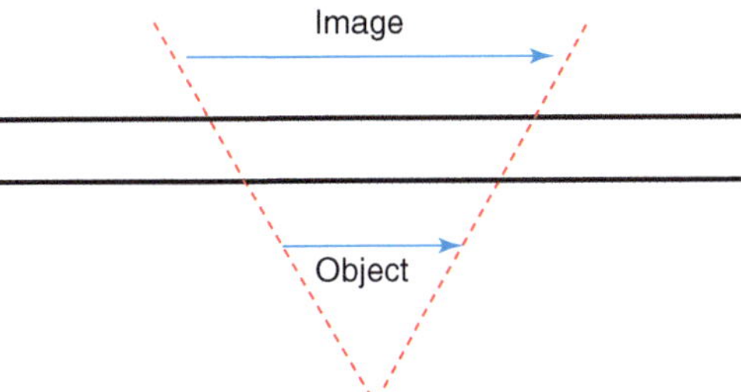

Fig. 5.7 Convergent collimator

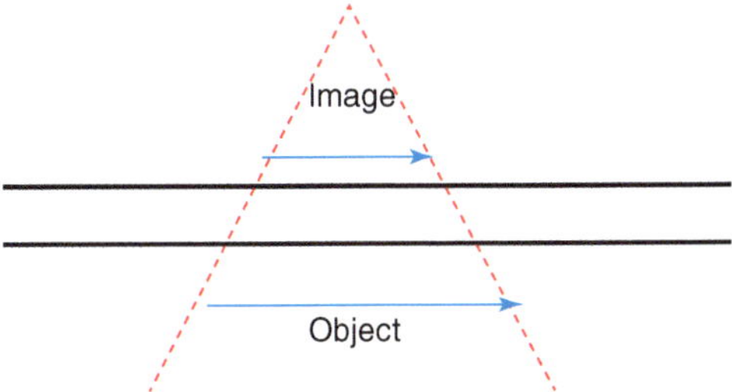

Fig. 5.6 Divergent collimator

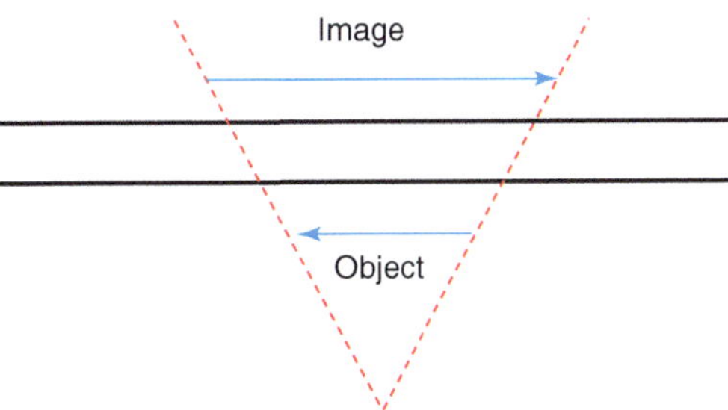

Fig. 5.8 Pinhole collimator

(b) Convergent collimator: The size of the object in the image from gamma camera's crystal is bigger than the original object (Fig. 5.7).

(c) Pinhole collimator

This collimator acts just like a pinhole camera and produces a magnified and inverted image of the object. This is typically used to examine small objects such as the thyroid gland and the hip joint (Fig. 5.8).

The level of energy of the radionuclide, which will be used for testing, dictates the thickness of lead from the collimator selected for examination. The septa and the hole's size influence the resolution of the collimator (Table 5.1).

It is very important to underline that the resolution of the gamma camera degrades severely with the distance between the testing body and collimator.

Briefly, higher sensitivity means bigger holes of the collimators, while higher resolution means smaller holes or longer septa between the holes.

Table 5.1 The selection of different types of collimator according to the energy level of the radionuclide

Type of collimator	Energy (keV)
Low-energy high sensitivity (LEHS)	140
Low-energy general (all) purpose (LEGP/LEAP)	140
Low-energy high resolution (LEHR)	140
Medium-energy general purpose (MEGP)	250
High-energy general purpose (HEGP)	364
Low-energy pinhole (LEP)	140

Regarding the performance of gamma camera, there are some characteristics determined by collimator proprieties and also by the intrinsic camera proprieties. All together, they express the following camera characteristics:

- Resolution is the ability to determine two separate sources of radioactivity as different entities. Thus, it is a measure of the amount of blurring of these sources by the camera.
- Sensitivity is the ability to register a certain fraction of gamma rays emitted by the source.
- Uniformity is the ability of the instrument to faithfully reproduce an image of a uniformly distributed radioactive source.

Choosing the collimator is the first step in preparing the examination. A careful changing of the equipment leads to an accurate diagnostic test and better results in the patient's management. In Fig. 5.9, the layout of three different collimators ready to be used is presented.

5.1.2 Crystals

The crystal is the "heart" of a gamma camera. This is a core of sodium iodide (NaI) doped with an activator (frequently thallium—Tl). The scintillations produced by the ionizing radiation from the patient's body occur in this core. A gamma photon enters the crystal; the energy given to this crystal is released as light photons. Not all the photons are detected; in most cases, three light photons are detected for every 1 keV of energy absorbed.

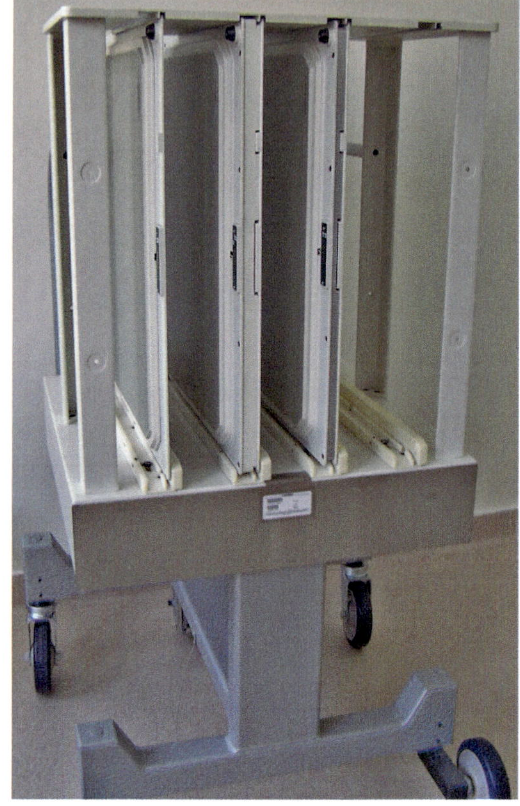

Fig. 5.9 Collimators in their deposit trolley

The crystal is very fragile; therefore, damage and shocks could be harmful for the performance of the gamma camera. This is the reason why the crystal is the most protected part of the equipment, being carefully maintained in proper conditions of mechanical injury avoidance, controlled humidity, and temperature of the area. It is encapsulated, and the lead shielding prevents the entrance of the photons, except through the collimator.

The crystal degenerates during time. The most common period of viability is about 7–10 years; after this period, the camera is no longer able to handle all events input to it, and there is a rapid loss in apparent sensitivity. Resolution is degraded as camera errors increase.

An interface optically couples the crystal to the front face of the photomultiplier tubes (PMT). It leads the light photons to the front surfaces of the PMT, which is as close as possible to the crystal for obtaining the best resolution.

5.1.3 The Photomultiplier Tubes

The PMT turns the light photons into detectable electric currents. The number of electrons is proportional to the original energy of the photon. Inside the tube, there are a number of positively charged dynodes (metal plates) coated with cesium antimonide. The cathode and each successive dynode have voltage gaps of about 200 V. The number of dynodes increases the current by millions. There is proportionality between this current and the characteristic energy of the photon. These bursts of current are converted into voltage pulses and shaped into the preamplifier. They all need to be multiplied by the same factor before sorting and positioning. Pulses from a gamma event arriving at the end of the amplifier part of the circuit are then examined. If the size of the pulse corresponds to the characteristic energy of the chosen nuclide, it is passed on to the positioning electronics. A normal distribution is when the characteristic energy of the nuclide is at a median value. The upper and the lower level discriminators form the energy window that determines which events are accepted as part of the image. The narrower the window, the less scatter will be included, and more genuine photons will be rejected.

The signals from those PMT that have detected the light are compared. The signals are digitized, and the x and y values determine to which pixel they should be ascribed to. When enough events have been detected for an image, the acquisition is ended.

5.1.4 Imaging and Processing

In imaging, a pixel constitutes a sample. If there is less statistical variation between pixels, there is less statistical "noise" and better diagnosis accuracy.

A matrix is an array of picture cells or pixels. Each pixel should be square, and each signal is assigned or digitized to a pixel.

Choice of the matrix size depends on the organ to be examined. There are sizes from 64 × 64 up to 521 × 512, and sometimes the matrix is not square, for example, 1024 × 256.

The following table can be clinically useful for a quick overview (Table 5.2).

Different types of color scale are available and are useful to show particular information of the test.

The data storage must be safe, accessible, and economical, and also it must protect the patient's information.

Nowadays, there are gamma cameras designed to satisfy different clinical purposes.

The gamma cameras with one head or double heads (Fig. 5.10) are dedicated to general purposes, especially for whole-body scanning in oncology, because of their rapid time of examination. These cameras are moving over the patient's whole body obtaining two incidences in only one passage (anterior-posterior and posterior-anterior views) or in multiple separate passages for all the views that are necessary.

The triple- or quadruple-headed camera is designed mainly for brain examinations; the angular double-headed camera is used for cardiac scanning (Fig. 5.11). In endocrinology, the quadruple-headed camera has a special use for the evaluation of orbitopathy in Basedow-Graves' disease (Fig. 5.12).

In all cases, the quality control is defined as the assessment, maintenance, and optimization of the equipment, and it is mandatory for obtaining accurate results.

The tested parameters are daily, weekly, or monthly scheduled and consist in checking the

Table 5.2 Choice of the matrix size

Matrix	64 × 64	128 × 128	256 × 256	1024 × 256
Indication	Rapid dynamic studies Small organs	In most cases of indication just about adequate	For low-count images	Whole-body scans

uniformity, the resolution, the sensitivity, the count rate performance, the collimator, and the angle variations.

The single-headed camera specially designed for thyroid scanning is presented in Fig. 5.13. It is a camera with less versatility, but with an easy installation, fact that does not require special features of the examination room.

Only with title of information in the next Fig. 5.14 is presented the former scanning instrument, linear scanner, with limited use in nowadays. Actually, this one was among the first equipment used in nuclear medicine, with important place in thyroid imaging, before the approach of these pathologies being definitively modified.

Almost every gamma camera used in our days has a special feature, which is named SPECT (single-photon emission tomography); in fact, it is the propriety of the instrument to acquire images in tomographic way and to process the sectional images in a more accurate modality.

In planar imaging, contrast is often low because of radioactivity in front of and behind the area of interest. Emission computer tomography removes this superimposition, thus vastly improving the detectability of abnormal areas.

Special attention in data acquisition is accorded to matrix size and to the arc of rotation, while in reconstruction the correct filter, back projection, attenuation, and uniformity are essential. The matrix determines spatial resolution; spatial resolution degrades with distance between the camera and the object.

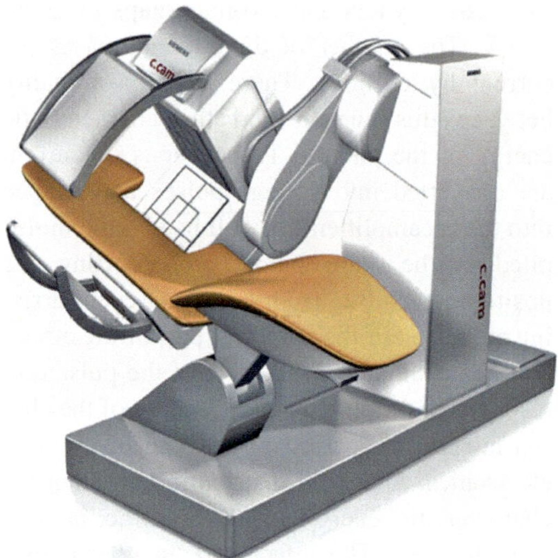

Fig. 5.11 Double-headed gamma camera cardiac purpose (Model Siemens, with courtesy)

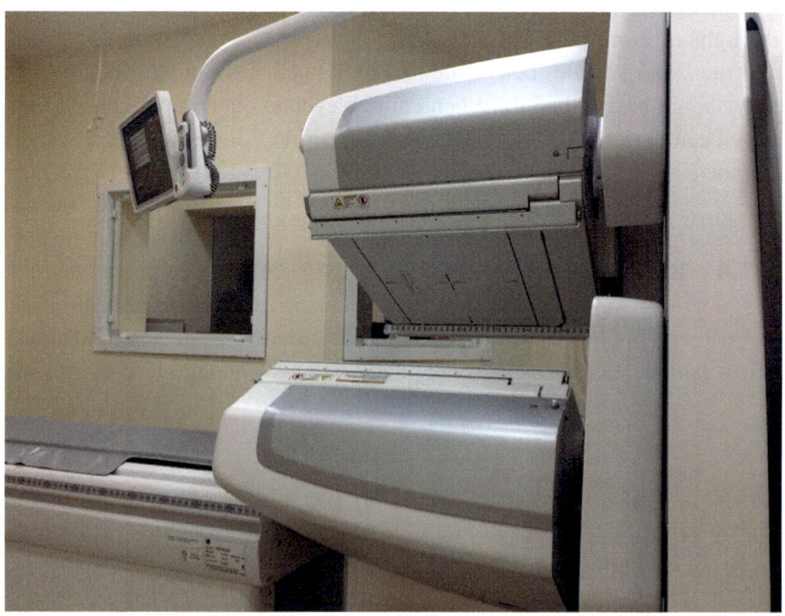

Fig. 5.10 Double-headed gamma camera (Model GE, with courtesy)

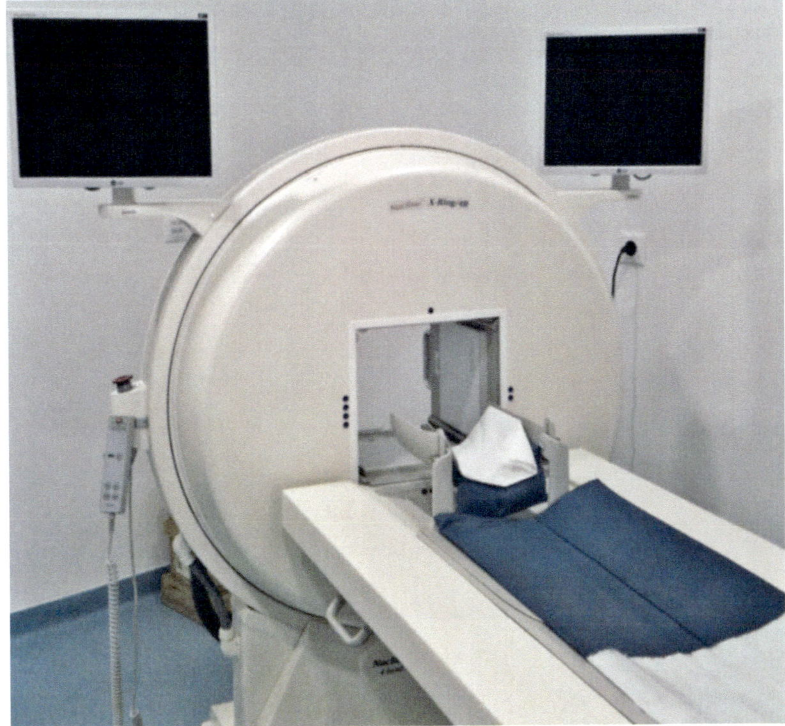

Fig. 5.12 Quadruple-headed camera (Model Mediso, with courtesy)

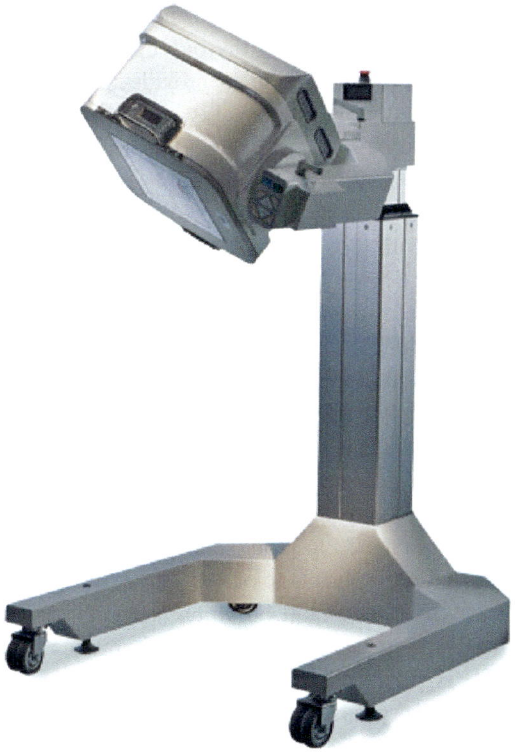

Fig. 5.13 Thyroid gamma camera (Model Mediso, with courtesy)

More delicate than in the case of planar acquisition of gamma cameras is the reconstruction of the images, which involves a series of special precautions. For accurate reconstruction, the number of views taken over the 360° arch should equal the image matrix. The answer lies in the use of filters to extract and enhance the diagnosis information and at the same time to minimize the noise component that results from scattering and the back projection process. The planes (sagittal, coronal, and oblique) will be processed for obtaining a three-dimensional image, suitable for more details. It is necessary to be able to generate high-quality projections and reconstructions in order to have a view of the effect on contrast and spatial resolution.

There is an increasing tendency to use fusion images obtained in equipment like SPECT/CT (Fig. 5.15) and SPECT/CT/PET. All these techniques are trying to improve the accuracy of the diagnosis in nuclear medicine, increasing the level of sensitivity, and providing essential structural information together with the functional ones.

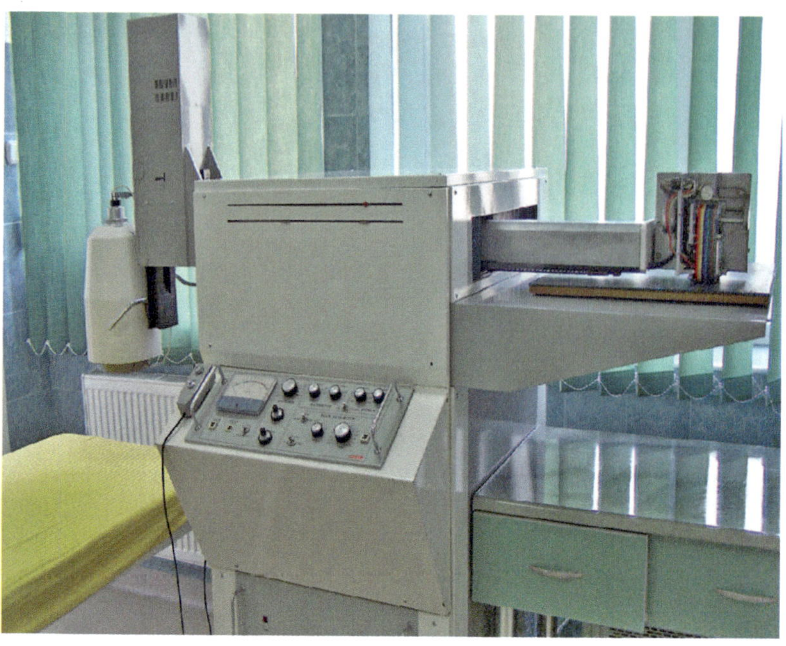

Fig. 5.14 Linear scanner

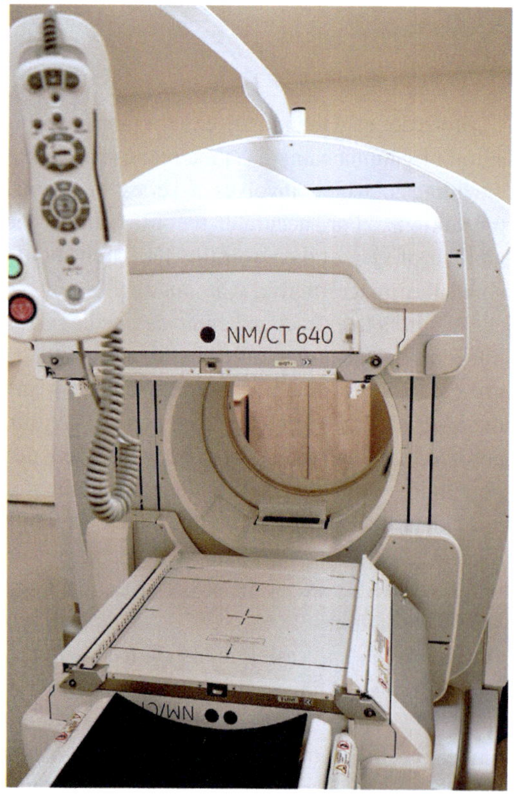

Fig. 5.15 SPECT/CT (Model General Electric, with courtesy)

5.2 Instruments for Thyroid Uptake Evaluation

Before the determination of thyroid hormonal level being a routine, thyroid uptake was an extensive modality able to provide information related to thyroid functionality.

The probe system designed for measuring the radioactive activity in the thyroid gland is called thyroid uptake system. This probe is more or less similar with the anterior-described gamma camera, with a lower level of complexity, but keeping the same principle of examination based on scintillation.

Thallium-doped sodium iodide NaI (TI) is the most widely used scintillation material. The reasons of its great light output among scintillators are convenient emission range, the possibility of large-sized crystal production, and their low prices compared to other scintillation materials. The main disadvantage of NaI (TI) is the hygroscopicity, on account of which NaI (TI) can be used only in hermetically sealed assemblies. NaI (TI) is produced in two forms: single crystals and polycrystals. The optical and scintillating characteristics of the material are the same in both states.

The uptake system consists of scintillation crystal of NaI (TI), collimator, photomultiplier tubes, analyzer, and computer (Fig. 5.16). The system uses a flat field collimator leading to an image of the thyroid with the same size as in reality.

As all other imaging instruments, in nuclear medicine it is mandatory to calibrate the system before use. There are three required tests:

- Accuracy test
- Linearity test
- Constancy test

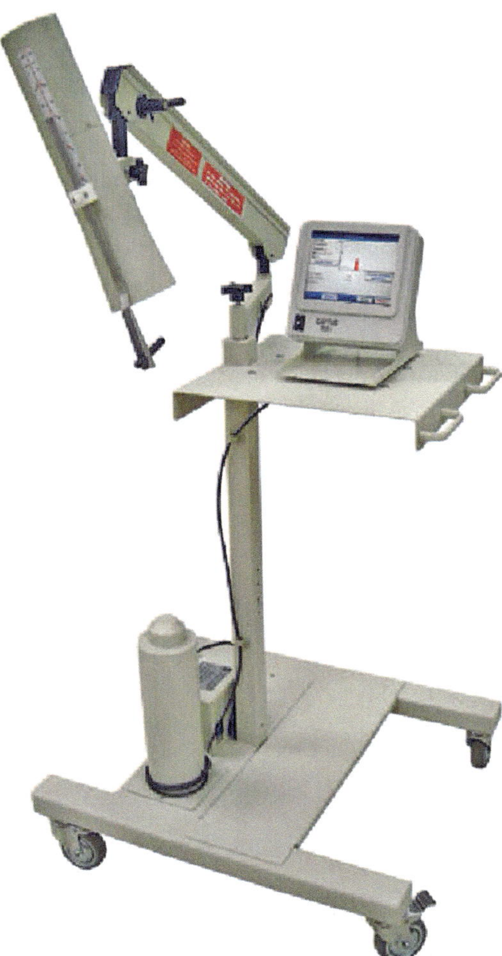

Fig. 5.16 Thyroid uptake system

Ingested radioiodine is absorbed into the bloodstream and then trapped by the thyroid gland. The principle of thyroid uptake is thyroid uptake determination is the measurement of the fraction of an administered amount of radioactive iodine that accumulates in the thyroid at selected times following ingestion.

Alternatively, intravenous (IV) administration of Tc-99m pertechnetate can determine thyroid uptake on a gamma camera. This procedure reflects the vascular compound, not the iodophilic pattern.

The diagnosis NaI-131 iodide capsule is firstly kept for measurements in a phantom, designed to have a geometric dimension similar to that of the neck. Then this capsule is given to that patient orally.

Radioactive iodine uptake is a ratio between the counting at thyroid level in different moments (2, 5, or 24 h) and the counts registered in the phantom, prior to ingestion.

There are published studies about the high correlation of thyroid uptake values obtained in the classic uptake systems and those obtained using measurements with gamma probes (instrument that will be describe in the following section).

5.3 Positron Emission Tomography (PET) and Fusion Images Equipments (PET/CT)

"The best of the two worlds" is a simple definition of what the PET/CT system represents in this moment; it creates images by merging functional and morphological images. Positron emission occurs in radionuclides with too many protons. The decay is by emission of a positive charge (positron). This is unstable in tissue.

PET is a molecular imaging technique, which measures the distribution of a radioactive tracer in vivo. After the radiotracer is administrated to the patient, it distributes among and within the organs. The emitted positron combines with an electron after traveling a distance up to several millimeters in tissue. The positron and electron are then converted into two photons, each one having energy of 511 keV, emitted in nearly opposite directions. PET image acquisition is based on the simultaneous (coincidence) detection of these two photons. A PET scanner consists of many photon detectors surrounding the patient. During a PET scan, millions of coincidence detections are collected, providing a piece of information about the distribution of the radiotracer in tissue.

The modern PET and PET/CT scanners are no longer equipped with collimators, the acquisition in 3D or 4D modes being now used (Fig. 5.17). PET measures coincidences, which are usually stored in sinograms. A sinogram contains the projections from all the angles of the activity distribution in the patient. The process of calculating the activity distribution in the body from the measured sinograms (correction for random, scatter, attenuation, normalization, and dead time) is called image reconstruction.

Image reconstruction algorithms can be classified into analytical and iterative methods.

In 2011, the first integrated CT and PET/CT system with time-of-flight (TOF) technology for exceptional speed and full fidelity PET imaging was produced. With improved contrast over non-TOF, this technology provides enhanced lesion detectability with high reconstruction speed.

5.4 Whole-Body Counting Systems

"Whole-body counting" (WBC) refers to the measurement of radioactivity within the human body. In general, the technique is only applicable to radioactive materials that emit gamma rays, although, in certain circumstances, beta emitters can also be measured. Usually, either a scintillation detector or a semiconductor detector would be used for such purposes. The person can be positioned for this measurement: sitting, lying, or standing. The detectors can be single or multiple, stationary or moving. The advantage of WBC is that it measures body contents directly. Disadvantages of WBC are that it can only be used for gamma emitters, except in special circumstances, and it is possible to misinterpret external contamination as an internal one. A well-designed counting system can detect levels of most gamma emitters at levels far below that would cause adverse effects on people's health.

A WBC is calibrated with phantom containing a known distribution and a known activity of radioactive material.

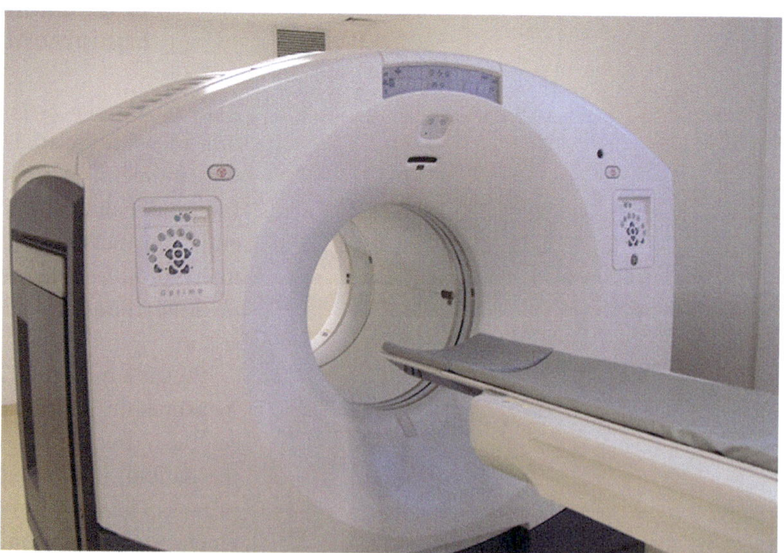

Fig. 5.17 PET/CT system (Model General Electric, with courtesy)

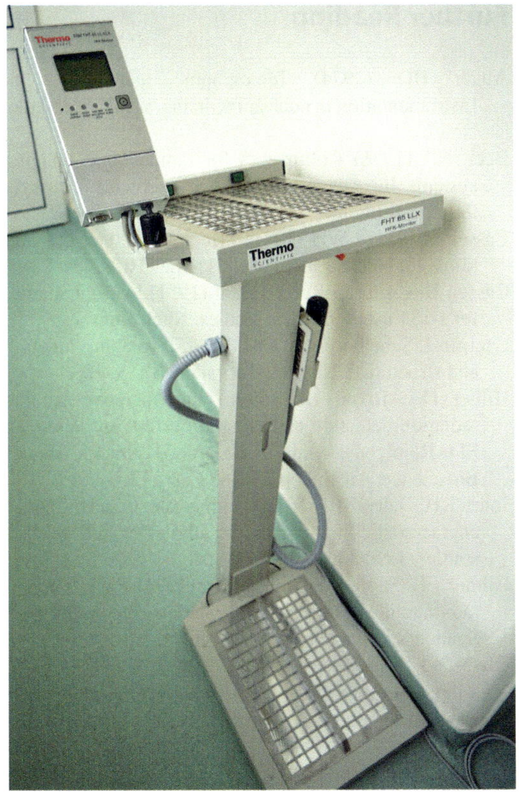

Fig. 5.18 The hand and foot monitor

In radionuclide therapy, WBC may be useful in monitoring the patient's status referring to radioprotection or to dosimetry approach.

In nuclear endocrinology, mainly in therapy departments, it is useful to set an equipment for the evaluation of possible, hazardous contamination, so-called "hand and foot" monitor (Fig. 5.18).

5.5 Gamma Probe Equipment

Gamma probe is a handheld device for intraoperative use following administration of radionuclide, having the purpose to locate sentinel lymph nodes by their radioactivity. It is primarily used for sentinel lymph node mapping and parathyroid surgery.

The sentinel node experienced high growth during the last 10 years, starting with melanoma sentinel node surgical search and breast cancer sentinel node staging; both are currently considered standards of care. In addition, it has been demonstrated to have potential in colorectal, gastrointestinal, lung, and head and neck cancers or in any other type of cancer that has the potential to spread via the lymphatic system.

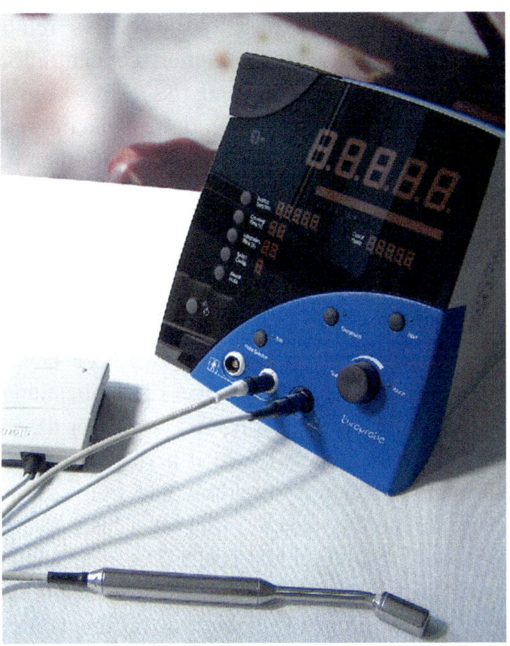

Fig. 5.19 Gamma probe

New applications are being developed for parathyroid direct detection and intraoperative detection of cancerous tissue using tumor-seeking radiopharmaceuticals.

Parathyroid detection is growing fast, while the intraoperative use of gamma probes for direct tumor detection is just emerging (Fig. 5.19).

The radiopharmaceutical Tc-99m labeled with specific albumin is injected near the tumor and flows to the local lymph nodes. Surgeons use the gamma probe to identify the first lymph node(s) in order to drain the tumor, the "sentinel lymph node." This node is excised and sent to the pathology department, where it is analyzed for the presence of metastasis from the tumor.

In the case of parathyroid surgery, the radiopharmaceutical Tc-99m MIBI is injected intravenously. The parathyroid glands retain the radioactivity, with higher concentration with respect to the thyroid tissue, between 1 and 3 h after the IV injection. This interval allows the imaging of parathyroid with gamma camera and the use of gamma probe during surgery. On the basis of the specific protocol adopted, minimally invasive radio-guided parathyroid surgery is started 30 min to 3 h after Tc-99m MIBI administration.

A wide selection of probes has been developed to meet a broad range of applications: angle-headed geometry, perfect for larger detection volume, especially when performing small incisions; radiation shielding and collimation, built around the detector, provide a high degree of spatial resolution and protection from scatter radiation while preserving significant sensitivity.

There are probes available with different range of energy suitable for using multiple types of radioisotopes: I-123, I-131, Tc-99m, and F-18, fact that permits their usage in many fields.

Further Reading

Anger HO (1974) Tomographic techniques. In: Instrumentation in nuclear medicine, vol II. Academic, New York

Beck NR (1976) Collimators for radionuclide imaging system. In: Diagnostic nuclear medicine. Waverly Press, Baltimore

Cassen B, Blahd WH (1971) Principles of instrumentations. In: Nuclear medicine. McGraw Hill, New York

Cassen B, Curtis L, Reed C et al (1951) Instrumentation for I-131 use in medical studies. Nucleonics 9:46

Czernin J, Schelbert H (2004) PET/CT: imaging function and structure. J Nucl Med 45(suppl 1):1S–103S

Hillier DA, Royal HD (1998) Intraoperative gamma radiation detection and radiation safety. In: Whitman ED, Reintgen D (eds) Radioguided surgery. Landes Bioscience, Austin, pp 23–38

Jones RH, Bates BB (1973) Gamma camera performance characteristics for dynamic quantitative radionuclide studies. J Nucl Med 14:413

Palmer EL, Scott JA, Strauss HW (1992) Radiation and radionuclides. In: Practical nuclear medicine. WB Saunders, Philadelphia, pp 27–57

Townsend DW, Carney JP, Yap JT et al (2004) PET/CT today and tomorrow. J Nucl Med 45(suppl 1):4S–14S

Radiopharmaceuticals

6

"Primum non nocere"

–First do not harm—Hippocrates

6.1 Introduction

The use of specific radiotracers called radio pharmaceuticals for imaging organ function and disease states is a unique capability of nuclear medicine. Unlike other imaging modalities, such as computed tomography (CT), magnetic resonance imaging (MRI), and ultrasonography (US), nuclear medicine procedures are able of mapping physiological or pathological activities and thereby giving more specific information about the organ function and dysfunction. The widespread utilization and growing demands for these techniques are directly attributable to the development and availability of a vast range of specific radiopharmaceuticals.

Radiopharmaceuticals are medicinal formulations containing radioisotopes that are safe for administration in humans, for diagnosis, or for therapy. The diagnosis radiopharmaceuticals usually have no pharmacologic effect because in most cases they are used in trace quantities; they should be sterile and pyrogenic-free. Although radiotracers were tried as a therapeutic medicine immediately after the discovery of radioactivity, the first significant applications came much later with the availability of cyclotrons for acceleration of particles to produce radioisotopes. Subsequently, nuclear reactors realized the ability to prepare larger quantities of radioisotopes. The most commonly used "reactor" to produce isotopes in medical applications is molybdenum-99 generator (for the production of technetium-99m).

The early use of cyclotron in radiopharmaceutical field was for the production of long-lived radioisotopes that can be used to prepare tracers for diagnosis imaging. For this, medium- to high-energy (20–70 MeV) cyclotrons with high beam currents were needed. With the advent of positron emission tomography (PET), there has been a surge in the production of low-energy cyclotrons (9–19 MeV) exclusively for the production of short-lived PET radionuclides such as fluorine-18 (F-18), carbon-11 (C-11), nitrogen-13 (N-13), and oxygen-15 (O-15). The majority of the cyclotrons worldwide are now used for the preparation of fluorine-18 for making radiolabeled glucose for medical imaging.

Currently there are over 100 radiopharmaceuticals developed using either reactor or cyclotron-produced radioisotopes which are used for the diagnosis of several common diseases and the therapy of a few selected diseases, including cancer.

Radiopharmaceuticals production involves handling of large quantities of radioactive substances and chemical processing.

The last decade has seen an increase in the use of PET in regular diagnosis imaging and a commensurate use of PET radiopharmaceuticals, particularly fluorine-18 in the form of fluorodeoxyglucose (18F-FDG). The associated 511 keV high-energy radiations need thicker shielding and more sophisticated handling devices. Regarding the short half-lives, the emphasis is also increasing on the validation process and strict adherence to

D. Piciu, *Nuclear Endocrinology*, DOI 10.1007/978-3-319-56582-8_6

Table 6.1 The ideal radiopharmaceutical

Radionuclide criteria	Radio pharmacokinetic criteria	Radiobiological criteria	Economic criteria
Gamma or X-ray emission detectable outside the body	Maximum ratio target organ/ surrounding tissues	In diagnostic tests, no corpuscular emission	Low cost
Optimal photonic energy (50–300 keV)	Optimal effective halftime ($T_{1/2}$); it must be eliminated from the body with a $T_{1/2}$ similar to the duration of the diagnostic test	Short halftime and effective halftime	Availability at hospital
Halftime ($T_{1/2}$) short, but sufficient till the end of the diagnostic test	The radionuclide should be chemically suitable for incorporating it into the pharmaceutical, without altering its biological behavior		Adequate equipment
Absence or as low as possible of alpha, beta particles, Auger electrons			Easy to prepare

approved procedures in handling all steps of the manufacture, rather than relying on the final quality control (QC) test results alone.

The specific features of the ideal radiopharmaceutical are summarized in Table 6.1. It must be emphasized, however, that there is no radiopharmaceutical that has all these properties. For the definition of this radiopharmaceutical, there are radionuclide criteria, radiopharmaceutical, radiobiological, and economical criteria.

Regarding the radiopharmaceuticals, the presence of radionuclide gives the level of radiotoxicity to the entire product. Radiotoxicity refers to radioactive materials that are toxic to living cells or tissues.

Radiotoxicity results from the:

- Type of radiation
- The radionuclide half-life
- The biological half-life in the tissues
- The dose absorbed in the organ

There are four groups of toxicity. The radiotoxicity of most commune radionuclides is presented as follows:

Group 1: Very High Radiotoxicity

Pb-210 Po-210 Ra-223 Ra-226 Ra-228 Ac-227 Th-230 Pa-231 Pu-238 Am-241 Am-243 Cm-242 Cm-243 Cm-244 Cm-245 Cm-246 Cf-249 Cf-250 Cf-252 Ra-226

Group 2: High Radiotoxicity

Na-22 Cl-36 Ca-45 Sc-46 Mn-54 Co-56 Co-60 Sr-89 Sr-90 Y-91 Zr-95 Ru-106 Ag-110m Cd-115m In-114m Sb-124 Sb-125 Te-127m Te-129m I-124 ***I-125*** I-126 ***I-131*** I-133 Cs-134 Cs-137 Ba-140 Ce-144 Eu-152 (13 y) Eu-154 Tb-160 Tm-170 Hf-181 Ta-182 Ir-192 Tl-204 Bi-207 Bi-210 At-211 Pb-212 Ra-224 Ac-228 Pa-230

Group 3: Moderate Radiotoxicity

Be-7 C-14 ***F-18*** Na-24 C1–38 Si-31 P-32 S-35 Ar-41 K-42 K-43 Ca-47 Sc-47 Sc-48 V-48 Cr-51 Mn-52 Mn-56 Fe-52 Fe-55 Fe-59 Co-57 Co-58 Ni-63 Ni-65 Cu-64 Zn-65 Zn-69m Ga-72 As-73 As-74 As-76 As-77 Se-75 Br-82 Kr-85m Kr-87 Rb-86 Sr-85 Sr-91 ***Y-90*** Y-92 Y-93 Zr-97 Nb-93m Nb-95 Mo-99 Tc-96 Tc-97m Tc-97 Tc-99 Ru-97 Ru-103 Ru-105 Rh-105 Pd-103 Pd-109 Ag-105 Ag-111 Cd-109 Cd-115 In-115m Sn-113 Sn 125 Sb-122 Te-125m Te-127 Te-129 Te-31m Te-132 I-130 I-132 I-134 I-135 Xe-135 Cs-131 Cs-136 Ba-31 La-140 Ce-141 Ce-143 Pr-142 Pr 143 Nd-147 Nd-149 Pm-147 Pm-149 Sm-151 Sm-153 Eu-152 Eu-155 Gd-153 Gd-159 Dy-165 Dy-166 Ho-166 Er-169 Er-171 Tm-171 Yb-175 ***Lu-177*** W-181 W-185 W-187 Re-183 Re-186 Re-188 Os-185 Os-191 Os-193 Ir-190 Ir-194 Pt-l91 Pt-193 Pt-197 Au-196 Au-198 Au-l99 Hg-197 Hg-197m Hg-203 Tl-200 Tl-201 Tl-202 Pb-203 Bi-206 Bi-212 Rn-220 Rn-222

Group 4: Low Radiotoxicity
H-3 O-15 Ar-37 Co-58m Ni-59 Zn-69 Ge-71 Kr-85 Sr-85m Rb-87 Y-9lm Zr-93 Nb-97 Tc-96m ***Tc-99m*** Rh-103m In-113m I-129 Xe-131m Xe-133 Cs-134m Cs-135 Sm-147 Re-187 Os-191m Pt-193m Pt-197m

Considering this fact, in nuclear endocrinology, there are not used radiopharmaceuticals with very high radiotoxicity; the iodine isotopes I-125 and I-131 belong to the group of high radiotoxicity (group 2), and this is important to keep in mind, in order to limit the unjustifiable indication of diagnostic tests. The most frequent used in diagnosis is Tc-99m, which is included in the group 4 of radiation toxicity, of low risk.

6.2 Radiopharmaceuticals in Endocrinology

In nuclear endocrinology, radiopharmaceuticals may be classified according to their purpose: diagnosis or therapy. Even if the compounds are multiple, the radionuclides which are linked to this substances are relatively limited, many of them laying on some physiological features and proprieties of the endocrine system (Table 6.2).

6.2.1 Fluorine-18 Fluorodeoxyglucose (18F-FDG)

Fluorine-18 is a positron-emitting radioisotope. The application of 18F-FDG was aimed for mapping glucose metabolism in tumors considered to be highly glucose consuming. The major use of 18F-FDG subsequently emerged in the detection, staging, and treatment response monitoring of various types of cancers. Currently, in PET studies, the use of 18F-FDG accounts for the majority of all images performed with radiopharmaceuticals. A number of other fluorine-18-labeled radiopharmaceuticals have been developed, and many more are under clinical investigations.

Table 6.2 The most common radiopharmaceuticals used in nuclear endocrinology

Radiopharmaceutical	Usage
F-18 fluorodeoxyglucose (18F-FDG)	Tracer for PET (thyroid, endocrine tumors)
F-18 choline (18-FCH)	Tracer for PET parathyroid
16α-(18F)Fluoro-17β-Estradiol (18F-FES)	Tracer for PET tumors expressing estrogen receptors
Gallium-67 citrate	Infection and inflammation
Gallium-68 DOTA (Ga-68 DOTA)	Neuroendocrine tumors
Iod-123 as sodium iodide (I-123 NaI)	Thyroid, adrenal glands
Iod-124 as sodium iodide (I-124 NaI)	Tracer for PET (thyroid, endocrine tumors)
Iod-125 as sodium iodide (I-125 NaI)	Thyroid
Iod-131 as sodium iodide (I-131 NaI)	Thyroid, adrenal glands
Iod-123 as metaiodobenzylguanidine (I-123 MIBG)	Thyroid, adrenal glands, neuroendocrine tumors
Iod-131 as metaiodobenzylguanidine (I-131 MIBG)	
Indium-111 pentetreotide (In-111 pentetreotide)	Endocrine tumors
Technetium-99m pertechnetate (Tc-99m Pt)	Thyroid
Technetium-99m sestamibi (Tc-99m MIBI)	Parathyroid
Technetium-99m tetrofosmin (Tc-99m tetrofosmin)	Parathyroid
Technetium-99m Tekrotyde	Neuroendocrine tumors
Technetium-99m dimercaptosuccinic acid (Tc-99m DMSA)	Thyroid
Thallium-201 chloride (Tl-201 chloride)	Thyroid
Other peptide receptor radiotracers (PRR)—(lutetium-177, yttrium-90, etc.)	Endocrine tumors

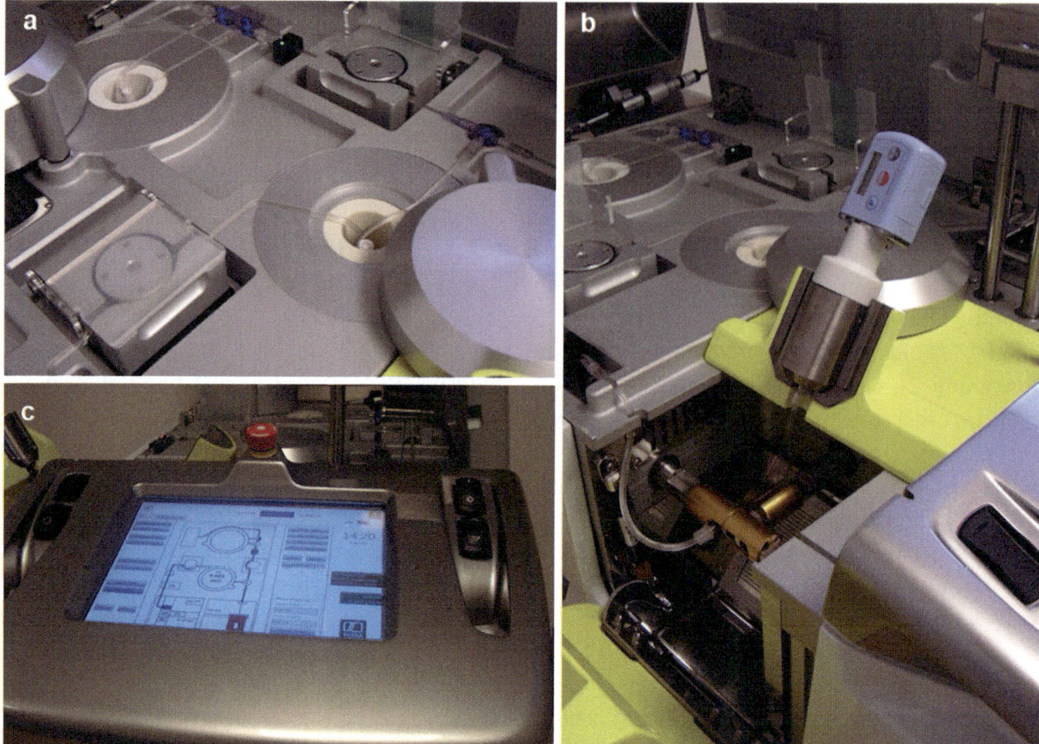

Fig. 6.1 The 18F-FDG calibrator used for loading and calibrating 18F-FDG for PET or PET/CT imaging, model *Karl 100 (Tema Sinergie)*: dispersing (**a**), loading in the syringe (**b**), and calibrating (**c**)

Increasing clinical demand for 18F-FDG has triggered technological advances in various fields such as accelerator technology, radiochemistry, automated processing modules, detector systems, and imaging software.

Dispensers and injectors perform the most critical steps in the radiopharmaceutical handling processes. In Fig. 6.1 the equipment for loading, dispensing, and calibrating the dose of F18-FDG ready for injection for PET/CT imaging is presented.

The use of 18F-FDG in endocrinology was not particularly interesting, until the experience brought the necessary knowledges, especially in endocrine cancers. Nevertheless PET studies are still indicated in well-defined clinical situations, due to some less invasive and more accessible methods that might be used in the frequent pathologies, such as those of the thyroid gland; regarding the diagnosis of the endocrine tumors, the role of PET/CT is clear and will be discussed in the following chapters of the book.

6.2.2 Fluorine-18 Fluorocholine (18F-FCH)

F18-Fluorocholine PET/CT appears to be a promising, effective imaging method for localization of hyperfunctioning parathyroid tissue. The performance of 18F-FCH PET/CT was superior to Tc-99m MIBI standard methods, particularly in patients with multiple lesions or hyperplasia. The tracer was first used in prostate cancer, where the mechanism consists in the following mechanism: FCH enters cell through choline transporters with accumulation in tumors in part due to malignancy-induced overexpression of choline kinase (CK) that catalyzes the phosphorylation of choline to form phosphorylcholine followed by generation of phosphatidylcholine in the tumor cell membrane.

The lack of availability and the costs are limiting seriously the use of this tracer in parathyroid pathology, being necessary larger studies to conclude on the superiority of the method, over the standard MIBI imaging.

6.2.3 Radiopharmaceuticals with Gallium-68 and Gallium-67

Gallium-67 is produced by bombardment of Zn-68 in a cyclotron. Ga-67 decays by electron capture to Zn-67, with a half-life of about 78 h. There are three gamma emissions at 93, 185, and 300 keV. Following intravenous injection, gallium distributes widely in the body. It binds to circulating proteins, fact that leads to long persistency in the plasma. Gallium has a wide normal distribution throughout the soft tissues, mainly in the liver, spleen, bone, bone marrow, and bowel. There is a rapid uptake in the zones with high rate of inflammation, due mainly to the increased capillary permeability occurring in these processes.

Somatostatin receptors are expressed by many neuroendocrine and non-neuroendocrine cells of the body, so different organs may be imaged by somatostatin receptor scintigraphy, including the liver, spleen, pituitary gland, thyroid, kidneys, adrenal glands, salivary glands, stomach wall, and bowel.

Ga-67 citrate was considered the master radiopharmaceutical for tumor imaging and detection of inflammatory sites. Its role is highly affected after the introduction of PET tracers.

Gallium-68 (halftime is 68 min) is available from the Ge-68/Ga-68 generator. In terms of radiochemistry, labeling with metallic nuclides is based on chelating systems which are coupled to biomolecules or which have interesting biological properties themselves. A new tracer is Ga-68 DOTA (Ga-68-labeled 1,4,7,10-tetraazacyclodode cane-*N*, *N*′,*N*″,*N*‴-tetraacetic acid). Ga-68 DOTA-conjugated peptides (DOTA-TOC, DOTA-NOC, DOTA-TATE) are rapidly cleared from the blood. Arterial activity elimination is bi-exponential, and no radioactive metabolites are detected within 4 h in serum and urine. Excretion is almost entirely through the kidneys.

Just recently the Ge-68/Ga-68 generators and the DOTA-conjugated peptide obtained a marketing authorization, until now, and they have to be prepared taking into account national regulations and good radiopharmaceutical practices (GRPP) as outlined in specific European Association of Nuclear Medicine (EANM) guidelines. PET with Ga-68-DOTA-conjugated peptides has brought dramatic improvement in spatial resolution and is being used more and more often in specialized centers. All of them can bind to some of the somatostatin receptors, and they also present different affinity profile for other somatostatin receptor subtypes. In particular, PET clearly offers higher resolution and improved pharmacokinetics as compared to somatostatin receptor scintigraphy, with promising results for the detection of somatostatin receptor expressing tumors, and provides prognostic information and selection for targeted specific treatments.

6.2.4 Radiopharmaceuticals with Radioiodine

6.2.4.1 Radioiodine I-123 Sodium Iodide (I-123 NaI)

The isotope iodine-123 (I-123) with a half-life of 13.22 h is used as a tracer, in order to evaluate the anatomic and physiologic function of the thyroid. It decays by electron capture to tellurium-123 and emits gamma radiation with predominant energies of 159 and 127 keV. This is the most suitable isotope of the iodine for the diagnosis study of thyroid diseases. The half-life of approximately 13.2 h is ideal for the 24-h iodine uptake test and also diagnostic scanning imaging of the thyroid tissue.

The energy of the photons, 159 keV, is ideal for the NaI (sodium iodide) crystal detector of current gamma cameras. It has a much higher photon flux than I-131. It gives approximately 20 times the counting rate of I-131 for the same administered dose. The radiation burden to the thyroid is far less (1%) comparing to I-131 mainly because of the absence of beta radiation compound. This is the reason why this isotope is reserved only for diagnosis, not being suitable for treatment.

Moreover, scanning a thyroid remnant or metastasis from differentiated thyroid carcinoma with I-123 does not cause "stunning" of the tissue (with loss of uptake) because of the low radiation burden of this isotope.

Iodine-123 is supplied as sodium iodide (NaI), sometimes in basic solution in which it has been dissolved as the free element. This is administered to a patient in capsule form, by intravenous injection, or (less common due to the risk of spilling) as a drinkable solution. Quantitative measurements of the thyroid can be performed to calculate the iodine uptake (absorption).

6.2.4.2 Radioiodine I-124 Sodium Iodide (I-124 NaI)

I-124 is a proton-rich isotope of iodine with a half-life of 4.18 days. Its modes of decay are 74.4% electron capture and 25.6% positron emission. I-124 decays to Te-124 and may be obtained by nuclear reactions in the cyclotron.

This radiopharmaceutical can be used to obtain a direct image of the thyroid using positron emission tomography (PET) or labeled to a pharmaceutical to form a positron-emitting radiopharmaceutical, which is injected into the body and imaged by PET scan.

In the recent years, the use of the radiopharmaceutical increased mainly in thyroid cancer dosimetry studies on PET/CT.

6.2.4.3 Radioiodine I-125 Sodium Iodide (I-125 NaI)

Radioiodine I-125 is a radioisotope of iodine, which has a half-life of 59.4 days and is used in biochemistry, in some radioimmunoassay tests, in nuclear endocrinology imaging, in radiotherapy for prostate, and in brain tumor treatments.

I-125 decays by electron capture while excited to tellurium-125. The relatively long half-life and the low-energy photon emissions are the main criteria, which determine I-125 to be suitable in the radioimmunoassay tests and brachytherapy, less for imaging. I-123 is preferably used, due to its shorter half-life and better penetration. The emission gamma rays are at 35.5 keV.

6.2.4.4 Radioiodine I-131 Sodium Iodide (I-131 NaI)

This iodine isotope is the most used radiopharmaceutical in nuclear endocrinology therapies. It is the "parent" of radionuclide therapies, and until now, there is no other specific treatment in differentiated thyroid carcinomas with better results than I-131.

I-131 has 78 neutrons and 53 protons with the atomic mass (*A*) of 131. Most I-131 production comes from nuclear neutron irradiation of natural tellurium target, Te-130. Its half-life is of 8.02 days.

Radioiodine I-131 decays with beta and gamma emissions. This is the major propriety of I-131, which makes it useful both in imaging and in therapy.

The I-131 decay is in two steps:

1. Firstly, the I-131 decay leads to unstable xenon and beta particles with energies of 606, 248, and 807 keV. In this decay occurs also an antineutrino (Eq. 6.1):

   $$^{131}_{53}\mathrm{I} \Rightarrow ^{131}_{54}\mathrm{Xe}^{*} + e^{-} + \nu \quad (6.1)$$

   e^- is the beta minus particle.
   ν is the antineutrino.
   $^{131}_{54}\mathrm{Xe}^{*}$ is the unstable xenon.

   Due to their high energy, the beta particles penetrate the tissues of 0.6–2 mm, fact that is suitable in therapy.
2. Secondly, the unstable Xe^{*} passes rapidly in stable Xe with gamma rays emission. Almost 90% of the gamma energy is of 364 keV, the rest being of 723 keV (Eq. 6.2).

$$^{131}_{54}\mathrm{Xe}^{*} \Rightarrow ^{131}_{54}\mathrm{Xe} + \gamma \quad (6.2)$$

These features make I-131 proper for diagnosis, due to the gamma energy able to be detected by the gamma cameras. For nuclear endocrinologists, it is important to remember that this level of energy imposes the use of collimators for medium energy, different from those used for Tc-99m. If the number of cameras is limited, the change of collimator is time consuming and needs a careful organization of both patients and examinations.

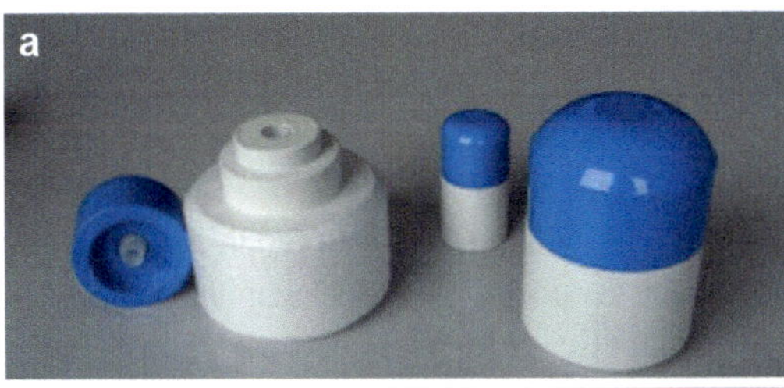

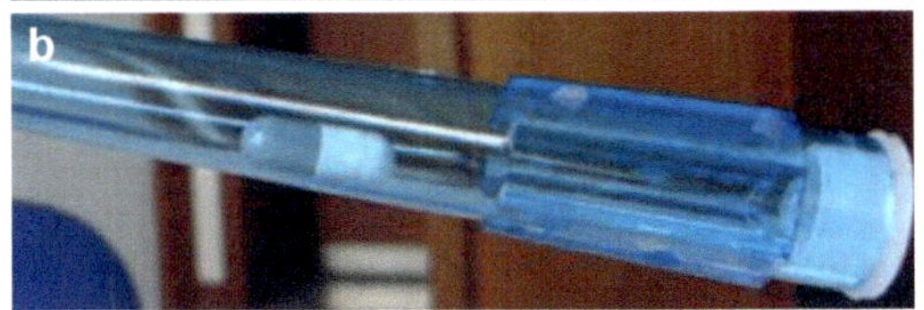

Fig. 6.2 The I-131 shielded container (**a**) and the capsule (**b**) ready to be used by patient for radioiodine therapy

One must keep in mind that the presence of beta particles limits the use of I-131 in diagnostic procedures, other than those recommended in the follow-up of thyroid carcinomas.

The beta particles produce the irradiation and destroy thyroid tissue, fact that justifies its use in treatment of some thyroid diseases.

It is important to underline that the penetration of beta particles of 0.6–2 mm in the narrowing tissues is the basis for using this radionuclide in the treatment of some situations of medullar thyroid carcinomas. In this particular thyroid cancer, the tumor occurs from C cells of the thyroid, which do not trap radioiodine. This penetration propriety justifies the irradiation of C cells from the surrounding follicular cells, which are iodine selective.

The pharmacological presentation is of I-131 sodium iodide. This sodium iodide I-131 may be a solution, as it has an activity strictly calibrated per volume unit, or gelatine capsules. The capsules have precise calibrated doses of I-131, ready to use according to the endocrinologist's prescription of dosage (Fig. 6.2)

6.2.4.5 Radioiodine I-123 Metaiodobenzylguanidine (I-123 MIBG)

I-123 metaiodobenzylguanidine (I-123 MIBG), or iobenguane, is a combination of an iodinated benzyl and a guanidine group labeled with I-123, especially developed for the diagnosis of tumors of neuroendocrine origin. MIBG enters neuroendocrine cells by an active uptake mechanism via the epinephrine transporter and is deposited in the neurosecretory granules, resulting in a specific concentration in contrast to the cells of the surrounding tissues.

MIBG scintigraphy is used to image tumors of neuroendocrine origin, particularly those of neuroectodermal origin (pheochromocytomas, paragangliomas, and neuroblastomas), and other neuroendocrine tumors (e.g., carcinoids, medullary thyroid carcinoma).

The 159 keV gamma energy of I-123 is more suitable for imaging (especially when using SPECT) than the 360 keV photons of I-131; with the latter, results are usually available within 24 h, whereas with I-131, MIBG-delayed images may be required for optimal target to background ratios.

I-123-labeled agent is to be considered the radiopharmaceutical of choice as it has a more favorable dosimetry and provides better image quality allowing an accurate anatomical localization by the use of SPECT/CT hybrid systems. Nonetheless, I-131 MIBG is widely used for most routine applications mainly in adult patients because of its rapid availability and the possibility of obtaining delayed scans.

The effective dose is of 0.013 mSv/MBq for adults, from an I-123 MIBG scanning.

The radioactive MIBG preparation is usually a ready-for-use licensed radiopharmaceutical, which is sold by specialized companies. The compound is radioiodinated by isotope exchange and distributed to nuclear medicine centers, where no additional preparation is required.

6.2.4.6 Radioiodine I-131 Metaiodobenzylguanidine (I-131 MIBG)

I-131 metaiodobenzylguanidine (I-131 MIBG) is a combination of an iodinated benzyl and a guanidine group labeled with I-131, both developed for the diagnosis and treatment of tumors mainly derived from adrenal medulla. Because of its energy of 364 keV and the presence of beta particles, this radiotracer is not one of the best radiopharmaceuticals for the diagnosis of these neuroendocrine tumors; the injuries to other surrounding tissues may occur due to beta particles penetration. In opposition, this particularity is the major feature that makes the I-131 MIBG the selective targeted treatment for the tumors of neuroendocrine origin.

Even if there are some disadvantages, like the high burden rate and the delay in obtaining the final results of the examination, this radiotracer is still very popular among the endocrinology centers mainly because of its large availability (half-life much longer than I-123) and more accessible price.

Regarding the I-131 MIBG for treatment, the indications are laying on the particular beta emission, which is able to destroy tumor tissues with the features of neuroendocrine tumors.

For I-123 and I-131, it is important to underline, both for diagnostic and therapy, the mandatory indication of blocking the thyroid, before any of these procedures is done, in order to protect the gland from the injuries caused by iodine trapping. The blocking starts 1 day before the procedure and continues 2–4 days afterward. As a special precaution in both cases, there are many drugs that may interfere with the uptake or with the vesicular storage of the tracers, fact that requires a special attention when preparing the patient for examination.

I-131 MIBG is also indicated in the evaluation of the response to treatment by analyzing the uptake of the radiopharmaceutical in the tumor.

The effective dose calculated for an adult in an I-131 MIBG procedure is of 0.14 mSv/MBq, which is ten times higher per MBq than in the case of I-123 MIBG.

6.2.5 Indium-111 Pentetreotide (In-111 Pentetreotide)

Indium In-111 pentetreotide is a diagnostic radiopharmaceutical with indication in the diagnosis of the neuroendocrine tumors.

Indium In-111 pentetreotide is an agent for the scintigraphic localization of primary and metastatic neuroendocrine tumors bearing somatostatin receptors.

The product is represented by two components:

1. The vial, which contains a lyophilized mixture ofpentetreotide[*N*-(diethylenetriamine-*N*,*N*,*N*′,*N*″-tetraacetic acid-*N*″-acetyl)-D-phenylalanyl-L-hemicystyl-L-phenylalanyl-D-tryptophyl-L-lysyl-L-threonyl-L-hemicystyl-L-threoninol cyclic (2→7) disulfide] (also known as octreotide DTPA), and other unspecific compounds. Prior to lyophilization, sodium hydroxide, or hydrochloric acid, may have been added for pH adjustment. The vial contents are sterile and non-pyrogenic. No bacteriostatic preservative is present.
2. A 10 mL vial of indium In-111 chloride sterile solution, which contains 1.1 mL of 111 MBq/mL (3.0 mCi/mL) indium In-111 chloride in 0.02 N HCl at the time of calibration. The vial contents are sterile and non-pyrogenic. No bacteriostatic preservative is present. Indium In-111 pentetreotide is prepared by combining the two kit components.

The indium In-111 pentetreotide solution is suitable for intravenous administration as it is, or it may be diluted to a maximum volume of 3.0 mL with 0.9% sodium chloride injection. The labeling yield of indium In-111 pentetreotide should be determined before administration to the patient by chromatography.

Indium In-111 decays by electron capture to cadmium-111 (stable) and has a physical half-life of 2.805 days (67.32 h). The biological half-life is of 6 h.

Pentetreotide is a form of octreotide, which is a long-acting analogue of the human hormone somatostatin. Indium In-111 pentetreotide binds to somatostatin receptors on the cell surfaces throughout the body. Within an hour from the injection, most of the dose of indium In-111 pentetreotide distributes from plasma to extravascular body tissues and concentrates in tumors containing a high density of somatostatin receptors. After background clearance, visualization of somatostatin receptor-rich tissue is achieved. In addition to somatostatin receptor-rich tumors, other organs are normally visualized, such as pituitary gland, thyroid gland, liver, spleen, and urinary bladder and also the bowel. Excretion is made almost exclusively via the kidneys.

Indium In-111 pentetreotide binds to cell surface receptors for somatostatin; the hormonal in vitro effect is one-tenth from the effect of the octreotide.

The recommended intravenous dose for planar imaging is of 111 MBq (3.0 mCi) of indium In-111 pentetreotide. The recommended intravenous dose for SPECT imaging is of 222 MBq (6.0 mCi) of indium In-111 pentetreotide.

The effective dose of In-111 pentetreotide in adults is of 13.03 mSv/111 MBq, dose used for one scan.

A better sensitivity and resolution is by using the SPECT/CT, mainly in the neuroendocrine tumor of the gastrointestinal tract.

The use of In-111 octreotide has the same basic principles as the therapeutic agents of somatostatin analogues, with the systemic action and special indication in the therapy of neuroendocrine tumors with somatostatin expression, so the imaging test might be a selection tool for the responder patients.

6.2.6 Radiopharmaceuticals with Techentium-99m

Technetium-99m (Tc-99m) is the radioisotope most widely used in nuclear medicine diagnosis. It is estimated that over 80% of the nearly 25 million nuclear medicine diagnostic studies carried out annually are done with this single isotope. This percentage share is expected to remain in the foreseeable future, notwithstanding the introduction of new diagnostic radiopharmaceuticals containing other radionuclides. The availability of the short-lived technetium-99m (a half-life of 6 h), as the daughter product of the long-lived molybdenum-99 (a half-life of 66 h), is one of the major factors, which have promoted the universal use of this radioisotope. The parent radionuclide molybdenum-99 (Mo-99) can be prepared in abundant quantities by the fission of uranium-235 in a nuclear reactor with a fission yield of about 6%.

There are only a limited number of industrial companies and national centers producing molybdenum-99 from fission products, but together they have the adequate capacity to meet the world's demands for molybdenum-99.

The generator is an automated, highly shielded system, allowing easy elution of a sterile and pyrogen-free Tc-99m sodium pertechnetate solution. This solution is eluted from an alumina chromatography column.

The device consists of the following parts (Fig. 6.3):

- Chromatography column which contains alumina, which absorbs molybdate ions but releases pertechnetate ions when eluted with saline solution.
- Inlet needle connected to the top of the column.
- Sterilization filter with hydrophobic spot; one of its ends is linked to the lower part of the column while the other one to an outlet needle.
- Lead shielding (minimum thickness, 41 mm; maximum thickness, 70 mm).
- The outer cylindrical cover is in plastic (diameter, 130 mm; maximum height, 278 mm).

The complete system weighs about 16 kg. Each generator is shipped ready to use and does not need to be assembled by the user. The generator of technetium is conceived to elute the whole available activity into 5 mL. It is possible, however, to elute larger volumes (10 or 15 mL) to obtain a different radioactive concentration. The elute must be used within 6 h from the elution. The Tc-99m pertechnetate (Tc-99m Pt) solution eluted from the generator is a clear, colorless, isotonic, sterile, and pyrogen-free solution with a pH ranging from 4.5 to 7.5, meeting the requirements of European and US Pharmacopoeias. The available generators have different activities, varying from 2.5 GBq (67.5 mCi) Mo-99, corresponding to 2.2 GBq (59.0 mCi) Tc-99m at calibration, up to 25.0 GBq (675.0 mCi) Mo 99m, corresponding to 21.9 GBq (591.0 mCi) Tc-99m at calibration. Recently, the available activities became much higher, going up to 175 GBq.

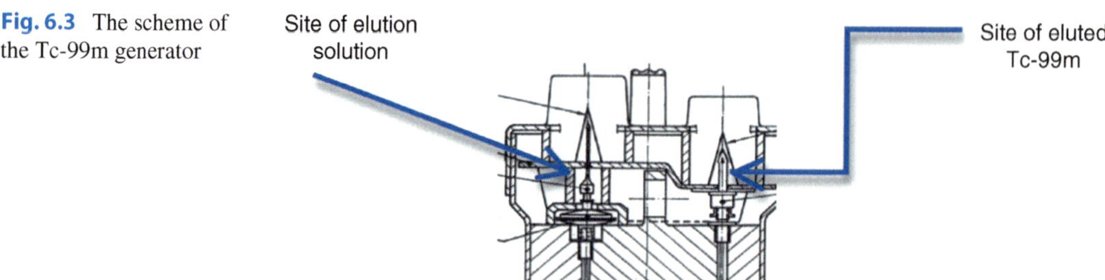

Fig. 6.3 The scheme of the Tc-99m generator

Intermediate doses are also available. Until now, no adverse reactions have been observed. Injectable Tc-99m sodium pertechnetate solution should not be administered to pregnant or breast-feeding women.

The generator of Tc-99m is delivered in the medical unit at the begging of each week or twice a month in a ready-to-use form. A total amount of activity is calculated for each type of generator, and it represents the life of the generator; in fact, these data establish how many days we are able to benefit from that generator, how many patients, and what kind of examinations may be proceeded until the decay will lead to a total consumption of the radiotracer. Usually, the process of preparation of radiolabeled compounds with Tc-99m is repeated every morning, starting with the elution of the generator. Figures 6.4, 6.5, and 6.6 show a brief presentation of this process. Figure 6.4 presents the vials (c, d, e, f), some of them specially designed for radioactive materials, made of materials such as lead (b) or tungsten (a). There is a series of special shielding, made on tungsten, for syringes of different sizes and types (g), which confers high protection during their manipulation.

Figure 6.5 presents the materials ready to be used under the sterile laminar flow hood. The next image (Fig. 6.6) presents the generator with the vials, one of sterile saline solution and the other shielded with the eluted technetium.

Figure 6.7 presents the next steps where the eluted Tc-99m is calibrated. The transfer takes place in a sterile area, and the measurement of the activity is performed with an instrument called calibrator (Figs. 6.8 and 6.9). This instrument must be adjusted according to the type of radionuclide that we intend to measure (attention to the energy!).

The early technetium radiopharmaceuticals were developed by taking advantage of the physiological properties, such as adsorption, distribution, metabolism, and excretion of various technetium-99m complexes, and were used for imaging the thyroid, the liver, the bone, the kidneys, etc.

Technetium-99m radiopharmaceuticals are often formulated from the so-called "cold" kits (they do not contain radioactivity). When treated with a sodium pertechnetate solution eluted from a technetium-99m generator, the final product used for patient injection is directly formed. Cold kits are prepared in such a manner as to have stability, ranging from several months to a few years, and may be transported at room temperature and then stored in a refrigerator to ensure stability. Large-scale preparation of cold kits requires special techniques and facilities, and it is

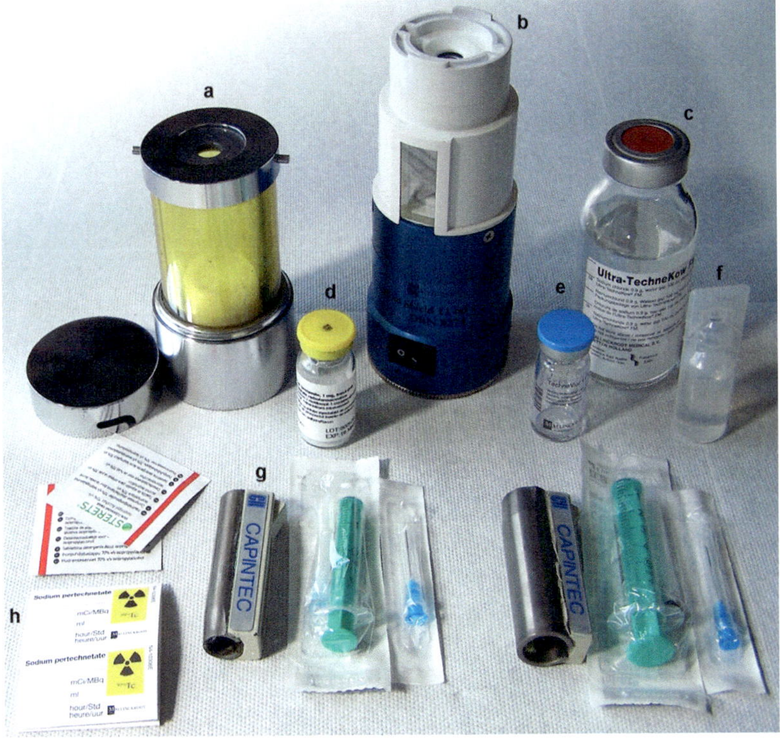

Fig. 6.4 Elution kit for Tc-99m generator

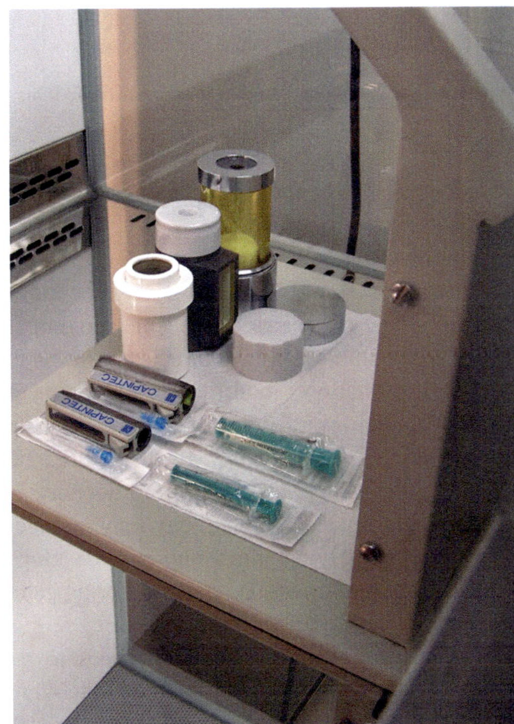

Fig. 6.5 Shielding for elution and injection preparation under sterile laminar flow

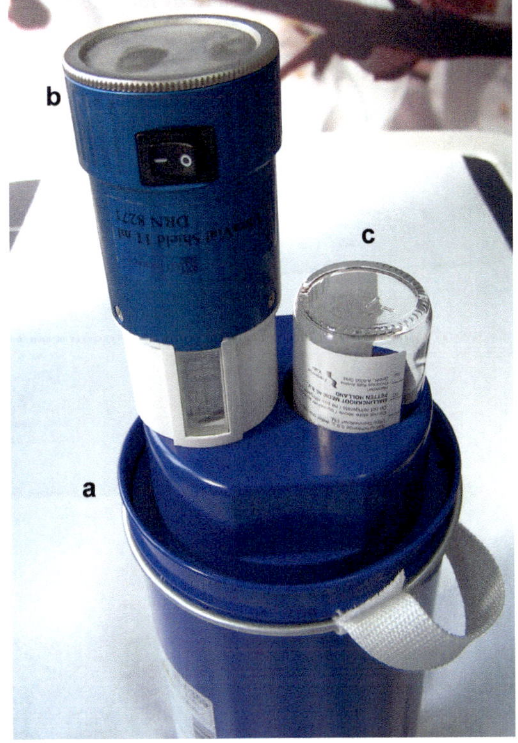

Fig. 6.6 The generator with eluted Tc-99m Pt ready to use

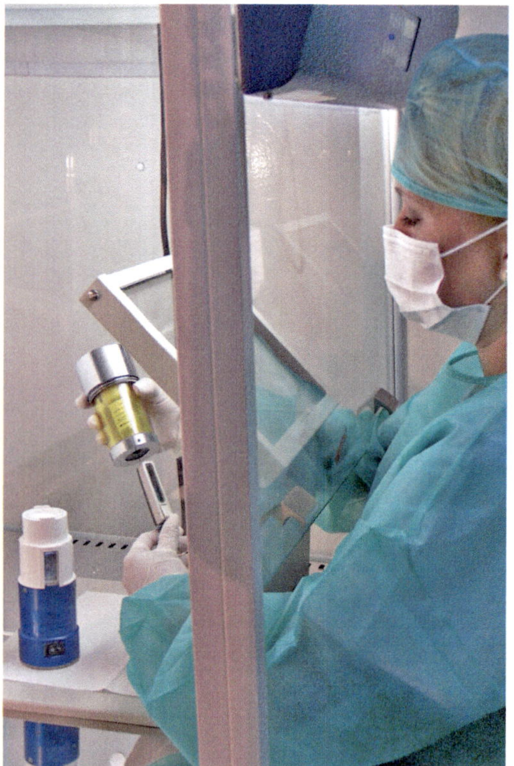

Fig. 6.7 The dose of Tc-99m Pt, ready for calibration

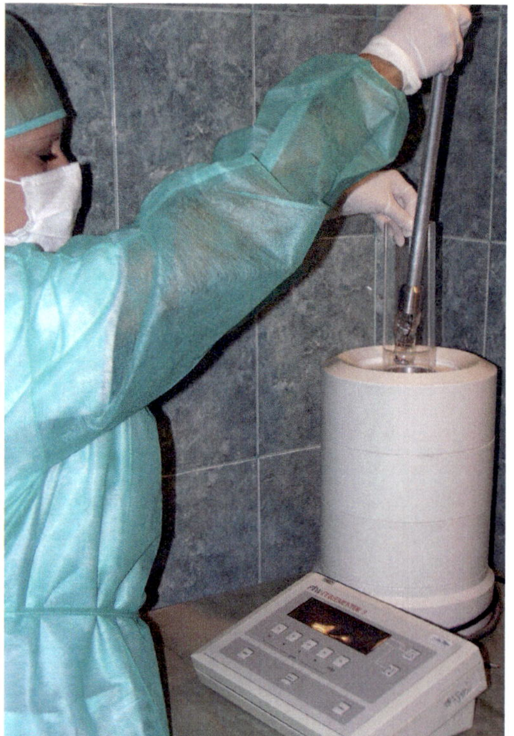

Fig. 6.8 Calibration of the dose

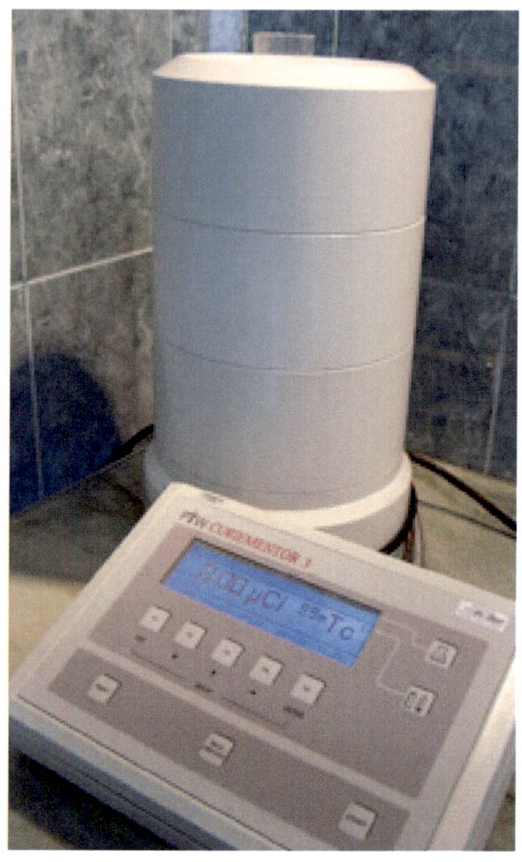

Fig. 6.9 The calibrator, adjusted for the use of Tc-99m

mostly performed by industrial companies and in national laboratories.

The investigations used for the development of cancer imaging agents mostly use peptides and antibodies as carrier molecules to target tumor sites. Radiopharmaceuticals can provide useful information about the function and molecular biology of the tumor, by measuring several of its causal factors. In the future, the specific roles of technetium-99m radiopharmaceuticals for imaging in oncology may include, for example, the lymphatic system, the development of new blood vessels, and monitoring gene therapy.

The most frequently used substances to be labeled with Tc-99m in nuclear endocrinology are presented in the next sections.

As a particular situation, the pure eluted technetium-99m is a ready-to-use radiopharmaceutical, so-called technetium-99m pertechnetate.

6.2.6.1 Technetium-99m Pertechnetate (Tc-99m Pt)

This is the simplest, cheapest, and easiest to prepare radiotracer in nuclear endocrinology, mainly used in thyroid imaging. This product, having the symbol Tc-99m Pt, is injected IV in order to evaluate the function, by thyroid uptake, and the structure of the thyroid, by scan (scintigraphy).

The pertechnetate of Tc-99m is actually the brut product from the generator being the pure eluate obtained without any labeling compounds. After the elution of the generator, the pertechnetate is just calibrated, and it is ready to be injected for scanning.

This Tc-99m Pt represents the most common radiotracer, used worldwide for thyroid scanning; all other radiopharmaceuticals based on Tc-99m use the Tc-99m Pt for labeling.

In thyroid imaging, the fundament of this procedure is to have an image of the thyroid gland obtained in direct relation with the blood flow and not with the main thyroid process of organification of iodine.

6.2.6.2 Technetium-99m MIBI (Tc-99m MIBI or Sestamibi)

This radiopharmaceutical is the most important tracer in parathyroid gland imaging. Initially being a product with indication in myocardial perfusion and breast imaging, its proprieties imposed the procedure of MIBI scan, as the imagistic "gold standard" in the diagnostic of primary hyperparathyroidism.

Composition of the kit:

- 2-Methoxyisobutylisonitrile (MIBI) copper (I) tetrafluoroborate
- Stannous chloride
- L-Cysteine hydrochloride monohydrate
- Sodium citrate dihydrate
- Mannitol

Tc-99m MIBI is administered intravenously after labeling the kit with a sterile, oxidant-free solution of eluate from a radionuclide generator of technetium. The radioactivity of a given dose should always be adjusted taking into account its usefulness in diagnosis.

Tc-99m MIBI is a lipophilic cation complex, which is accumulated in the cardiac muscle in proportion to the blood flow. Although the mechanism of uptake is not known, studies on cellular fractionation show that 84% of it is within the cytoplasm. The diffusion to the intracellular compartment occurs easily and in proportion to the blood flow. The process of washing the complex out from the cardiac muscle is slow. The effective half-life in the cardiac muscle is similar to the physical half-life of technetium-99m. The complex is redistributed in a small extent.

Tc-99m MIBI is accumulated within the cells through active transport and passive diffusion, a process facilitated by the lipophilic nature of tracer, and by the negative transmembrane potential found in metabolically hyperactive cells in hyperparathyroidism. As increased numbers of mitochondria have been found in hyperactive parathyroid cells, intramitochondrial sequestration may be an additional mechanism of Tc-99m MIBI tissue binding. This may account for slower Tc-99m MIBI washout from hyperactive parathyroid compared to normal thyroid and parathyroid tissues.

Tc-99m MIBI radiopharmaceutical may be used within 6 h since the end of the labeling procedure.

The safety regulations regarding work in the conditions of ionizing radiation exposure should be strictly respected during the preparation and administration of a radiopharmaceutical.

The labeling procedure consists of:

- The vial with lyophilisate is placed in a lead protective container.
- With a syringe (piercing the rubber stopper), introduce Tc-99m Pt with the desired activity supplemented with physiological saline solution into a vial containing lyophilised MIBI.
- Without withdrawing the needle, remove the volume of gas equal to the volume of solution introduced with the same syringe, in order to counteract the pressure.
- Shake the vial until the contents are fully dissolved (about 1 min).
- Take the vial out of the lead container, place it in a hot boiling water bath (the water should

be boiling during the procedure of labeling), and boil for 10–12 min. While boiling, do not allow contact between boiling water and an aluminum cap.

- Take the vial out of the boiling water bath; put it into a lead container and leave to cool down to room temperature (about 15 min).
- The resulted solution is a ready-to-use solution for injections.

The determination of radiochemical purity should be performed with ascending thin-layer chromatography. The sum of contaminations of unbound Tc-99m Pt and a reduced form of Tc-99m should not be higher than 5% of the total activity.

Tc-99m MIBI is also used in the evaluation of thyroid nodules. It was a method considered to be able to bring new data in relation to define the differential diagnosis between a benign and a malignant thyroid nodule. In a dual phase study (early and late scans), the behavior of a nodule, with respect to MIBI, was reported by some authors as being at least as sensitive as the genetic results from a fine needle aspiration biopsy.

6.2.6.3 Technetium-99m Tetrofosmin (Tc-99m Tetrofosmin)

Some centers use Tc-99m tetrofosmin to perform parathyroid scanning. Studies have shown that myocardial uptake of Tc-99m tetrofosmin is linearly related to coronary blood flow, confirming the effectiveness of the complex as a myocardial perfusion imaging agent. Additional studies concluded that Tc-99m tetrofosmin is taken up/retained by the mitochondria of parathyroid cells. This mechanism is dependent on the mitochondrial membrane potential in a manner similar to that of other lipophilic technetium cationic complexes.

In a critical manner, the use of sestamibi or tetrofosmin in the scanning of parathyroid is a subject that will not be discussed in this section, but it is important to underline that both tracers and methods were used in this endocrine pathology, and until nowadays, the clinical studies continue to establish the superiority of one of the tracer.

Each vial contains a pre-dispensed, sterile, non-pyrogenic, lyophilized mixture of tetrofosmin [6,9-bis(2-ethoxyethyl)-3,12-dioxa-6,9-diphosphatetradecane] and other excipients. The lyophilized powder is sealed under a nitrogen atmosphere with a rubber closure. The product contains no antimicrobial preservative. When technetium Tc-99m pertechnetate is added to tetrofosmin in the presence of stannous reductants, a lipophilic, cationic technetium Tc-99m complex is formed, the Tc-99m tetrofosmin. This complex is the active ingredient in the reconstituted drug product, on whose biodistribution and pharmacokinetic properties the indications for use depend. This product does not need boiling for labeling.

6.2.6.4 Technetium-99m (V) DMSA (Tc-99m (V) DMSA)

Dimercaptosuccinic acid (DMSA) pentavalent is used for the evaluation of the medullary thyroid carcinoma. Clinical trials showed improvement of patient management in this disease, succeeding to localize the recurrence in the presence of an increased serum level of calcitonin.

Technetium-99m (V) DMSA is prepared using the DMSA kit, but it requires the addition of a second component (bicarbonate buffer, 4.4%, pH 9.0) for adjusting the pH to 8–9 prior to labeling.

- The freeze-dried kit using 1.0 mL of bicarbonate buffer at pH 9.0 is well mixed.
- Add 2 mL of Tc-99m Pt solution containing a maximum of 3 mCi (1.11 MBq) of activity.
- Stir for 1 min and allow standing for 20 min. The Tc-99m (V) DMSA labeled in this manner should be stable for over 4 h after labeling.

Radiochemical purity is determined by ascending chromatography.

6.2.6.5 Technetium-99m Tektrotyde (Tc-99m Tektrotyde)

Tc-99m Tektrotyd (HYNIC-[D-Phe1,Tyr3-octreotide]·TFA) is a radiopharmaceutical indicated for diagnostics of pathological lesions in which somatostatin receptors are overexpressed (particularly subtypes 2 and 3, 5): gastro-entero-pancreatic neuroendocrine tumors (GEP-NET); pituitary adenomas; tumors originating in a sympathetic system; pheochromocytoma, paraganglioma, neuroblastoma, and ganglioneurinoma; and medullary thyroid carcinoma. It is also used in other tumors which may overexpress somatostatin receptors, beyond endocrinology area: breast cancer, melanoma, lymphomas, prostate cancer, non-small lung carcinoma, sarcoma, renal cell carcinoma, astrocytoma, meningioma, and ovarian cancer.

6.2.7 Thallium-201 Chloride (Tl-201 Chloride)

Thallium-201 has the atomic mass (*A*) of 201 and the proton number (*Z*) 81.

Tl-201 decays to mercury Hg-201 by electron capture with a half-life of 3.0408 days. The X-ray energies are 69 and 83 keV, and the γ-ray energies are 135, 166, and 167 keV.

Thallium-201 chloride is an isotonic sterile solution for IV administration, with a pH ranging from 4.0 to 7.0.

The main cardiac diagnostic indications are myocardial scintigraphy in the evaluation of coronary perfusion and cellular viability in ischemic heart disease, cardiomyopathies, myocarditis, myocardial contusion, and secondary lesions.

In endocrinology, it is used for parathyroid scintigraphy, but not as a standard investigation, and also in some special cases of thyroid tumors and metastases, like the differentiated thyroid tumors that are not iodine sensitive anymore.

The development of sophisticated molecular carriers and the availability of radionuclides in high purity and adequate specific activity are contributing toward the successful application of radionuclide therapy.

6.2.8 Radiopharmaceuticals for Targeted Radionuclide Therapy

Selective molecule-binding radionuclide therapy involves the use of radiopharmaceuticals to selectively radiation releases to a disease site, as this would potentially deliver the absorbed radiation dose more selectively to cancerous tissues.

Advances in tumor biology, recombinant antibody technology, solid-phase peptide synthesis, and radiopharmaceutical chemistry molecular vectors are being developed for targeted therapy. When labeled with therapeutic radionuclides, peptide molecules have the potential to destroy receptor-expressing tumors, an approach referred to as peptide receptor radionuclide therapy (PRRT).

Yttrium-90 and Lutetium-177 are frequently used as radionuclides in such PRRT studies.

Lutetium-177 (halftime is 6.71 days) is a radionuclide that has both beta particle emissions for therapeutic use and gamma emissions (113 and 208 keV) for imaging purposes. It has a short radius of penetration, which makes it suitable for the radioimmunotherapy of small and soft tumors. Both Y-90 and Lu-177-DOTA analogues were developed for targeted radiotherapy of neuroendocrine tumors.

Further Reading

Chilton HM, Witcofski RL (1986) Nuclear pharmacy. An introduction to the clinical applications of radiopharmaceuticals. Lea and Fiebiger, Philadelphia

Henkin RE, Boles MA, Dillehay GL et al (1996) The scientific basis of nuclear medicine; Part IIB: radiopharmacy. In: Nuclear medicine. Mosby, New York

Hung JC, Ponto JA, Hammes RI (1996) Radiopharmaceutical- related pitfalls and artifacts. Semin Nucl Med 26:208–255

IAEA (2007) Comparative evaluation of therapeutic radiopharmaceuticals. Technical reports series no. 458 STI/Doc/010/458

Ishibashi M et al (1998) Comparison of technetium-99m-MIBI, technetium-99m- tetrofosmin, ultrasound and MRI for localization of abnormal parathyroid glands. J Nucl Med 39:320–324

Campennì A, Giovanella L, Siracusa M, et al (2016) (99m)Tc-Methoxy-isobutyl-isonitrile scintigraphy is a useful tool for assessing the risk of malignancy in thyroid nodules with indeterminate fine-needle cytology. Thyroid 26(8):1101–1109

Khalil MM (2011) PET chemistry. Radiopharmaceuticals. In: Basic sciences of nuclear medicine. Springer, Berlin, pp. 103–116

Kowalsky RJ, Perry JR (1987) Radiopharmaceuticals. In: Nuclear medicine. Appleton & Lange, Norwalk

Palmer EL, Scott JA, Strauss HW (1992) Radiation and radionuclides. In: Practical nuclear medicine. WB Saunders, Philadelphia, pp 57–71

Rubello D, Mariani G, Pelizzo MR, Giscris A (2007) Minimally invasive radio-guided parathyroidectomy on a group of 452 primary hyperparathyroid patients – refinement of preoperative imaging and intraoperative procedure. Nuklearmedizin 46:85–92

Rubow SM, Ellmann A, Leroux J, Klopper J (1991) Excretion of Tc-99m hexakismethoxyisobutylisonitrile in milk. Eur J Nucl Med 18:363–365

Saha GB (1992) Fundamentals of nuclear pharmacy, 4th edn. Springer, New York

Sampson CB (1999) Textbook of radiopharmacy: theory and practice, 3rd edn. Gordon and Breach Science, Amsterdam

Sharp PF, Gemmell H, Murray A (eds) (2005) Practical nuclear medicine, 3rd edn. Springer, New York, pp 113–143

Thakur ML (2003) New radiopharmaceuticals in oncologic diagnosis and therapy. Cancer Biother Radiopharm 18:276

Williams LE (2010) Radiopharmaceuticals – introduction to drug evaluation and dose estimation. CRC Press/ Taylor & Francis, Boca Raton

Part II

Nuclear Endocrinology

7 The Thyroid Gland

Madman with Goiter: Medieval Painting

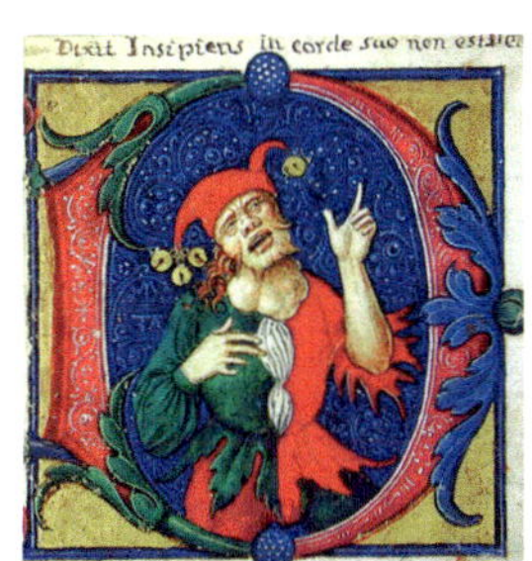

7.1 Anatomy of the Thyroid Gland

The thyroid gland is located beside the trachea, just below the larynx. It has two oval lobes, one of each side of the trachea. The thyroid isthmus lies at about half distance between the thyroid cartilage and the sternal notch.

Laterally, from the anterior to posterior, the internal jugular vein, the vagus nerve, and the common carotid artery are in close relation to the thyroid, as it is possible to observe in the intraoperatory image of the thyroid bed, obtained after the removal of the thyroid gland (Fig. 7.1).

The parathyroid glands are also located in the posterior part; usually there are four: two in the upper bilateral part and two in the lower part of the thyroid.

The recurrent laryngeal nerves are also found in the posterior part, between the trachea and the thyroid. These are very important and delicate elements during the surgery of the thyroid (Fig. 7.2).

The thyroid gland consists of two lobes (right and left) linked by a common part, the isthmus. From the upper margin of the thyroid isthmus may exist sometimes another accessory lobe, named Lalouette pyramid. This particular shape frequently associated with a "butterfly" will be easy to recognize during many of the nuclear imaging procedures.

As a special attention regarding the anatomy details, it is important to underline that, during intrauterine evolution, the thyroid gland descends from its upper position under the tongue, until it reaches the normal pretracheal position. Sometimes, there is a leftover structure in the thyroglossal duct, a failure in descend, which is able to lead to different pathologies involving thyroid tissues in this area.

The thyroid gland is highly vascularized, being mainly supplied from the superior and inferior thyroid arteries, which lie between capsule and pretracheal fascia (false capsule). All thyroid arteries anastomose with one another on and in the substance of the thyroid, but there is little anastomosis across the median plane (except for branches of the superior thyroid artery).

The superior thyroid artery belongs to the first branch of extern carotid artery, it descends to the superior pole of the gland, it pierces the pretracheal fascia, and then it divides into 2–3 branches. The inferior thyroid artery is a branch of the thyrocervical trunk, it runs superomedially posterior to the carotid sheath, it reaches the posterior aspect of the gland, and it divides into several branches, which pierce pretracheal fascia to supply the inferior pole of the thyroid gland. In approximately 10% of the people, the thyroid IMA artery arises from the aorta, the brachiocephalic trunk, or the internal carotid artery, and it ascends anterior to the trachea to supply the isthmus.

Usually, there are three pairs of veins that drain the venous plexus on the anterior surface of the thyroid: the superior thyroid veins drain its superior poles, the middle thyroid veins drain its lateral parts, and the inferior thyroid veins drain its inferior poles.

D. Piciu, *Nuclear Endocrinology*, DOI 10.1007/978-3-319-56582-8_7

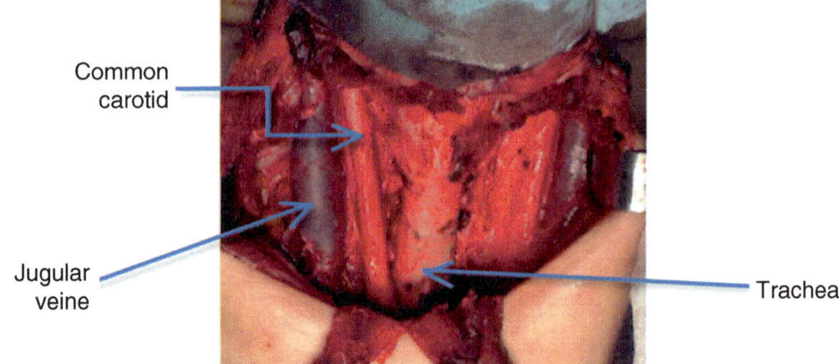

Fig. 7.1 Thyroid bed, after surgical thyroid removal (With the courtesy of A. Irimie, from the Institute of Oncology "Prof. Dr. I. Chiricuță" Cluj-Napoca)

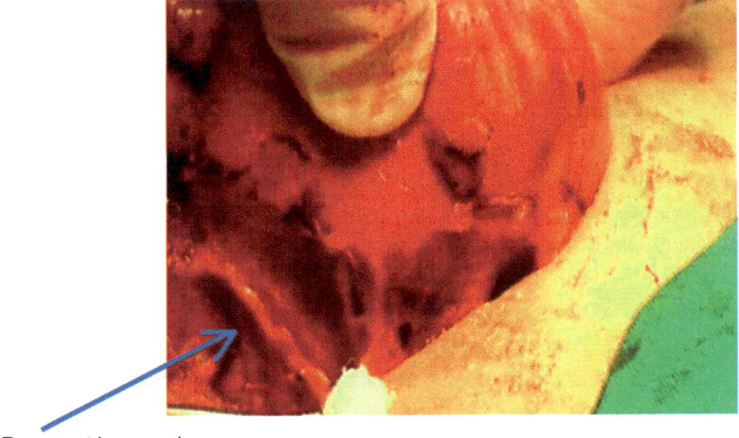

Fig. 7.2 Recurrent laryngeal nerve posterior of thyroid gland (With the courtesy of Dr. A. Irimie, Institute of Oncology "Prof. Dr. I. Chiricuță" Cluj-Napoca)

Lymphatics run in the interlobular connective tissue, often around arteries, communicate with a capsular network of lymph vessels, and after that pass to the prelaryngeal lymph nodes and to the pretracheal and paratracheal lymph nodes. Lateral lymphatic vessels along the superior thyroid veins pass to deep cervical lymph nodes.

The nerves derived from the superior, middle, and inferior cervical sympathetic ganglia reach the thyroid through the cardiac and laryngeal branches of the vagus nerve, which accompanies the arterial vessels; postganglionic and vasomotor fibers have indirect action on the thyroid by regulating the blood vessels.

The thyroid gland is made up of a large number of individual units, called thyroid follicles, and a number of larger cells, called parafollicular cells, which are responsible for the secretion of calcitonin.

Each follicle consists of a layer of follicular cells surrounding the colloid content, which gives a special histological appearance to the thyroid tissue.

The colloid has a variable content, according to the functional status of the thyroid gland. The size of the thyroid gland is largely variable in the range of normal values, being influenced by age, gender, area of residence, and iodine content of environment. Usually, in the case of adults, a thyroid lobe is 4–5 cm high, 2 cm wide, and 2 cm thick, and the thyroid can weigh about 20–30 g. The pathologies affecting the gland may enlarge it considerably, sometimes reaching a weight of 500 g.

7.2 Physiology of the Thyroid Gland

The role of the thyroid gland is the synthesis and release of the thyroxine (T4) and triiodothyronine (T3) thyroid hormones. Circulating iodide is actively transported into the cytosol, where a thyroid peroxidase oxidizes it and iodinates tyrosine residues on the thyroglobulin (Tg) molecule; iodination occurs mostly at the apical plasma membrane. A rearrangement of the iodinated tyrosine residues of thyroglobulin in the colloid produces the iodothyronines T4 and T3. Thyroid-stimulating hormone binding to receptors on the basal surface stimulates follicular cells to become columnar and to form apical pseudopods, which engulf the colloid by endocytosis. After the colloid droplets fuse with lysosomes, controlled hydrolysis of iodinated thyroglobulin liberates T3 and T4 into the cytosol.

These hormones are released into the bloodstream and lymphatic vessels. These processes are promoted by the thyroid-stimulating hormone (TSH), which binds to G-protein-linked receptors on the basal surface of follicular cells.

Parafollicular cells are also called clear (C) cells because they stain less intensely than thyroid follicular cells. They synthesize and release calcitonin, a polypeptide hormone, in response to high blood calcium levels.

The regulation of the thyroid function follows up the hypothalamic-pituitary-thyroid axis negative feedback mechanism (Fig. 7.3):

Thyrotropin-Releasing Hormone (TRH)

- TRH is produced by the hypothalamus.
- Release is pulsatile, circadian.
- Travels through the portal venous system to the adenohypophysis.
- Stimulates thyroid-stimulating hormone (TSH) formation.

Thyroid-Stimulating Hormone (TSH)

- Upregulated by TRH
- Downregulated by thyroid hormones
- Travels through the portal venous system
- Stimulates iodine uptake, colloid endocytosis, and growth of the thyroid gland
- Produced by adenohypophysis

Biosynthesis of T4 and T3 Includes

- Dietary iodine (I) ingestion.
- Active transport and uptake of iodide (I−) by the thyroid gland.
- Oxidation of I− and iodination of thyroglobulin (Tg) tyrosine residues.
- Coupling of iodotyrosine residues to form T4 and T3; the iodination of tyrosyl residues forms monoiodotyrosine (MIT) and diiodotyrosine (DIT), which are then coupled to form either T3 or T4.

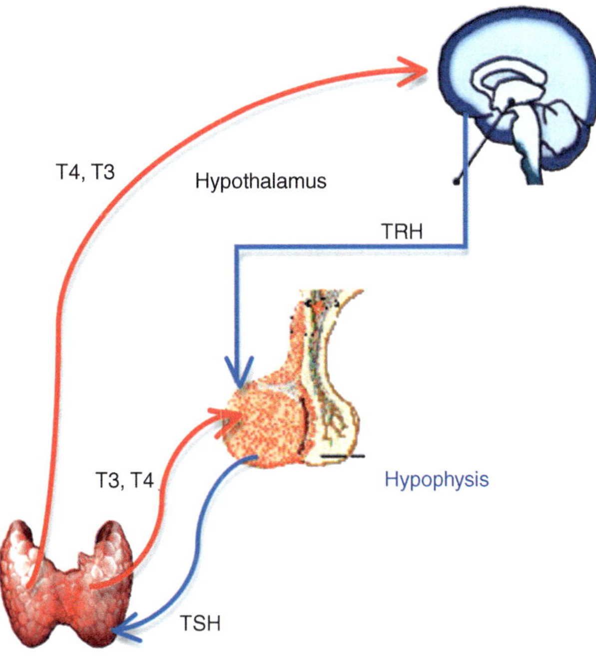

Fig. 7.3 The hypothalamic-pituitary-thyroid axis negative feedback mechanism

- Proteolysis of Tg with release of T4 and T3 into the circulation.

Active Transportation and I– Uptake by the Thyroid

- Dietary iodine reaches the circulation as iodide anion (I–).
- The thyroid gland transports I– to the sites of hormone synthesis.
- Accumulation in the thyroid is an active transportation process stimulated by the TSH.
- Must be oxidized to be able to iodinate tyrosyl residues of Tg.
- Both reactions are catalyzed by TPO.

Thyroperoxidase (TPO)

- TPO catalyzes the oxidation steps involved in I– activation, iodination of Tg tyrosyl residues, and coupling of iodotyrosyl residues.
- TPO acts in the proteolysis of Tg with release of T4 and T3.

Production of T4 and T3 and Conversion

- T4 and T3 are synthesized and stored within the Tg molecule.
- To liberate T4 and T3, Tg is resorbed into the follicular cells in the form of colloid droplets, which fuse with lysosomes to form phagolysosomes.
- Tg is then hydrolyzed to T4 and T3, which are then secreted into the circulation.
- T4 is the primary secretory product of the thyroid gland, being the only source of T4. The thyroid secretes approximately 70–90 μg of T4 per day; the total daily production rate of T3 is about 15–30 μg (80% of circulating T3 comes from deiodination of T4 in peripheral tissues, and 20% comes from direct thyroid secretion).
- T4 is biologically inactive in target tissues until converted to T3; T3 then becomes the biologically active hormone responsible for the majority of thyroid hormone effects.

Sites of T4 Conversion

- The liver is the major extrathyroidal T4 conversion site for the production of T3.
- Some T4 to T3 conversions also occur in the kidney and other tissues.

Hormonal Transport

- More than 99% of the circulating T4 and T3 is bound to plasma carrier proteins: thyroxine-binding globulin (TBG) binds about 75%; transthyretin (TTR), also called thyroxine-binding prealbumin (TBPA), binds about 10–15%; albumin binds about 7%; and high-density lipoproteins (HDL) bind about 3%.
- The only unbound (free) hormone has metabolic activity and physiologic effects.

Free Hormones

- Free hormones (FT3, FT4) are a tiny percentage of the total of hormones in the plasma (about 0.03% T4; 0.3% T3).
- Increased TBG: increased levels of total serum thyroid hormones T4 and T3; free T4 (FT4) and free T3 (FT3) concentrations remain unchanged.
- Decreased TBG: decreased levels of total serum T4 and T3—FT4 and FT3 levels remain unchanged.
- From the above, it is apparent that the plasma concentrations of T4 and T3 are a function of TRH, TSH, thyroid production of T4 and T3, TBG, peripheral deiodinative conversion of T4 to T3, and deiodinative clearance of T3. Perturbation in any of these determinants may lead to changes in others, and these changes may be reflected by changes in thyroid function studies.

The Functions of the Thyroid Hormones

- The thyroid hormone initiates or sustains differentiation and growth: it stimulates the formation of proteins; it is essential for normal brain development and essential for childhood growth; untreated congenital hypothyroidism or chronic hypothyroidism during childhood can result in incomplete development and mental retardation.
- The thyroid hormone influences cardiovascular hemodynamics: increased cardiac output, increased heart rate and stroke volume, increased systolic pressure, and decreased systemic vascular resistance.
- The thyroid hormone-mediated thermogenesis (increased expression of mitochondrial uncoupling proteins).

- The thyroid hormone influences the female reproductive system.
- The thyroid hormone is critical for normal bone growth and development.
- The thyroid hormone regulates mitochondrial activity.
- The thyroid hormones stimulate metabolic activities in most tissues: increased basal metabolic rate, increased oxygen consumption, and increased protein turnover.

With its features, the thyroid gland is the "internal clock" for all the functions of the body, a normal thyroid function being reflected in the whole equilibrium of the human organism. If we consider that an adult thyroid gland weighs about 30 g, this represents in a healthy 70 kg adult about 0.05% of all his body; but without a normal development of the thyroid gland, without this minimal quantity of special tissue, the passage from primitive human being to *Homo sapiens* would not be possible.

7.3 Diagnosis of the Thyroid Gland

7.3.1 Clinical Examination

Among other endocrine glands, the thyroid gland has a particular advantage related to its easy accessible situation. As previously mentioned, the malfunction of the thyroid gland may be reflected in every organ or system of the body, covering a multitude of signs and symptoms. This is the reason why every physician of any specialty must be prepared at least in performing a physical examination and in doing a careful anamnestic interview.

7.3.1.1 History

Since the thyroid pathology may have genetic determinism, the history is one of the first steps in the evaluation of the patient.

Nowadays, a special attention is given to patient history, due to severe increasing of nodular goiter, in order to have or not an aggressive approach of the nodule.

The history will bring information related to:

- Age (elder patients need special attention firstly because of the evident difference in cancer evolution, age being an important staging factor)
- Gender (even if female patients are more frequently affected by thyroid diseases, the male ones are related to a more aggressive evolution)
- Exposure to radiation (in this case, a nodular goiter must be very carefully investigated for the exclusion of cancer)
- Signs/symptoms of hyper-/hypothyroidism
- Rapid change in volume or size of the nodule
  - The pain may indicate hemorrhage into nodule.
  - The lack of pain may indicate a malignant pathology.

The history may report the association of thyroid pathology with other syndromes:

- Gardner's syndrome (familial adenomatous polyposis)
  - Association with thyroid cancer.
  - Mostly in young women.
  - Thyroid cancer preceded the diagnosis of polyposis in 1/3 of cases.
- Cowden syndrome (mucocutaneous hamartomas, keratosis, fibrocystic breast changes, and gastrointestinal polyps)
  - Association with thyroid cancer
- Familial medullary thyroid carcinoma (MTC)
  - Familial MTC or multiple endocrine neoplasia (MEN II)
- Family cases of other thyroid cancers

History elements suggestive for malignancy:

- Rapid progressive enlargement
- Hoarseness
- Dysphagia
- Dyspnea
- Lymph nodes

7.3.1.2 Physical Examination

The situation of the thyroid gland in the anterior neck region gives a unique chance to this organ to be very easily inspected and to signalize the presence of diseases.

The thyroid gland can be seen easily by tilting the patient's head backward. This position raises the thyroid up from the supraclavicular region and throws it into relief against the structures of the neck. Because the thyroid is fixed to the pretracheal fascia, it moves with the trachea when the patient is swallowing. This fact is very important in the differential diagnosis, with other structures that may appear in the anterior cervical area (e.g., adipose tissue). The large goiter may deviate the trachea, and this is the reason why it is mandatory to palpate it.

The palpation of the thyroid gland facing the patient and standing behind him gives the physician the necessary information regarding the structure of the gland and its relation with the surrounding tissues. The palpation of the lymph nodes situated on the neck should be carefully done, undergoing the known pathways of lymphatic drainage: lateral-cervical, supraclavicular, and submental.

The gland and the lymph nodes:

- Inspection (enlargement, asymmetry, color, pulsation).
- The patient drinks a glass of water so the physician can observe the swallowing (mobility of the gland, difficulties in swallowing, etc.).
- Palpation.
  - Texture—soft/firm
  - Surface—smooth/seedy/lumpy
  - Volume—increased in different grades (diffuse, unilateral/nodular) and decreased/atrophic
  - Presence of regional pathologic lymph nodes
  - Spontaneous pain or pain at palpation
  - Mobility over the neck structures and with swallowing

The eyes and the face:

- Presence of ophthalmopathy, grade, and evolution
- Puffy face, facial, or general edema
- Tongue edema and thyroid ectopy behind the tongue base

The general signs:

- Tremor
- Sweating
- Diarrhea/constipation
- Anxiety, depression, and lethargy
- Heat/cold intolerance
- Coarse skin
- Weight loss/weight gain
- Pretibial edema
- Muscle weakness
- Increased/reduced heart rate
- Dry hair

All these signs and symptoms come to design a clinical presentation that may very seriously affect the patient status.

A complete clinical exam is able to suggest the diagnosis of the thyroid pathology, but the positive diagnosis of the type of thyroid disease is sometimes very difficult and energy consuming.

There are many evaluation guidelines continuously published, and many scientists have huge interest in the optimization of the procedures.

7.3.2 Laboratory Serum Testing

7.3.2.1 Thyroid-Stimulating Hormone

The first generation of TSH assays was based on radioimmunoassay (RIA) methodology, with limited functional sensitivity. Currently, most TSH testing is performed on automated immunoassay platforms employing non-isotopic technology. Serum TSH normally exhibits a diurnal variation with a peak between midnight and 4:00 a.m.; TSH testing is not usually influenced by the time of day of the blood draw.

Current guidelines worldwide recommend that serum TSH be used as the first-line test for detecting both overt and subclinical hypo- or hyperthyroidism in ambulatory patients with stable thyroid status and intact hypothalamic/pituitary function.

The current standards of care necessitate that laboratories use third-generation TSH assays, with the possibility of detecting serum TSH values lower than 0.1 mIU/L. This level of sensitivity is necessary for detecting differing degrees of TSH suppression.

In addition, targeting the degree of TSH suppression plays a critical role in the management of thyroid cancer.

- In general, a normal reference range for TSH for adults is between 0.4 and 5.0 mIU/L, but values vary slightly among different types of analyzers.
- TSH values in thyroid pathology may be:
  - Under lower limit establishing the diagnosis of clinical or subclinical hyperthyroidism
  - In normal range—euthyroid status (normal)
  - Over higher limit establishing the diagnosis of clinical or subclinical hypothyroidism

7.3.2.2 Thyroid Hormones (T4, T3, FT4, FT3)

- Total thyroxine (T4). Most of the thyroxine (T4) in the blood is attached to a protein called thyroxine-binding globulin. Less than 1% of the T4 is unattached. A total T4 blood test measures both bound and free thyroxine. Free thyroxine affects tissue function in the body, but bound thyroxine does not. Normal range is between 57 and 148 nmol/L.
- Free thyroxine (FT4). Free thyroxine (T4) can be measured directly (FT4) or calculated as the free thyroxine index (FTI). The FTI tells how much free T4 is present compared to the bound T4. The FTI can help tell if abnormal amounts of T4 are present because of abnormal amounts of thyroxine-binding globulin. Normal values of FT4 are 10–26 pmol/L.
- Triiodothyronine (T3). Most of the T3 in the blood is attached to thyroxine-binding globulin. Less than 1% of the T3 is unattached. A T3 blood test measures both bound and free triiodothyronine. T3 has a greater effect on the way the body uses energy than T4 even though T3 is normally present in smaller amounts than T4. Normal values are 80–200 μg/L (1.2–3.1 nmol/L). For FT3, the normal values are 260–480 ng/L (3.4–6.8 pmol/L).
- Thyroid hormone tests are done to find out what is causing an abnormal thyroid-stimulating hormone (TSH) test, to check how well treatment of thyroid disease is working, and for screening newborns, to find out if the thyroid gland function is normal.
- In practice, measurement of free thyroxine and free triiodothyronine is a more reliable test of thyroid function than measurement of total hormone levels.

7.3.2.3 Antithyroid Peroxidase Antibodies/Anti-thyroperoxidase (Anti-TPO) Antibodies

- Anti-TPO is a large, dimeric, membrane-associated, and globular glycoprotein that is expressed on the apical surface of thyrocytes.
- Anti-TPO can be detected using complement fixation, agglutination test, or immunofluorescence on thyroid tissue sections, but concentrations are most commonly estimated using enzyme-linked immunosorbent assay or other sensitive and specific (manual or automated) immunoassays.
- Anti-TPO prevalence is significantly higher in dietary iodine-sufficient countries like the USA and Japan as compared with iodine-deficient areas. The prevalence of anti-TPO is higher in women of all age groups and ethnicities and increases with age.
- Anti-TPO measurement may serve as a useful prognostic indicator for future thyroid dysfunction. It may have an important clinical application to employ the presence of serum anti-TPO as a risk factor for developing thyroid dysfunction in patients receiving amiodarone, interferon alpha, interleukin-2, or lithium therapies.
- Serial anti-TPO measurements are not recommended for monitoring treatment for autoimmune thyroid diseases. This is not surprising since the treatment of these disorders addresses the consequence (thyroid dysfunction) and not the cause (autoimmunity) of the disease.
- Normal values are considered below 34 IU/mL.

7.3.2.4 Thyroglobulin

- The tissue-specific origin of Tg has also led to its widespread use as a tumor marker for differentiated thyroid cancers (DTC).
- Over the last 10 years, laboratories have adopted the more rapid, automated Tg immunometric assays (IMA) to replace the older isotopic radioimmunoassay (RIA). However, some laboratories still retain a Tg RIA because this methodology appears less prone to interferences from Tg autoantibodies (TgAb) and heterophilic antibodies (HAMA).

- Unfortunately, serum Tg measurement is technically challenging. There are five methodologic problems that impair the clinical utility of the test:
  - Between-method biases
  - Insensitivity
  - Suboptimal inter-assay precision
  - "Hook" problems (IMA methods)
  - Tg autoantibody (TgAb) interference
- For these and other reasons, current guidelines of treatment of DTC stress the critical importance of maintaining the same Tg method for serial monitoring of patients with DTC because a change in Tg method is very likely to produce misleading results. The American Thyroid Association and European Thyroid Association guidelines for managing patients with DTC state that an undetectable basal and recombinant human TSH (rhTSH)-stimulated Tg should be used as a parameter for the absence of disease. Specifically, a basal (unstimulated) Tg measurement below 0.1 μg/L predicts a negative rhTSH (recombinant human TSH) test (rhTSH-stimulated Tg below 2.0 μg/L) with a high degree of confidence.
- Thyroglobulin values measured by immunometric methods have more pronounced variation than those determined by radioimmunology methods. This difference is probably due to the use of polyclonal antibodies with broad epitope specificity for radioimmunological determinations. This enables them to measure a wider range of abnormal tumor-derived thyroglobulin isoforms than immunometric assay methods that use monoclonal antibodies with limited epitope specificity.
- Current guidelines do not routinely recommend preoperative serum Tg measurement.
- Serum Tg measurements performed even as early as 6–8 weeks after surgery have been shown to be of important prognostic value. The serum Tg half-life approximates 3 days, and the acute injury-related Tg release resulting from the surgical procedure should largely resolve within the first 2 months.
- The trend in serum Tg, measured over time and under constant TSH conditions, has proven to have a higher diagnostic sensitivity than using a fixed serum Tg cutoff value, especially when measured using a sensitive second-generation assay.
- Because Tg protein is tissue specific, the detection of Tg in non-thyroidal tissues or fluids (such as pleural fluid) indicates the presence of metastatic thyroid cancer (Mazzaferri 2003). Struma ovary is the only (rare) condition in which the source of Tg in the circulation does not originate from the thyroid.

7.3.2.5 Antithyroglobulin Antibodies

- Antithyroglobulin antibodies interfere with the accurate measurement of serum thyroglobulin. Serial antithyroglobulin antibody monitoring necessitates the use of the same method each time because assays vary in sensitivity, specificity, and absolute values. Current guidelines recommend that a sensitive TgAb immunoassay rather than an exogenous Tg recovery test be employed for this screening because a Tg recovery assessment has been shown to be an unreliable tool for detecting interfering TgAb.
- There has been a growing recognition that serial TgAb measurements can serve as a surrogate tumor marker postoperatively. Supporting this view is the finding that patients who have serum TgAb detected at the time of initial surgery and who are rendered disease-free show a progressive decline in serum TgAb levels that become undetectable over a median period of 3 years. In contrast, patients with persistent/recurrent disease typically maintain detectable and often exhibit rising TgAb concentrations in association with tumor recurrence.
- The use of a reference range derived from normal subjects is not recommended. Laboratories and manufacturers should determine and quote the minimum detection limit of their assays.

7.3.2.6 Calcitonin and Carcinoembryonic Antigen

- Calcitonin is a marker for medullary thyroid cancer (MTC). Elevated serum calcitonin levels are highly suggestive for MTC; calcitonin levels may also be increased, although infrequently, in other clinical conditions such as C-cell hyperplasia, pulmonary and pancreatic neuroendocrine tumors, renal failure, and hypergastrinemia. Depending on the method used, smoking may either increase or decrease calcitonin concentration.

- At present, the infusion of pentagastrin (0.5 μg/kg over 5 s), with determination of calcitonin levels at 0, 1, 2, 5, 10, and 15 min, appears to be the best test but is limited to countries where pentagastrin is available.
- Basal calcitonin values are normally under (depending on the laboratory) 30 ng/L. Values of 30–100 after pentagastrin indicate hyperplasia, and values over 100 typically indicate the presence of cancer. Calcitonin should drop to levels of <30 ng/L if the tumor is completely removed surgically. It should be noted that excess production of calcitonin is not unique for medullary cancer but can occur with granulomatous diseases and other cancers. Patients with the syndrome should also be studied with parathyroid hormone and catecholamine assays in order to determine the presence of other components of the syndrome.
- Calcium infusion, although less sensitive than pentagastrin, is a practical and attractive alternative.
- Calcitonin and calcium/pentagastrin-stimulated calcitonin are used as tumor markers to screen relatives and to monitor patients who have been treated for MTC.
- The C cells also produce carcinoembryonic antigen (CEA) in large amounts; it does not offer any obvious advantage and lacks the specificity of CT determinations. Tumor dedifferentiation is associated with a fall of CT and increasing CEA.

7.3.2.7 RET Oncogenes and Medullary Thyroid Cancer

- Serum calcitonin measurement, which was once the mainstay in the diagnosis of familial MTC, has been replaced by sensitive polymerase chain reaction (PCR) assays for germline mutations in the *RET* proto-oncogene.
- Studies on patients with MEN I and MEN II indicated linkage to chromosomes 11 and 10, respectively. Subsequent studies demonstrated that the RET oncogene is present at 10q11.2. RET is a cell membrane receptor of the growth factor family, with tyrosine kinase function. In up to 97% of patients with MEN IIA, mutations are found in codons 609, 611, 618, 620, and 630 in exons 10 and 11. These all involve substitutions of other amino acids for cysteine and are thought to cause activation of the gene by aberrant disulphide bonding causing dimerization. Similar changes are seen in familial MTC.

7.3.2.8 TSH Receptor Autoantibodies (TRab)

- Circulating TSH receptor subunits have been implicated as a potential antigen in the autoimmune disease process.
- TRab tests are useful in the differential diagnosis of various causes of hyperthyroidism but are particularly relevant in predicting fetal and neonatal thyroid dysfunction due to transplacental passage of maternal TRab from mothers with active or previously treated Graves' hyperthyroidism.
- A TRab measurement prior to radioiodine therapy may also be useful in predicting the risk for exacerbating Graves' opthalmopathy (GO).

7.3.2.9 Mutations for KRAS, HRAS, NRAS, and BRAF and Translocations of PAX8/PPARγ and RET/PTC

- Mutations in BRAF have been found in 40–45% of papillary thyroid cancer and also in anaplastic thyroid cancer (30–40%) and poorly differentiated tumors (20–40%). The vast majority (98%) of BRAF mutation are V600E (valine to glutamic acid).
- The AKAP9-BRAF rearrangement is another mechanism of BRAF activation in thyroid cancers. This translocation, which fuses the first eight exons of the A-kinase anchor protein 9 (AKAP9) gene with the C-terminal region (exons 9–18) of BRAF, is found in up

to 11% of tumors associated with radiation exposure but in less than 1% of sporadic tumors.

- *RAS* mutations (HRAS, NRAS, and KRAS) are found in all thyroid carcinomas; *RAS* mutations are identified in 10–20% of papillary carcinomas, 40–50% of follicular carcinomas, and 20–40% of poorly differentiated and anaplastic carcinomas. HRAS mutations are also found in ~25% of sporadic medullary thyroid cancers. *RAS* point mutations are mutually exclusive with other thyroid mutations such as BRAF, RET/PTC, or TRK rearrangements in papillary thyroid cancers. In follicular carcinomas, RAS mutations are mutually exclusive with PAX8-PPARγ rearrangements.
- Approximately 10–20% of sporadic papillary thyroid cancers (PTCs) harbor RET fusions. The prevalence of RET rearrangements is higher in patients irradiated and in pediatric populations. Multiple different RET rearrangements have been described in PTCs, but RET/PTC1, RET/PTC2, and RET/PTC3 account for the vast majority of cases.

Nowadays there are available software which combine specialized cytopathology with validated, proven genomic analysis to deliver greater understanding of a patient's thyroid nodule diagnosis. These can help doctors identify benign nodules when cytopathology is indeterminate, thereby reducing the number of unnecessary thyroid surgeries, and also provide valuable additive information that may help guide decisions on the appropriate surgery.

7.3.3 Fine Needle Aspiration Biopsy

Fine needle aspiration biopsy has become the standard first-line test for diagnosis because it is safe, efficacious, and cost-effective and permits individualized therapy and monitoring. Fine needle aspiration biopsy (FNAB) is the most important diagnostic tool in evaluating thyroid nodules, and it should represent the first intervention.

Indication:

- To make a diagnosis of a malignant thyroid nodule
- To help select therapy for a thyroid nodule
- To drain a cyst that may be causing pain
- To inject a medication to shrink a recurrent cyst

Technique:

- 21–25-gauge needle (21–25G)
- Multiple passes
- Ideally from the periphery of the lesion
- Re-aspirate after fluid drawn
- Immediately smeared and fixed

Extend the patient's neck slightly and palpate the nodule. Clean the skin with alcohol and place a 21- to 25-gauge needle on the end of a syringe.

There is also an available technique using 21G 10 cm modified Menghini-type needle for cytologic and histologic biopsy sampling. The needle has a Menghini-type cannula and trocar point stylet, which is combined with a 10 mL syringe. By the help of a spring mechanism, the syringe plunger, which is connected to the stylet, can be charged and released automatically. After the punction, the material is smeared, and the slide is fixed in alcohol for Papanicolaou and hematoxylin-eosin staining. Some slides can be air-dried and stained with Romanowsky stain (Diff-Quick).

Successful diagnosis by the cytologist depends on accurate sampling of the nodule and specimen cellularity. Ultrasonographic guidance can help to increase the accuracy of FNAB.

The combination of cytology and serum Tg determination in the aspirate fluid increases sensitivity. In cases of lymph node metastases, the Tg concentration in the aspirate fluid is often elevated (>10 ng/mL), and concentrations above this level are highly suspicious. A Tg concentration in the aspirate fluid between 1 and 10 ng/mL is moderately suspicious for malignancy, and comparison of the Tg measurement in the aspirate fluid and the serum should be considered in these patients.

The possible results from FNAB are presented in Fig. 7.4:

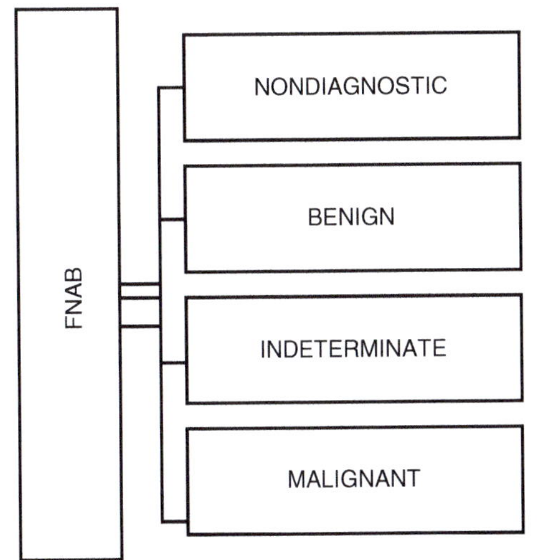

Fig. 7.4 FNAB cytology, according to the Bethesda System for Thyroid Cytology Classification

Bethesda System for Reporting Thyroid Cytopathology (Ali and Cibas 2010)

I. Nondiagnostic or unsatisfactory
  - Cyst fluid only
  - Virtually acellular specimen
  - Others (obscuring blood, clotting artifact, etc.)

II. Benign
  - Consistent with a benign follicular nodule (includes adenomatoid nodule, colloid nodule, etc.)
  - Consistent with lymphocytic (Hashimoto) thyroiditis in the proper clinical context
  - Consistent with granulomatous (subacute) thyroiditis
  - Other

III. Atypia of undetermined significance (AUS) or follicular lesion of undetermined significance (FLUS)

IV. Follicular neoplasm (FN) or suspicious for a follicular neoplasm (SFN)
  - Specify if Hurthle cell (oncocytic) type

V. Suspicious for malignancy
  - Suspicious for papillary carcinoma
  - Suspicious for medullary carcinoma
  - Suspicious for metastatic carcinoma
  - Suspicious for lymphoma
  - Other

VI. Malignant
  - Papillary thyroid carcinoma
  - Poorly differentiated carcinoma
  - Medullary thyroid carcinoma
  - Undifferentiated (anaplastic) carcinoma
  - Squamous cell carcinoma
  - Carcinoma with mixed features (specify)
  - Metastatic carcinoma
  - Non-Hodgkin lymphoma
  - Other

Another classification for FNAB results (Collins 2015), frequently used in clinical practice, is the British system.

British Thyroid Association (BTA 2007) *classifies FNAB results in*:

- *Thy 1*—Nondiagnostic and insufficient sample. Cyst containing colloid or histiocytes only, in the absence of epithelial cells. The following act: to repeat FNAB. Ultrasound guidance may help. If cyst aspirated to dryness with no residual swelling, clinical/ultrasound follow-up alone may be sufficient.
- *Thy 2*—Benign and nonneoplastic. Cyst containing benign epithelial cells.
- *Thy 3*—Follicular or Hurthle cell lesion/suspected follicular or Hurthle neoplasm. Repeat FNAC in 3–6 months. Two nonneoplastic results 3–6 months apart should exclude neoplasia.
- *Thy 4*—Suspicious of malignancy.
- *Thy 5*—Diagnostic of malignancy.

British Thyroid Association **(BTA 2014)** *classifies FNAB results in*:

The BTA updated in 2014 the terminology and introduced some subcategories. The Royal College of Pathologists publication should be followed for the terminology and is summarized below.

Thy1—nondiagnostic. This will include samples reflecting poor operator or preparation technique such as insufficient epithelial cells (the target is six groups each of at least ten well-visualized follicular epithelial cells) or only poorly preserved cells, as well as those reflecting the lesion such as cysts. The suffix Thy1c is used for cyst fluid samples with insufficient colloid and epithelial cells.

Thy2—nonneoplastic. These samples are adequately cellular and suggest a nonneoplastic lesion such as normal thyroid tissue, a colloid nodule, or thyroiditis. Cyst samples containing abundant colloid, even if less that the target number of epithelial cells, can be categorized as Thy2c.

Thy3—neoplasm possible. This is subdivided into:

Thy3a—when there are atypical features present but not enough to place into any of the other categories. The cytological interpretation should be clearly stated in the report and may include situations such as inability to exclude a follicular neoplasm or papillary carcinoma. Many Thy3a cases reflect suboptimal specimens and can be reallocated on repeat cytology.

Thy3f—when a follicular neoplasm is suspected. The histological possibilities then include a hyperplastic nodule, follicular adenoma, or follicular carcinoma. These cannot be distinguished on cytology alone, and a histology sample (lobectomy) will be required for diagnosis. Follicular variant of papillary thyroid carcinoma will also sometimes fall into this category.

Thy4—suspicious of malignancy but definite diagnosis of malignancy is not possible. The type of malignancy suspected should be stated in the report and is usually papillary carcinoma.

Thy5—diagnostic of malignancy. The type of malignancy should be stated, for example, papillary, medullary, or anaplastic thyroid carcinoma, lymphoma, or metastatic disease.

The likelihood of a malignancy on subsequent histology increases with increasing Thy category. There is also a false-negative rate for benign (Thy2, Thy1) cytology results, a fact that needs to be known.

Results of FNAB determine the next step in managing the thyroid nodule. Patients whose findings are nondiagnostic despite repeated biopsy can undergo surgery for lobectomy for tissue diagnosis, or they can be clinically monitored.

In these circumstances, radioiodine/technetium scans can be useful for determining the functional status of the nodule, as most hyperfunctioning nodules are benign (Piccardo et al. 2016).

Malignant diagnostics require surgical intervention. Papillary thyroid carcinoma and MTC are often positively identified on the basis of FNAB results alone. In patients with these carcinomas, definitive surgical planning can be undertaken at the outset. However, it is nearly impossible to distinguish a follicular adenoma from a follicular carcinoma on the basis of FNAB findings. Patients with follicular neoplasm, as determined with FNAB results, should undergo surgery for thyroid lobectomy for tissue diagnosis. These patients require complete thyroidectomy if a malignancy is discovered on review of the pathology.

Complications

The FNAB complications are few and generally minor. The most common complications are minor hematoma, ecchymosis, and local discomfort. Clinically significant hematoma and swelling are exceedingly rare. Inadvertent puncture of the trachea, carotid artery, or jugular vein usually does not cause clinically significant problems and is managed with the application of local pressure.

The results of FNAB will decide the following diagnostic and/or therapeutic strategies. Considering the recommendation of the latest American Thyroid Association thyroid nodule and differentiated thyroid carcinoma guidelines (ATA 2015), the algorithm for evaluation and management of patients with thyroid nodules based on US pattern and FNA cytology is presented in Fig. 7.5.

7.3.4 Imagistic Diagnostic

7.3.4.1 Plain Films

Not routinely ordered, but these films may show:

- Tracheal deviation
- Pulmonary metastasis
- Calcifications (suggests papillary or medullary carcinoma)

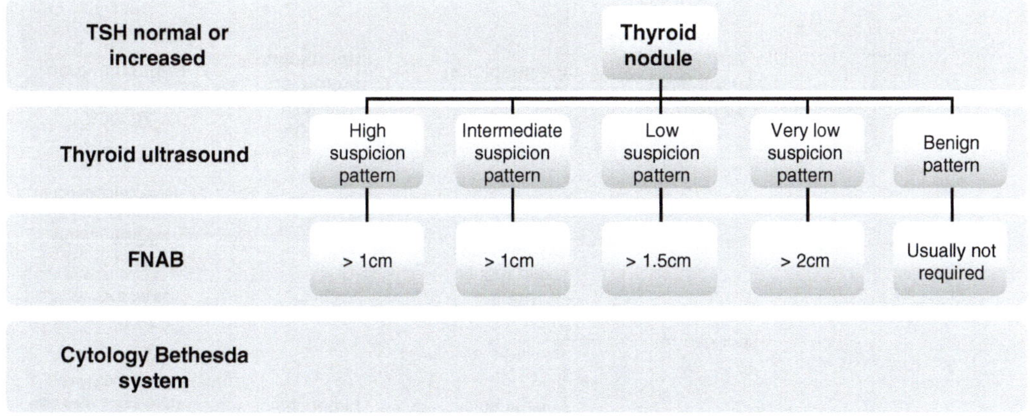

Fig. 7.5 The algorithm for FNAB evaluation and management of patients with thyroid nodules based on US patterns (ATA 2015)

7.3.4.2 Ultrasonography

Ultrasonography (US) is the simplest, noninvasive test for the evaluation of thyroid gland. US should evaluate the following: thyroid parenchyma (homogeneous or heterogeneous) and gland size; size, location, and sonographic characteristics of any nodule(s); and the presence or absence of any suspicious cervical lymph nodes in the central or lateral compartments. The US report should convey nodule size (in three dimensions) and location (e.g., right upper lobe) and a description of the nodule's sonographic features including consistency (solid, cystic proportion, or spongiform), echogenicity, margins, presence and type of calcifications, and shape if taller than wide, and vascularity. The pattern of sonographic features associated with a nodule confers a risk of malignancy and, combined with nodule size, guides FNA decision-making (ATA 2015).

Thyroid ultrasound should be used for:

- Screening for thyroid presence in children
- Differential diagnostic of cystic nodule vs solid nodule
- Localization for FNAB or injection
- Serial exam of nodule size
- 2–3 mm lower end of resolution
- May distinguish solitary nodule from multinodular goiter
- Nodule risk evaluation, mainly in Doppler mode or elastography

Findings suggesting for malignancy:

- Presence of halo.
- Irregular border.
- Presence of cystic components.
- Presence of calcifications.
- Heterogeneous echo pattern.
- Extrathyroidal extension.
- Enlarged lymph nodes with specific patterns.
- No findings are definitive.
- Anarchic vascularity.
- Rigidity at elastography.

The risk of malignancy is strongly correlated with some US patterns; many authors worldwide are being challenged to find the most appropriate criterion to be used in the differential diagnosis of benign/malignant thyroid nodules.

A schematic overview of some of the most important US parameters is presented in Fig. 7.6. The author's experience notes that the character of the blood flow distribution within the nodule is an important factor that should be considered and carefully analyzed.

The intense vascularity inside a thyroid nodule is more likely to add negative prognostic than a peripheral distribution, and even if as a single factor, it is not considered the most powerful criterion for the diagnosis of malignancy.

The results of the multicenter studies published by specialists in the latest years summarize

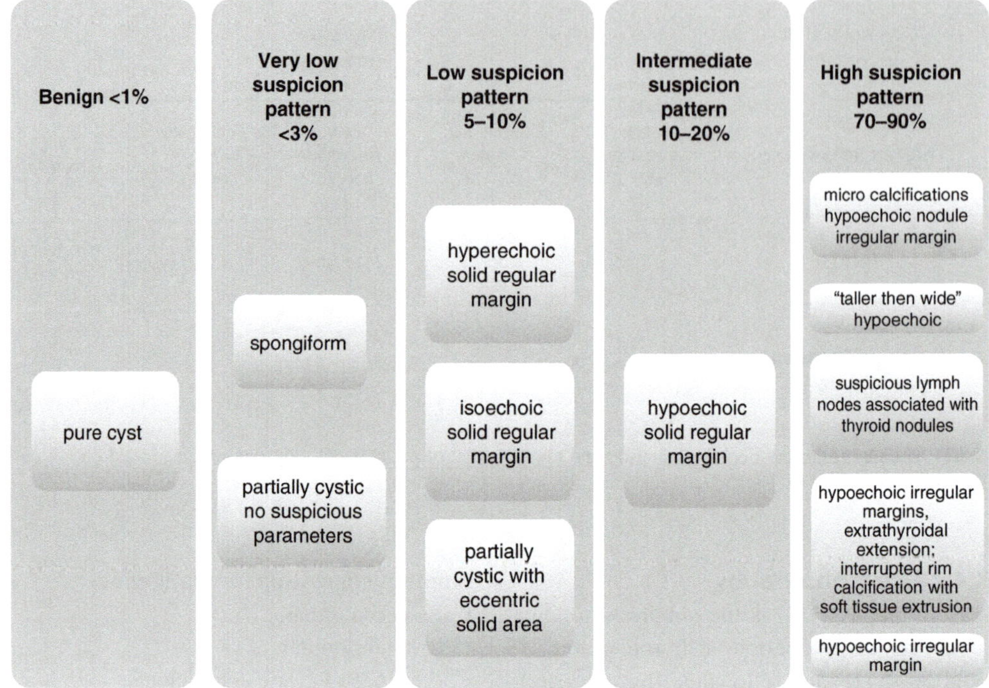

Fig. 7.6 The risk of malignancy of thyroid nodules based on US patterns (ATA 2015)

the most significant parameters to be linked to malignancy as the following ones:

- Marked hypoechogenicity
- Microcalcifications
- "Taller-than-wide" shape in transverse view
- Infiltrative, irregular margins
- Abnormal cervical lymph nodes

Considering the mentioned features, in order to have a common reporting system about the risk of malignancy in thyroid nodules, ATA proposed the TIRADS system, which is presented in Table 7.1

The role of modern techniques adjuvants to gray scale or Doppler ultrasound is controversial. An example is ultrasound elastography (USE) which is a measurement of tissue stiffness; initially it was considered to be an interesting additional tool in the diagnosis of malignancy in the thyroid (Bojunga et al. 2010). More recently, larger trials have reported substantially different results and lack of clear recommendation, mainly due to differences between the experience of the operators. Moon et al. (2016) showed that the performance of USE was inferior to that of gray-scale US assessment. The largest prospective study of 706 patients with 912 thyroid nodules was recently published by Azizi et al. (2013). In this study, the positive predictive value (PPV) of USE was only 36%, comparable to that of microcalcifications. Thus, at present, USE cannot be widely applied to all thyroid nodules in a similar fashion to gray-scale or Doppler US examination (Koh et al. 2016; Russ et al. 2013).

7.3.4.3 Computed Tomography Scanning, Magnetic Resonance Imaging, and Positron Emission Tomography Scanning

Computed tomography (CT) scanning or magnetic resonance imaging (MRI) is generally not cost-effective in the initial evaluation of the thyroid gland. Such studies may be useful in the

Table 7.1 ATA 2015 TIRADS

Pathology	TIRADS	Thyroid ultrasound
Normal	1	Normal
Benign	2	Typical thyroiditis
		Pure cyst
		Spongiform nodule
		Isolated macrocalcification
Most probable benign	3	Isoechogenic/hyperechogenic
		None of the high suspicious aspects
Low suspicious malignant	4A	Moderately hypoechogenic
		None of the high suspicious aspects
Highly suspicious malignant	4B	One or two signs of high suspicious aspects and NO adenopathy
Highly suspicious malignant	5	More than three signs of high suspicious aspects and/or adenopathy

High suspicious aspects: taller-than-wide shape, marked hypoechogenicity, microcalcifications, and irregular margins

assessment of thyroid masses that are largely substernal or in the assessment of the extension of a known thyroid tumor.

CT and MRI are indicated if there is presence of a fixed thyroid mass or of patients with hemoptysis, indicating potential involvement of surrounding structures. Other important indications include cervical lymph adenopathy or when limits of the goiter cannot be clinically determined. CT or MRI can demonstrate involvement of the larynx, pharynx, trachea, esophagus, or major blood vessels. It is important to avoid iodine contrast media in CT scan to ensure subsequent radioiodine treatment uptake. This difficulty may be overcome by requesting for gadolinium-enhanced MRI scan.

Positron emission tomography (PET) scanning with 18F-fluorodeoxyglucose is not an investigational tool with role in the primary evaluation of the thyroid nodule. Since the first edition of this book, the last 5 years demonstrated a crucial role of PET/CT F18-FDG mainly in the management of differentiated thyroid carcinoma, with detectable Tg and negative I-131 whole-body scan (WBS). There will be a special part dedicated to this topic.

In the past, nuclear imaging studies of the thyroid, often combined with ultrasonography, were routinely performed in initial assessment of thyroid nodules. Because only 10% of solitary thyroid nodules are hot and because 90% of cold nodules are not malignant, nuclear imaging with or without ultrasonography typically offers a low yield of cancer diagnosis in surgical specimens when their results are used as the main guides for referral to a surgeon.

Any incidental nodule detected on US should be assessed using the criteria discussed above. Incidental nodules detected on computed tomography (CT) can be more problematic; no CT feature reliably distinguishes benign from malignant lesions. The incidentaloma detected on PET/CT F18-FDG should be evaluated with special attention.

7.3.5 Nuclear Imaging Tests

7.3.5.1 Thyroid Scintigraphy with Tc-99m Pertechnetate (Tc-99m Pt) Gamma Camera

Radiopharmaceutical:

- Technetium-99m pertechnetate (Tc-99m Pt)

Principle:

- Tc-99m Pt is trapped from the bloodstream into the thyroid gland but without organification.

Technique:

- Patient preparation: No special preparation needed.
  - No need for fasting
  - No need for thyroid hormone withdrawal
  - No significant influence caused by other drugs
  - No influence caused by recent procedures with iodine contrast substances

- Attention to breastfeeding patients, children, and potential fetal exposure
- Dose: 74–200–370 MBq/patient of Tc-99m Pt obtained from generator of Tc-99m in the department, respecting the quality control rules.
- Dose calibration.
- Injected I.V.
- 15–30 min are necessary for waiting, after injection.
- Patient position: Supine, slight neck extension.
- Gamma camera:
  - Daily calibration and valid quality control tests
  - Small-field rectangular/pinhole collimator
  - Low-energy high-resolution (LEHR) collimator
- Incidence: Anterior-posterior (AP) over the patient's neck, as close to the neck as possible, avoiding the influence of resolution by an inadequate distance. At 10 cm from the neck, this distance gives a magnification factor of 2–2.5.
- Acquisition:
  - Static acquisition.
  - Selected energy 140 keV.
  - Window 15–20%.
  - 128 × 128 matrix; 64 × 64 might be used also in special situations.
  - Minimum 250,000 counts/image.
  - Mark the suprasternal notch, with a point source of Tc-99m Pt or Cobalt-57; this mark will be registered on the images. This is important mainly in case of ectopy of the thyroid gland or in case of important enlargement and retrosternal position.
  - Lateral or oblique-lateral images may be also obtained.
  - Any palpable nodule should be marked on the images, during the acquisition, giving to the physician the facility to position the nodule.
- Processing: There is no need of special PC programs; an additional may be used in the analysis of counts in different regions of interest (ROI); image interpretation criteria are detailed below.

Clinical applications:

- The diagnosis of hyperthyroidism in:
  - Hyperfunctional nodular goiter
  - Autonomously hyperfunctioning adenoma ("hot" nodule)
  - Hyperfunctional diffuse goiter (Basedow-Graves' disease)
- The diagnosis of hypothyroidism in:
  - Primary congenital hypothyroidism (myxedema)
  - Secondary hypothyroidism
- Thyroid cancer (cold nodule)
- de Quervain thyroiditis and chronic thyroiditis (Hashimoto's disease)
- Thyroid cysts and other causes of nodules
- Thyroid anatomical variants: Retrosternal goiter, thyroid sublingual, left or right lateral-cervical thyroid, accessory lobe (Lalouette's pyramid), and agenesis of a lobe or of the entire gland

Necessary additional examinations:

- Clinical examination; remember to discuss and to examine the patient *before* the injection, in order to limit the hazardous radiation exposure.
- Thyroid ultrasound.
- Serologic tests: TSH, FT4, FT3, anti-TPO antibodies, anti-Tg, calcitonin, thyroglobulin, TRab, etc.
- Fine needle aspiration biopsy (FNAB).

Comments:

- The place of scintigraphy in the assessment of thyroid diseases, especially of thyroid nodules, is well established by the national and international algorithms of diagnostic and treatment of thyroid nodules and availability of tracers (Velzen et al. 2005).

Reports:

- The reports respect the general format of the department with all the identification data of the patient, the institution, and the physician. The report will include the technical data related to the radiopharmaceutical, the used dose, the type of gamma camera, and the acquisition data. The report will note the estimation of the absorbed dose due to this examination. These data are available in predefined forms calculated for the majority of tracers and investigations.
- The report will include a description of the:
  - Shape
  - Position
  - Size
  - Contour

- Presence or absence of nodules in the thyroid area; the distribution of the radiotracer in the entire gland, in each lobe and in the nodules
- Presence of any special findings on scintigraphy

The normal image of thyroid scan with Tc-99m Pt is shown below (Figs. 7.7 and 7.8)

The thyroid scan will show:

- The typical "butterfly" shape.
- The normal dimensions according to laboratory standard (these must be seated in relation with the area particularities and respecting the age variations).
- The position in the anterior neck area, above the sternal notch, in the region of the thyroid cartilage.
- The regular contour, without any interruption or mismatches.
- The homogenous distribution of the radiotracer; with intense color in the middle of each lobe related to the thickness of the thyroid tissue; the margins will have a less intense color, due to the decreasing quantity of the thyroid tissue. The image must present the color scale used in processing, so the physician will be able to correlate the percent of activity with the color.
- The absence of nodules with different metabolic activities.

There is a normal visualization on the scan of the salivary glands. Physiologically the right lobe may be larger than the left one.

We need to give special attention to technical details: the matrix, the color adjustment, and the image zoom; these may significantly modify the final presentation of the thyroid's images.

In the next two images, there is an example of important differences in the thyroid's images due to different details of acquisition:

- An inadequate 256 × 256 in Fig. 7.9
- Respectively a matrix of 64 × 64 in Fig. 7.10

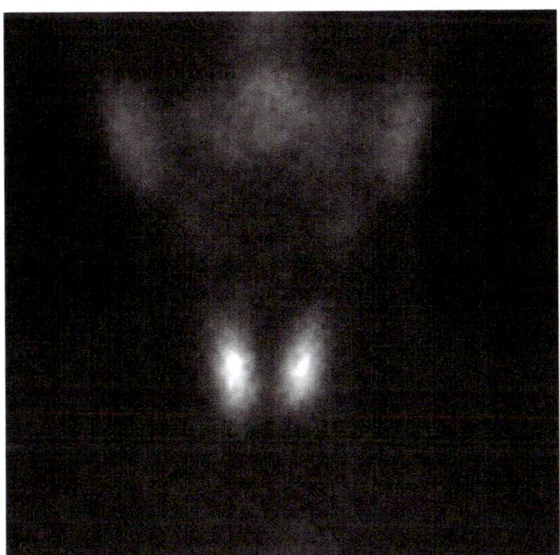

Fig. 7.7 Normal thyroid scan with Tc-99m Pt. Color scale—gray

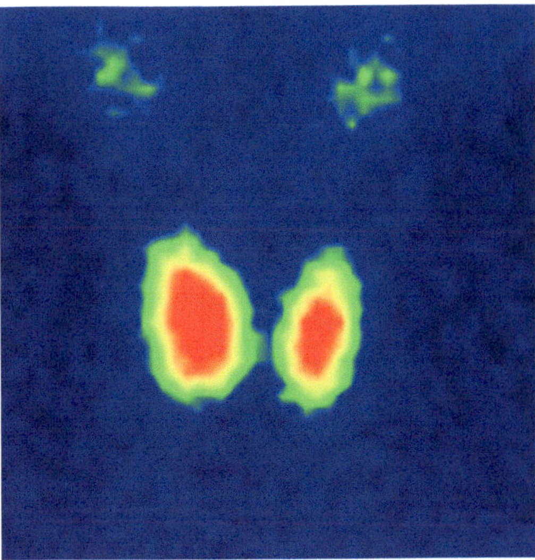

Fig. 7.8 Normal thyroid scan with Tc-99m Pt. Color scale—Sopha Rainbow

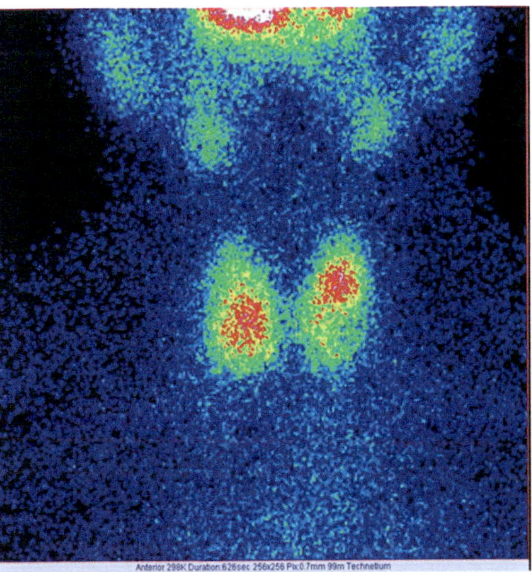

Fig. 7.9 Thyroid scan Tc-99m Pt obtained with a matrix of 256 × 256

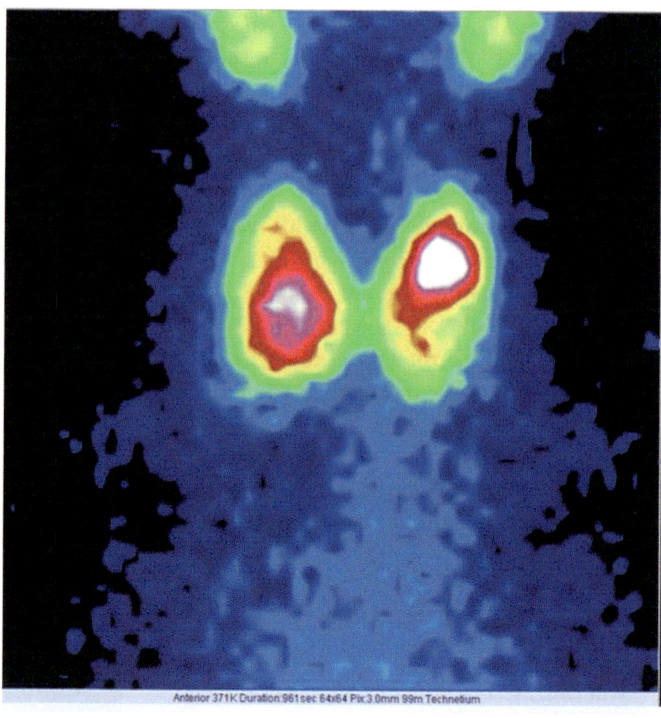

Fig. 7.10 Thyroid scan Tc-99m Pt obtained with a matrix of 64 × 64

Case 1: Autonomously Functioning Thyroid Nodule

History:

A 57-year-old male, with previous history of irradiation of the neck for a larynx neoplasm, 8 years before, returns for evaluation.

Clinical examination:

Symptoms: tremor, weight loss of 12 kg in 2 months, sweating, insomnia, and tachycardia.

The neck examination revealed a tumor mass in the anterior neck area, not very firm, with elastic structure, ascending when the patient is swallowing, developed quickly in the last 5 weeks. No clinical evidence of lymph nodes. The heart rate was 120/min. No signs of exophthalmia.

Examinations:

The ultrasound revealed a solid, hypoechogenic nodule involving almost the entire left lobe of the thyroid. The nodule has regular contour and intense vascularity. No pathologic lymph nodes.

TSH—0.15 mIU/L (N.V. 0.4–4.5 mIU/L), low

Findings:

The scintigraphy with Tc-99m Pt showed an intense uptake of the radiotracer in the entire left lobe of the thyroid ("hot" nodule), corresponding to the ultrasound finding.

The rest of the gland did not trap the tracer, due to the suppression of the tissue, by the dominant nodule; the rest of the gland did not appear on the image (Fig. 7.11).

Conclusion:

Autonomously hyperfunctioning left thyroid nodule (toxic adenoma)

Similar cases: Figs. 7.12, 7.13, and 7.14:

Key Points

- In the context of previous neck neoplasm and history of irradiation, it was mandatory to make the differential diagnosis of autonomously functioning adenoma with larynx neoplasm recurrence or primitive thyroid cancer.
- The frequency of thyroid cancer appearing in autonomous adenoma is worldwide communicated as being very low, but it does exist.
- It is important to keep in mind that even in this situation, to rule out the cancer is essential. Careful posttherapy follow-up of the patient and of the structure must be done. Increasing the volume or special patterns in ultrasound must indicate the FNAB.
- Several cases of autonomously hyperfunctioning "hot" nodule of differentiated thyroid carcinoma were published in the literature.
- The initial FNAB in this particular case is not recommended.

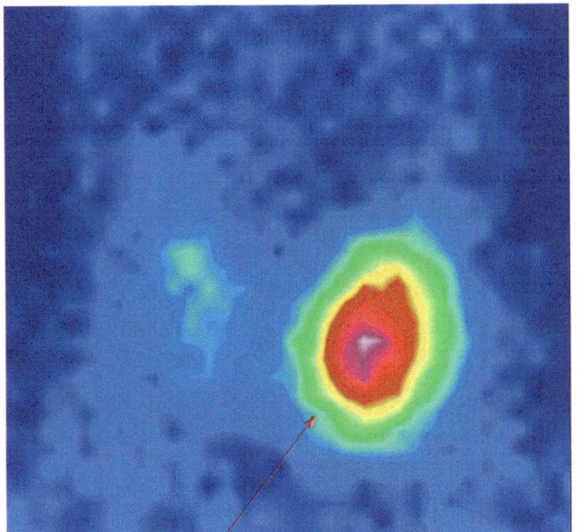

Fig. 7.11 Left thyroid lobe completely "hot" nodule

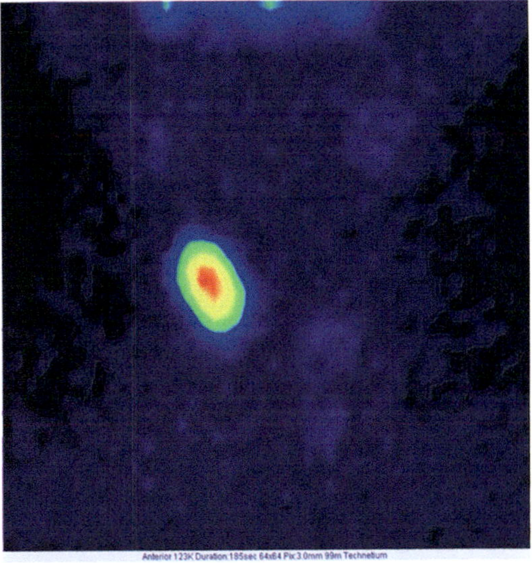

Fig. 7.12 "Hot" nodule in the upper pole of the right thyroid lobe; suppression of the surrounding thyroid tissue

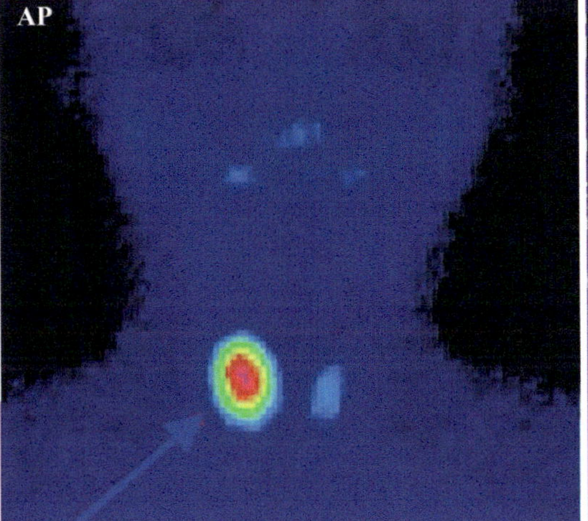

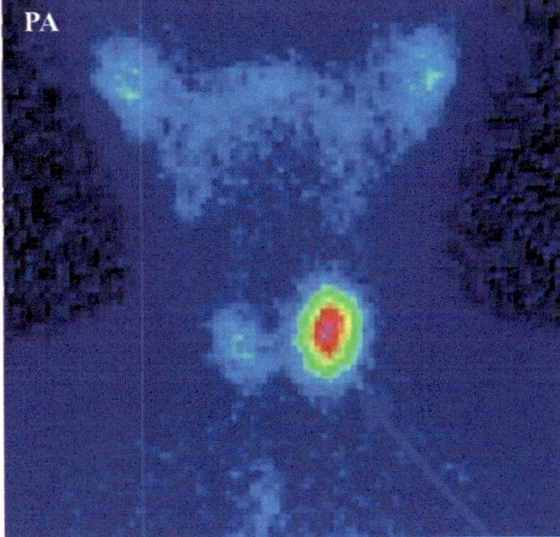

Fig. 7.13 "Hot" nodule in the right lobe—toxic adenoma. Incidence AP and PA

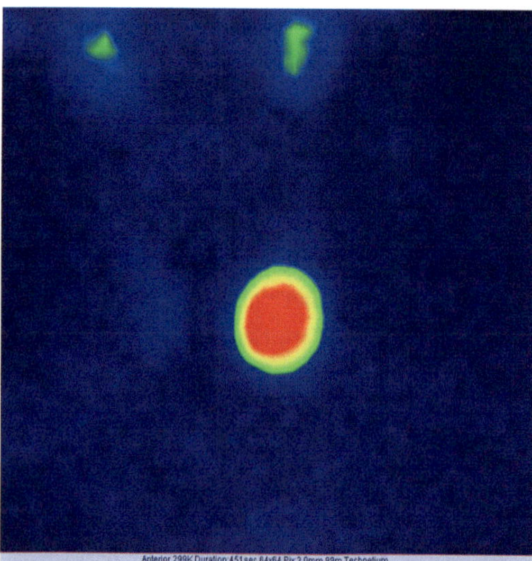

Fig. 7.14 "Hot" nodule involving the entire left thyroid lobe; suppression of the surrounding thyroid tissue

Case 2: Papillary Thyroid Carcinoma

History:

A 36-year-old female, with family history of thyroid cancer (father died with papillary thyroid carcinoma), is referred.

Clinical examination:

Insomnia and anxiety; swallowing difficulties.

The neck examination revealed enlargement of the thyroid gland, with a tumor mass of about 2.5 cm in the maximum diameter, in the central and left anterior neck area, with firm structure, ascending when the patient is swallowing.

The cervical tumor developed slowly in the last 3 years. No medication was administered for this pathology during this time. No clinical evidence of lymph nodes. No other signs or symptoms to be mentioned.

Examinations:

The ultrasound revealed a solid, hypoechogenic nodule 1.4/2.2 cm in the lower part of the left thyroid lobe, extended to the isthmus, regular contour but anarchic vascularity mainly in the periphery of the lobe. There were no calcifications.

The presence of another hypoechogenic nodule in the 1/3 medium to the lower part of the left lobe has been observed. This nodule is in the strict vicinity of the thyroid capsule and measures 1.3/1.9 cm. The nodule had regular contour and intense vascularity, mainly in the interior of the nodule. The right lobe was homogenous. No pathologic lymph nodes (Fig. 7.15).

TSH—2.31 mIU/L (N.V. 0.4–4.5 mIU/L), normal.

Anti-TPO < 34 (N.V. <34 mIU/L), normal.

FNAB previously performed 8 months ago—benign cytology (Thy 2)

Findings:

The scintigraphy with Tc-99m Pt showed a diffuse inhomogeneity of the uptake in the entire left thyroid lobe and isthmus.

There are two different metabolic nodular structures: the first is situated in the upper position, at the junction of medium to the lower third of the lobe, with less uptake of radiotracer, hypoactivity, and in some area even lack of the tracer uptake ("cold" nodule); the second is situated in the inferior part extended to the isthmus, with metabolic activity almost normal, corresponding to the surrounding thyroid tissue.

The rest of the gland has a normal tracer distribution (Fig. 7.16).

Conclusion:

Multiple left macronodular goiter. Family history of thyroid cancer. FNAB recommended (Fig. 7.17). The results of FNAB will establish the type of surgical intervention (left lobectomy or total thyroidectomy).

Similar cases: Figs. 7.18, 7.19, 7.20, and 7.21

The oblique incidence permits a more accurate visibility of the nodule, mainly situated in the posterior part of the left lobe.

These supplementary incidences may be useful especially in differential diagnosis of parathyroid adenoma or thyroid nodule.

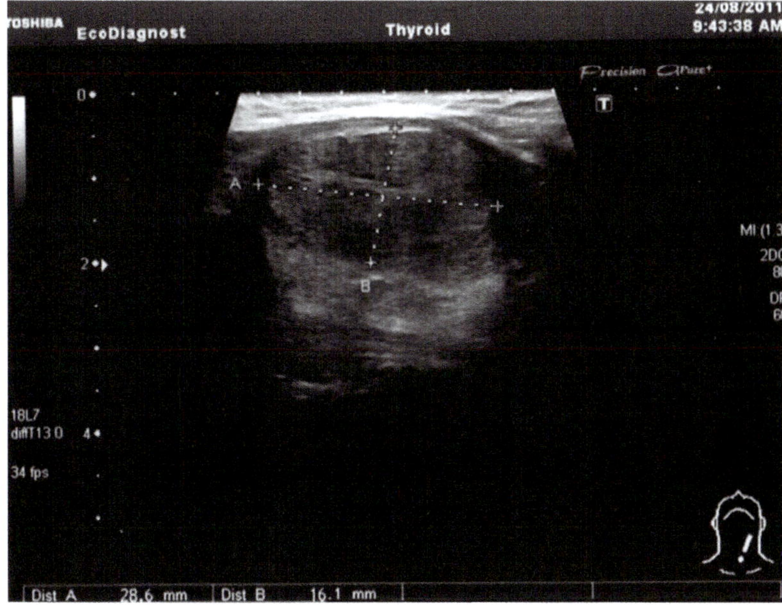

Fig. 7.15 Thyroid ultrasound (With the courtesy of Dr. H. Branda—Ecodiagnost Cluj-Napoca)

Key Points

- The family history of thyroid cancer makes from this case an example of the special attention to be given to the evaluation of thyroid nodules appearing in such families.
- The evolution in time, the significant growth of both nodules in a short period, marked an alert and imposed an aggressive approach.
- The ultrasound showed the two nodular structures, both of them larger than 1 cm in the maximum diameter.
- The result of previous FNAB was benign, but the physician aspirated only one nodule from the lower part, without knowing the difference between the metabolic behaviors of the two left nodular structures.
- The second FNAB was targeted to the "cold" nodule as is shown in the scintigraphy, and the result was highly suspicious for papillary thyroid carcinoma.
- The patient was referred to surgery and underwent total thyroidectomy with central pretracheal lymph node removal; the final histology report confirmed the papillary thyroid cancer, invasive in the adipose tissue near the thyroid gland.
- The presence of a thyroid nodule, in strict relation with the thyroid capsule, needs special attention, with the intention to rule out the cancer; penetrating the capsule, the tumor cells will be invasive in the surrounding soft tissues and will change the patient's group of risk.

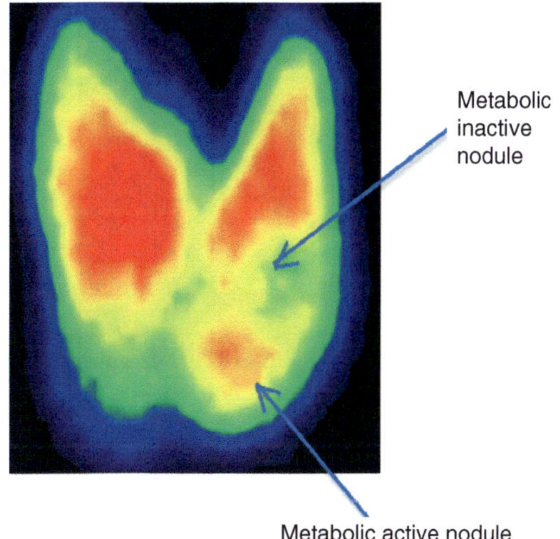

Fig. 7.16 Thyroid scintigraphy Tc-99m Pt, AP incidence, showing the left thyroid lobe with multiple macronodules

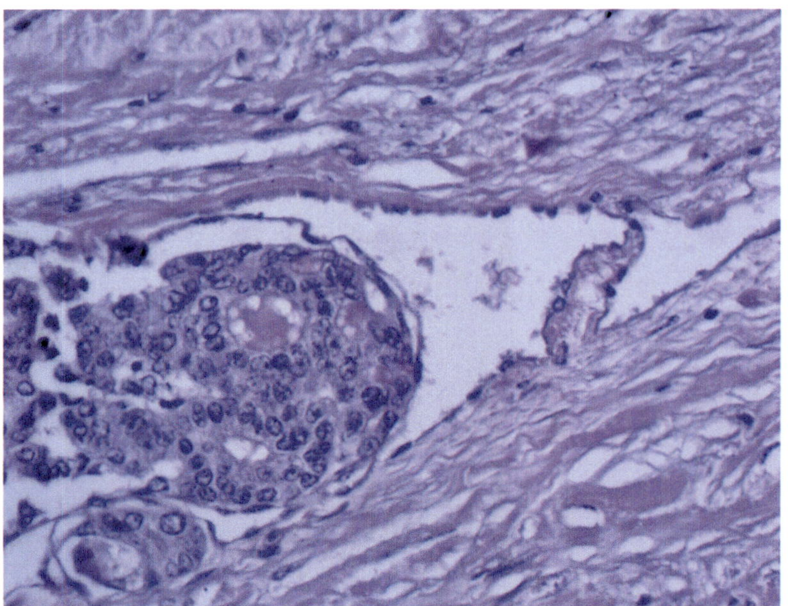

Fig. 7.17 Papillary thyroid carcinoma. Hematoxylin-eosin staining ×200 (With the courtesy of the Pathology Department of the Institute of Oncology Prof. Dr. Ion Chiricuţă Cluj-Napoca)

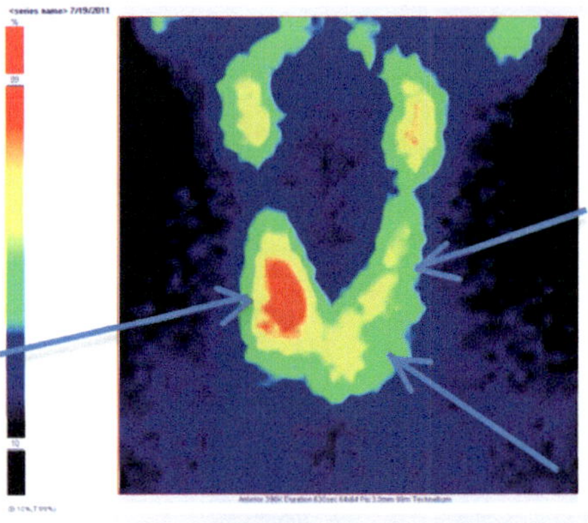

Fig. 7.18 Thyroid scintigraphy Tc-99m Pt, AP incidence, showing "cold" nodule in the lower pole of the left thyroid lobe extended to the isthmus. Similar structures appear in the superior left lobe and inferior pole of the right lobe

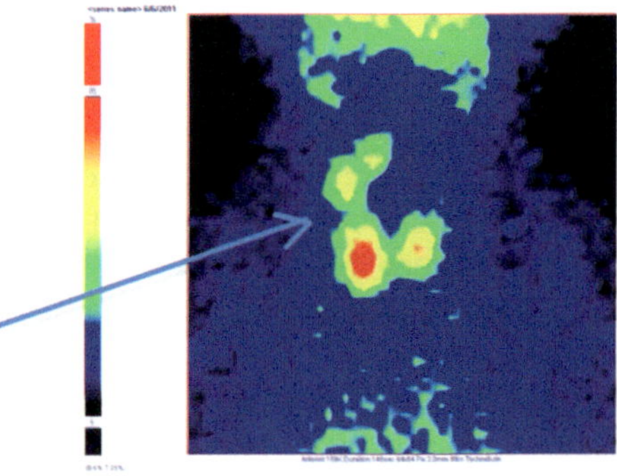

Fig. 7.19 Thyroid scintigraphy Tc-99m Pt, AP incidence, showing "cold" nodule in the upper pole of the right thyroid lobe

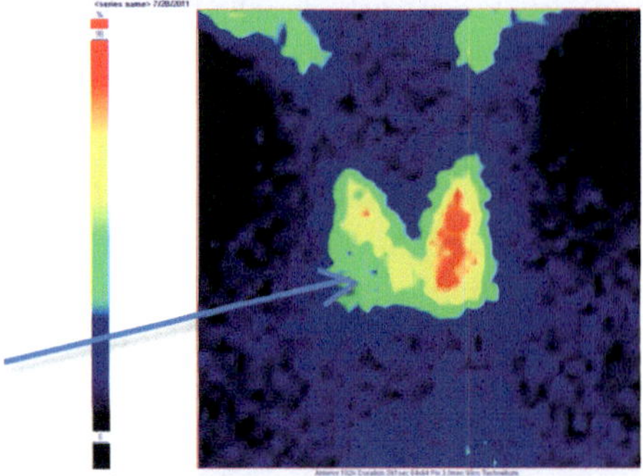

Fig. 7.20 Thyroid scintigraphy Tc-99m Pt, AP incidence, showing "cold" nodule in the lower pole of the right thyroid lobe

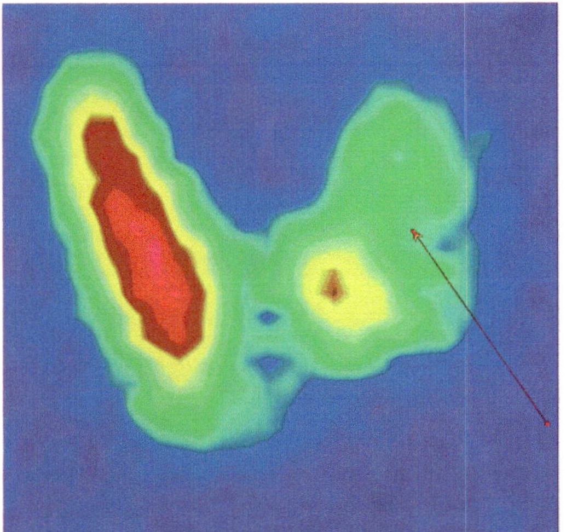

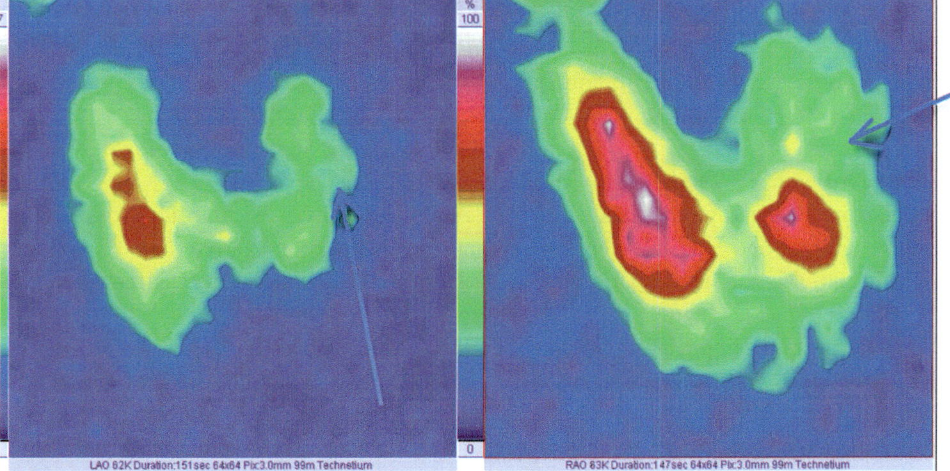

Fig. 7.21 Thyroid scintigraphy Tc-99m Pt showing left "cold" nodule. Images in AP incidence (*top* of image); left anterior oblique (*LAO*) and right anterior oblique (*RAO*)—*bottom* of the image

Case 3: Retrosternal Nodular Goiter

History:

A 29-year-old female, without history of risk (no irradiation, no family history of thyroid cancer or other cancers), is referred.

Clinical examination:

Swallowing difficulties, mainly at physical efforts.

Breathing distress related to emotional situations, efforts, and high environmental temperature.

The neck examination does not reveal anything pathologic. No enlargement of the thyroid gland and no tumor in the neck area; no changes while patient has deglutition.

No clinical evidence of lymph nodes. No other signs or symptoms to be mentioned.

Examinations:

The ultrasound revealed that the thyroid gland had no nodules. It had regular contour and normal vascularity. No pathologic lymph nodes. It had an entirely homogenous appearance.

TSH—1.7 mIU/L (N.V. 0.4–4.5 mIU/L), normal.

Anti-TPO < 34 (N.V. <34 mIU/L), normal.

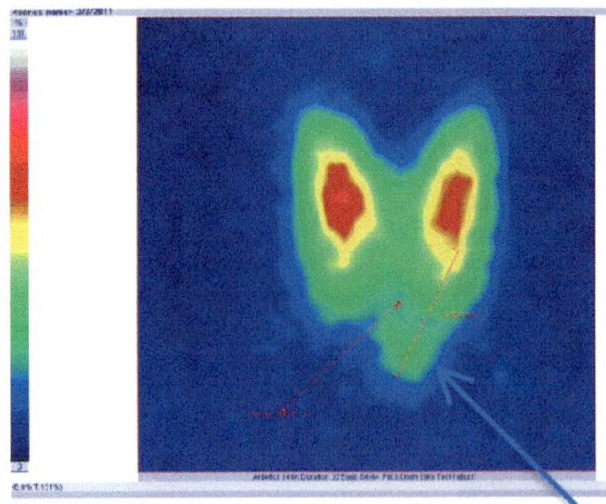

Fig. 7.22 Thyroid scintigraphy with Tc-99m Pt, AP incidence, which reveals nodular goiter with retrosternal position

FT4—16.4 pmol/L (N.V. 12–22 pmol/L), normal.

Findings:

The scintigraphy with Tc-99m Pt showed a diffuse enlargement of the thyroid gland. The lower pole of the left lobe and especially the isthmus were significantly larger. These parts were descended in the upper mediastinum.

The tracer was distributed highly none homogenously in the mentioned area, with some zones of lack of the tracer's uptake.

The rest of the gland has a normal tracer distribution (Fig. 7.22).

Conclusion:

Macronodular goiter with retrosternal position. Patient underwent surgical removal (Fig. 7.23).

Key Points

- The thyroid ultrasound is not able to detect the thyroid tissue beyond the sternal notch.
- In the situation of a goiter having a retrosternal position, the radiography may detect trachea deviation or compression.
- Scintigraphy is able to confirm the thyroid origin of the mediastinum mass.
- Tumors may be developed frequently, with an insidious evolution.

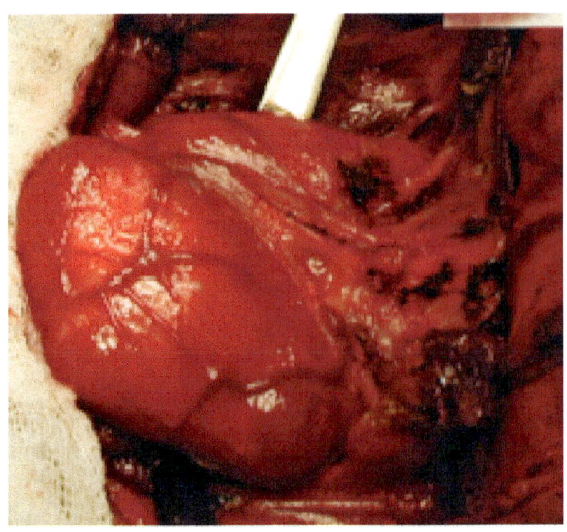

Fig. 7.23 Left thyroid lobe. Surgical specimen (With the courtesy of Prof. Dr. A. Irimie-Institute of Oncology "Prof. Dr. I. Chiricuţă" Cluj-Napoca)

Case 4: Remnant Thyroid Tissue Postlobectomy

History:

A 42-year-old female with total right lobectomy 2 years before is referred to the department. Nodular goiter histology revealed no malignant suspicion.

Clinical examination:

No complaints; routine check of the thyroid function after the partial thyroidectomy. The neck examination does not reveal anything pathologic.

No enlargement of thyroid gland, no tumor in the neck area; no changes while patient is swallowing.

No clinical evidence of lymph nodes. No other signs or symptoms to be mentioned.

Examinations:

The ultrasound revealed that the remnant left thyroid gland had no nodules. It had regular contour and normal vascularity.

No pathologic lymph nodes. It had an entirely homogenous appearance.

In the right part of thyroid bed, an irregular structure of 1/1.2 cm, without vascularity, intensely hypoechogenic.

TSH—1.1 mIU/L (N.V. 0.4–4.5 mIU/L), normal.

Anti-TPO < 34 (N.V. <34 mIU/L), normal.

FT4—13.2 pmol/L (N.V. 12–22 pmol/L), normal.

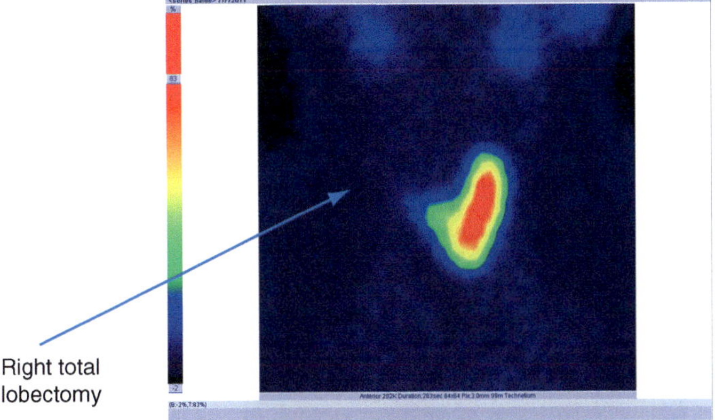

Fig. 7.24 Thyroid scintigraphy with Tc-99m Pt showing the absence of the radiotracer in the right area; right total lobectomy

Hormone values obtained under replacement dose of levothyroxine 50 µg/daily

Findings:

The scintigraphy with Tc-99m Pt showed a discrete diffuse enlargement of the left thyroid lobe.

The tracer was distributed homogenously in the lobe, without any inefficient metabolic zones.

There is no tracer uptake in the right area; existence of a total right lobectomy (Fig. 7.24).

Conclusion:

Right thyroid lobectomy. Normal left lobe. No nodular recurrence.

Key Points

- After the surgical intervention in the thyroid area, thyroid ultrasound may detect abnormal structures, due to fibrosis, sutures, or hematoma.
- Scintigraphy is able to confirm the presence or absence of metabolic active tissues.

Case 5: Subacute Thyroiditis

History:

A 22-year-old female is referred. The family history reveals mother with Hashimoto's thyroiditis.

Clinical examination:

Symptoms: fine tremor of extremities, weight loss of 4 kg in 3 weeks, swelling, insomnia, and fatigue.

The neck examination revealed a discrete enlargement of the thyroid gland, with an elastic structure, ascending while patient has deglutition.

Multiple lymph nodes were palpable in the bilateral neck area, having the maximum diameter of 1.5 cm. The heart rate was 120/min. No signs of exophthalmia.

She presented important headache and minimal fever of 37.6 °C 3 weeks before, apparently with no connection with the thyroid disease.

Examinations:

The ultrasound revealed that the thyroid gland has regular contour and very intense diffuse vascularity. The entire gland has multiple micronodules in the structure, with no dominant nodule and no calcifications.

Pathologic multiple lymph nodes detected in the bilateral lateral-cervical area. Lymph nodes had inflammatory presentation on ultrasound.

TSH < 0.001 mIU/L (N.V. 0.4–4.5 mIU/L), very low, and undetectable

Anti-TPO > 600 mIU/L (N.V. <34 mIU/L), very increased

Anti-Tg—1280 kIU/L (N.V. <115 kIU/L), very increased

FT4 > 100 pmol/L (N.V. 12–22 pmol/L), very increased

EBR—12 mm/h, normal

TRab negative

Findings:

The scintigraphy with Tc-99m Pt showed a very low uptake, with inhomogeneity in the neck area.

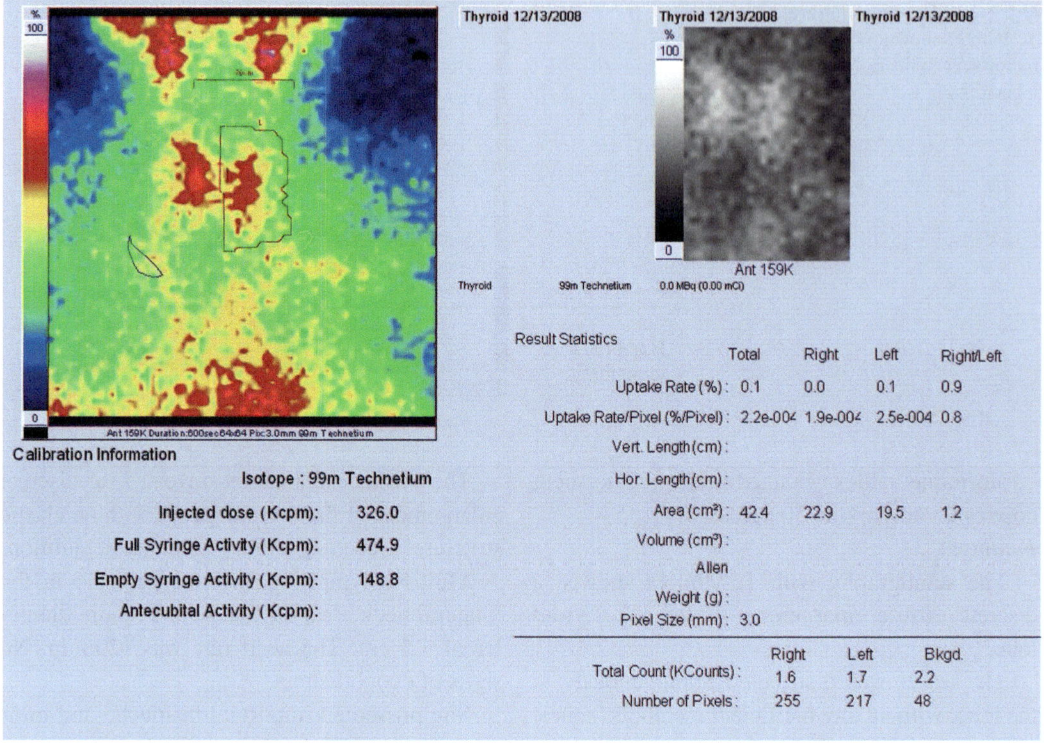

Fig. 7.25 Thyroid scintigraphy Tc-99m Pt and uptake values

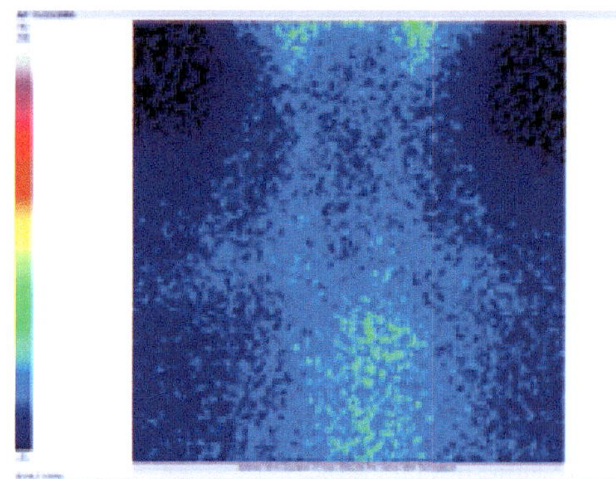

Fig. 7.26 Blank scintigraphy without any tracer uptake in the thyroid area

There was a very low Tc-99m Pt uptake (0.1%), while the normal values are 0.7–1.4% (Fig. 7.25).

Conclusion:

Subacute thyroiditis. There was a thyroid attack of an infectious mononucleosis disease (serologic confirmed in the next evaluation sequences).

There is also a possibility to have a complete blank scintigraphy, without any tracer uptake in the thyroid area (Fig. 7.26).

Key Points

- The scintigraphy features in acute or subacute inflammatory pathology of the thyroid gland are specific; the total or near-total absence of the tracer's uptake in the neck area is the characteristic presentation and may establish the diagnosis.
- Also, it is important to have the uptake sequences, which will confirm the blockage of the tracer's uptake (very low uptake values).
- Regarding the correlation with the serum hormonal values, we must give special attention to the phase of the disease; in an early phase, due to tissue destruction, there may be a hyperfunctional context; the scintigraphy will set the differential

diagnosis between thyroiditis and goiter with hyperthyroidism.
- Sometimes the clinical evaluation is nearly normal, highly discordant with the serum hormonal values and nuclear metabolic tests.
- Infectious diseases may affect the thyroid gland.

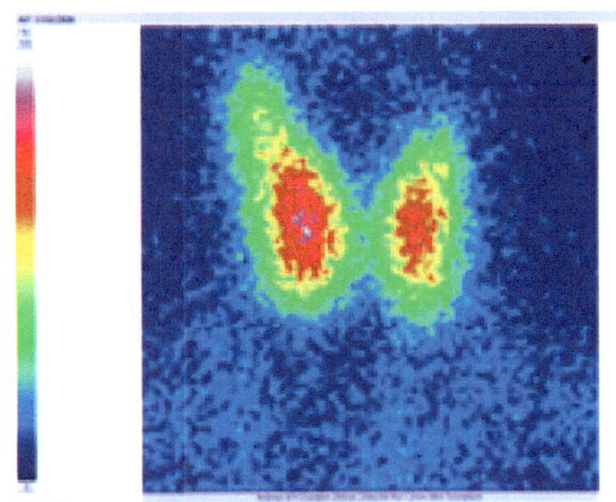

Fig. 7.27 Thyroid scintigraphy with Tc-99m Pt, AP incidence, which reveals inhomogeneous distribution of the tracer, suggestive for Hashimoto's thyroiditis

Case 6: Hashimoto's Thyroiditis

History:

A 58-year-old female, menopause installed 11 years before. Weight of 11 kg gained in 8 months.

Clinical Examination:

She presented fatigue, insomnia, depression, diffuse muscle pain and periodic contracture, swallowing difficulties, "globus hystericus," and postprandial pain in the right hypocondrium.

The neck examination does not reveal anything pathologic. No enlargement of thyroid gland, no tumor in the neck area.

No clinical evidence of lymph nodes. No other signs or symptoms to be mentioned.

Examinations:

The ultrasound revealed that the thyroid gland has a very important diffuse hypoechogenicity, with a multinodular structure in both lobes; micronodules (less than 1 cm in the largest diameter) with an important increase of vascularity. The thyroid had an irregular contour.

No pathologic lymph nodes.

TSH—14.1 mIU/L (N.V. 0.4–4.5 mIU/L), high

Anti-TPO > 600 (N.V. <34 mIU/L), high

FT4—7.31 pmol/L (N.V. 12–22 pmol/L), low

Hormone values obtained without any hormonal intake

Findings:

The scintigraphy with Tc-99m Pt showed a discrete diffuse enlargement of the entire gland.

The tracer was distributed without homogeneity in the gland, with some inefficient metabolic zones (Fig. 7.27).

Conclusion:

Hashimoto's thyroiditis

Key Points
- The presence of nodules in the area of a lymphatic thyroiditis suggests a very careful evaluation, with cytology description, in order to rule out the possible association with thyroid carcinoma.
- Thyroid cancer is frequently developed in Hashimoto's thyroiditis.
- There is the possibility to develop hyperthyroidism associated to Hashimoto's thyroiditis; this fact justifies the evaluation by nuclear tests, regarding a prospective radioiodine therapy.

Case 7: Thyroid Adenoma

History:

A 31-year-old male. No family history of irradiation or thyroid cancers.

Clinical examination:

Clinical evidence of left lateral-cervical lymph nodes, with elastic consistency and with a maximum diameter of 1.2 cm.

No complaints; routine check of thyroid gland during the evaluation of lymph nodes origin.

No enlargement of the thyroid gland and no tumor in the neck area; no changes while the patient has deglutition.

No other signs or symptoms to be mentioned.

Examinations:

The ultrasound revealed that the thyroid has regular contour and normal vascularity.

Pathologic enlargement of left lateral-cervical lymph nodes in the medial area of the neck, with characteristic pattern of inflammatory disease.

In the left part of the thyroid gland, we observed the presence of an intense hypoechogenic irregular structure of 2.41/1.2 cm, having an intense vascularity (Fig. 7.28).

TSH—1.8 mIU/L (N.V. 0.4–4.5 mIU/L), normal.

Anti-TPO < 34 (N.V. <34 mIU/L), normal.

FT4—17.2 pmol/L (N.V. 12–22 pmol/L), normal.

Findings:

The scintigraphy with Tc-99m Pt showed the distribution of the "cold" nodule in the 1/3 part of the thyroid gland's left lobe. This metabolic feature was very discordant with the thyroid ultrasound, which concluded the diagnosis of thyroid adenoma (Fig. 7.29).

Conclusion:

Left "cold" thyroid nodule. FNAB recommended.

In the case of thyroid adenomas, the uptake is normal, similar with that of the surrounding thyroid tissue (Fig. 7.30).

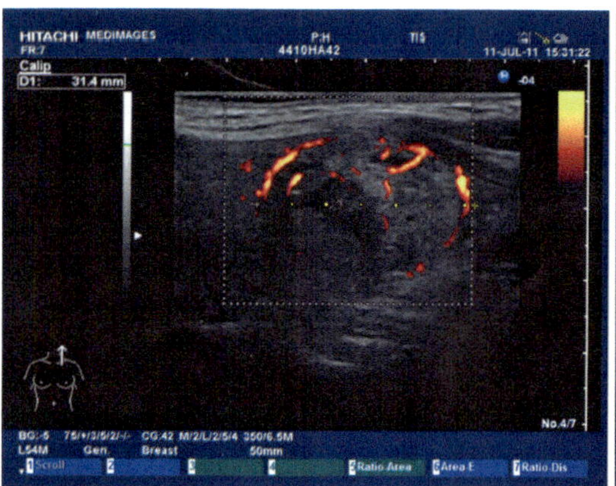

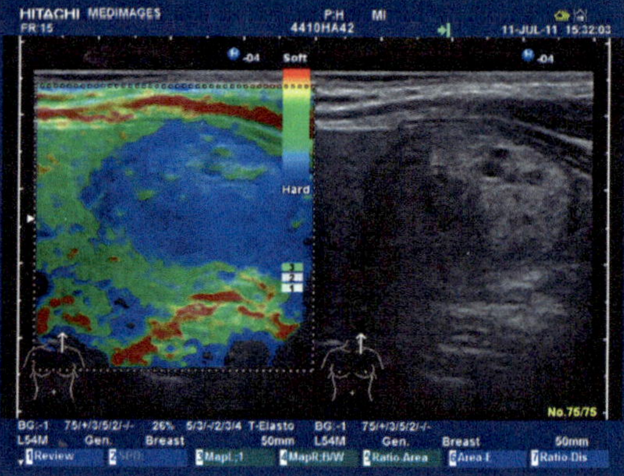

Fig. 7.28 Ultrasound elastography (With the courtesy of Dr. Angelica Chiorean—Medimages)

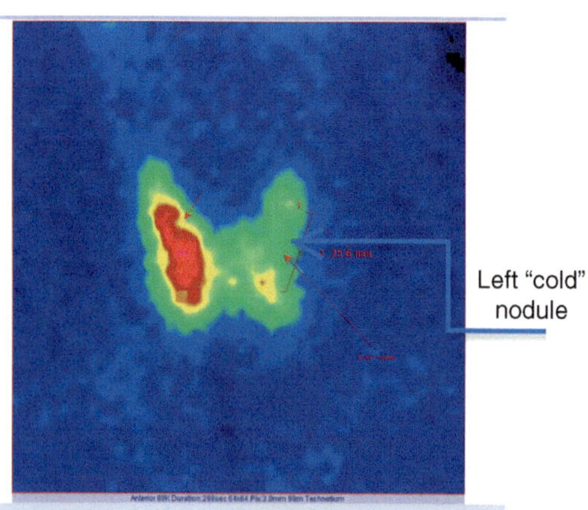

Fig. 7.29 Thyroid scintigraphy with Tc-99m Pt, AP incidence, showing the left thyroid lobe with "cold" nodule

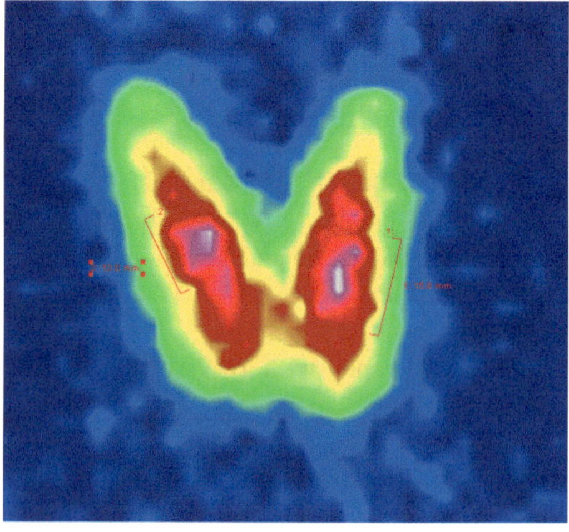

Fig. 7.30 Thyroid scintigraphy with Tc-99m Pt, AP incidence, with homogenous uptake nodules in both thyroid lobes. Thyroid adenomas

Key Points

- Even if the ultrasound is very improbable to suggest cancer, do not hesitate to do the best in excluding cancer, especially if there are also other criteria of risk (familial history, irradiation, gender, age, or lymph nodes).
- In these situations, scintigraphy may help to orient the physician to take an aggressive procedure and to perform FNAB.
- Except the pathologist, nobody has the right to affirm or infirm with clear and maximum accuracy the diagnosis of cancer; based on images, there may be a high probability but not certitudes.

Case 8: Thyroid Cyst

History:

A 32-year-old female. No family history of irradiation or thyroid cancers. She recently experienced a very intense physical effort, during childbirth.

Clinical examination:

Clinical evidence of a cervical tumor in the right part of the anterior neck, developed in a few days after the birth travail. The tumor had an elastic consistency and a maximum diameter of 6.2 cm.

She was referred for the second opinion at 5 months after that moment, presenting an enlargement of the thyroid gland, discrete tension, and slight pain in the tumor area, ascending while patient has deglutition. Multiple right-side lateral-cervical lymph nodes detected at palpation. Previous FNAB with evacuation performed at the begging of the disease (4 months ago) was negative for malignant cells.

No other signs or symptoms to be mentioned, except for breastfeeding.

Examinations:

The ultrasound revealed an important enlargement of the right thyroid lobe, due to an intense hyperechogenic nodule, but with some interior areas of hypoechogenic structures with low vascularity. No calcification detected.

Multiple lymph nodes in the right lateral area of the neck, highly probable with inflammatory character.

The rest of the thyroid gland presented an irregular structure, but without delimited nodules. The conclusion was thyroid cyst with a possible hemorrhagic interior or organized hematoma.

TSH—2.91 mIU/L (N.V. 0.4–4.5 mIU/L), normal.

Anti-TPO < 34 (N.V. <34 mIU/L), normal.

FT4—12.2 pmol/L (N.V. 12–22 pmol/L), normal.

Findings:

The scintigraphy with Tc-99m Pt showed the distribution of a "cold" nodule in the lower part of the thyroid gland's right lobe. Not all the nodule was completely metabolic inactive; there were some areas with tracer uptake, anarchically distributed in the nodule (Fig. 7.31).

In pure thyroid cyst, the nodule at scintigraphy appears complete metabolic inactive (Fig. 7.32).

Conclusion:

Right "cold" thyroid nodule. FNAB and cyst evacuation recommended.

The place of the thyroid Tc-99m Pt scan in the protocol of evaluation of thyroid nodules is nowa-

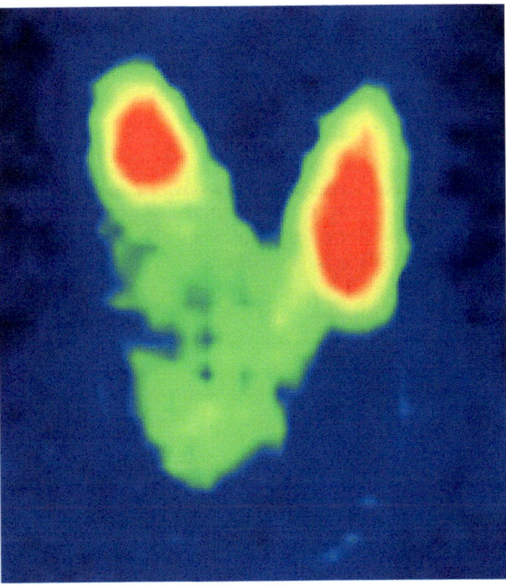

Fig. 7.31 Thyroid scintigraphy with Tc-99m Pt, AP incidence, showing a cyst of the right thyroid lobe with interior metabolic activity, due to papillary excrescences

days very well established, being clearly reserved to specific clinical situations. The very large availability of noninvasive, highly sensitive thyroid US and the performance of the FNAB, of cytogenetic studies, lead to a more conservative approach with respect to the use of routine scintigraphy. The main indications are summarized in Fig. 7.33.

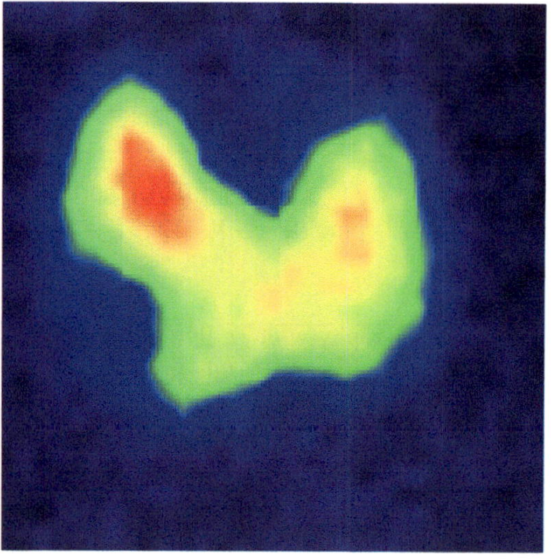

Fig. 7.32 Thyroid scintigraphy with Tc-99m Pt, AP incidence, which reveals a simple cyst of the right thyroid lobe, with no radiotracer uptake

Key Points

- The cystic structure of a thyroid nodule is easily confirmed at thyroid ultrasound, a fact that does not recommend the necessity of thyroid scintigraphy furthermore.
- In the case of a thyroid cyst, the FNAB has the role of diagnosis and also of therapy, with the evacuation of the cyst being performed in the same medical act.
- The presence of some hypoechogenic patterns in the cystic structure leads to other associated processes: hemorrhage in the cyst, organization of hematoma with fibrosis, or the appearance of hemorrhage in a thyroid tumor nodule. In this situation, the scintigraphy may help to orient the physician to perform the

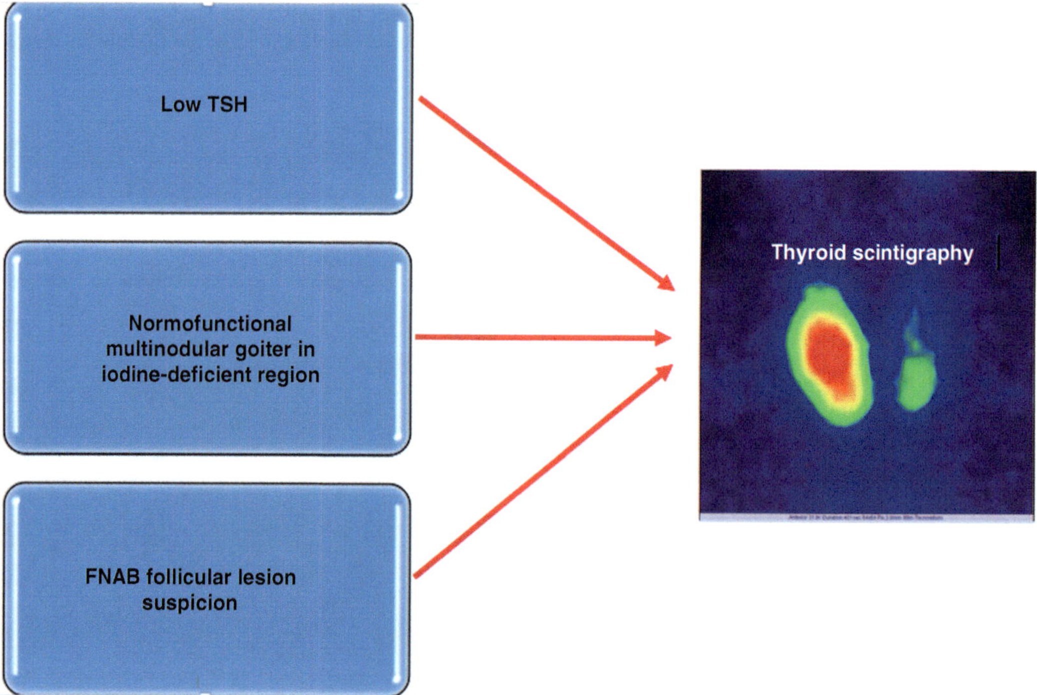

Fig. 7.33 Main indications of thyroid scintigraphy in the evaluation of thyroid nodules

FNAB. *The nuclear test is not the first-line indication*; in fact FNAB will set the differential diagnosis.

- *The indication of scintigraphy at a breastfeeding female is limited.*
- In the particular case described above, the indication of scintigraphy was related to the initial FNAB, which was negative (normal hematic cells and colloid). The increasing size and the appearance of lymph nodes suggested that it was not a simple cyst. The image obtained at nuclear test showed the intra-cystic tissue. The next sequence was the lymph node, and the FNAB showed metastatic papillary malignant cells.
- The procedures related to breastfeeding were as follows: before the examination, the milk was taken off and kept for use after the test; after the tracer injection, the milk was expressed for the next 12 h but not used for the child nourishment. The breastfeeding continues normally after that interval.

7.3.5.2 Thyroid Scintigraphy with Tc-99m DMSA-Tc-99m (V) DMSA Gamma Camera

Radiopharmaceutical:

- Technetium-99m pentavalent dimercaptosuccinic acid

Principle:

- Tc-99m Pt is trapped from the bloodstream and fixed by the tissues with high metabolic activity, for example, the malignant cells.

Technique:

- Patient preparation: No special preparation needed.
  - No need for fasting
  - No need for thyroid hormone withdrawal
  - No influence caused by other drugs
  - No influence caused by recent procedures with iodine contrast substances
  - Attention to breastfeeding and childbearing-age patients
- Dose: 5–10 mCi (185–370 MBq)/patient of Tc-99m (V) DMSA.
- Injected I.V.
- 1 h is necessary for waiting, after the injection for the first image.
- Patient position: Supine.
- Gamma camera.
  - Low-energy general-purpose (LEGP) collimator
- Acquisition:
  - Whole-body planar acquisition.
  - First image after 1 h and the next after 4 h.
  - Anterior and posterior position.
  - 1024 × 256 matrix.
  - Min 500,000 counts/image.
  - Also, spot images on the region of interest may be obtained.
- Processing: There are special PC programs for image processing; additional may be used for the analysis of counts in different regions of interest (ROI); image interpretation

Clinical applications:

- Diagnosis and follow-up of medullary thyroid carcinoma
- Follow-up in non-avid iodine differentiated thyroid carcinoma

Necessary additional examinations:

- Thyroid ultrasound
- Serologic tests: Calcitonin in medullary thyroid carcinoma and thyroglobulin and antithyroglobulin in differentiated thyroid cancer
- Fine needle aspiration biopsy (FNAB)
- CT and MRI
- PET/CT with specific neuroendocrine tracer

Comments:

- It is a complementary method in the evaluation of persistent disease, which failed to be localized by other classic techniques.

Reports:

- The reports respect the general format of the department with all the identification data of the patient, the institution, and the physician.

- The report will include the technical data related to the radiopharmaceutical, the used dose, the type of gamma camera, and the acquisition data.
- The report will include a description of the presence or absence of pathologic uptakes.

7.3.5.3 Thyroid Scintigraphy with Tc-99m MIBI Gamma Camera

Radiopharmaceutical:

- Technetium-99m MIBI
- Other names: Tc-99m-Sestamibi, Tc-99m-Hexamibi, Tc-99m 2 Methoxy 2 methylpropyl-isonitrile, Tc-99m Methoxy 2 isobutyl isonitrile, Tc-99m Sestamibi Chloride, and Cardiolite

Principle:

- Tc-99m MIBI is a well-known lipophilic monovalent cation that shows an increased uptake in epithelial cells containing high numbers of mitochondria. For this reason, increased retention of MIBI is currently employed to detect hyperfunctioning parathyroid tissue and may be observed in benign or malignant thyroid tumors, especially of oncocytic nature.
- Increased MIBI retention has also been described in hyperfunctioning thyroid tissue (toxic adenoma or toxic diffuse goiter), and this phenomenon is believed to be the consequence of increased mitochondria number in hypermetabolic cells. On the other hand, MIBI accumulation is reduced, or absent, in apoptotic or necrotic processes involving mitochondrial membrane potential collapse.

Technique:

- Patient preparation: No special preparation needed.
  - No need for fasting
  - No need for thyroid hormone withdrawal
  - No influence caused by other drugs
  - No influence caused by recent procedures with iodine contrast substances
  - Attention to breastfeeding and childbearing-age patients (see chapter of Radioprotection)
- Dose: 5–10 mCi (185–370 MBq)/patient of Tc-99m MIBI.
- Injected I.V.
- Early images at 1, 2, 5, and 15 min and delay at 1 h.
- Patient position: Supine.
- Gamma camera.
  - Low-energy general-purpose (LEGP) collimator
- Acquisition:
  - Thyroid spot view or whole-body planar acquisition.
  - Anterior and posterior images.
  - Spot images on the region of interest may also be obtained.
  - 1024 × 256 matrix in WBS or 128 × 128 in spot views.
  - Min 200,000 counts/image.
- Processing: There are special PC programs for image processing; additional analysis of counts in different regions of interest (ROI) may be used.

Clinical applications:

- Diagnosis and follow-up of medullary thyroid carcinoma
- Follow-up in non-avid iodine differentiated thyroid carcinoma
- Differential diagnosis between amiodarone-induced thyrotoxicosis type I (AIT I), amiodarone-induced thyrotoxicosis type II (AIT II), and amiodarone-induced thyrotoxicosis type III (AIT III).
- Differential diagnosis of indeterminate FNAB results of thyroid nodules

Necessary additional examinations:

- Thyroid ultrasound
- Serologic tests: Calcitonin in medullary thyroid carcinoma and thyroglobulin and antithyroglobulin in differentiated thyroid cancer, TSH, FT4, and TRab
- Fine needle aspiration biopsy (FNAB)
- CT and MRI
- PET/CT with specific neuroendocrine tracer

Comments:

- It is a complementary method in the assessment of AIT I, AIT II, and AIT III and treatment decision.

- Due to different patterns of action of amiodarone in AIT, Tc-99m MIBI scans will show a normal/intense uptake of the tracer in AIT I and a decreased/lack of activity in AIT II. There is also a very rare AIT type III, mixt, where the MIBI scan is also essential: early images show low/no uptake and delayed images also low or a very faint uptake. Even if AIT is considered a rare complication of the frequently used antiarrhythmic drug, the disease is very difficult to be managed in many situations. The MIBI scan is a noninvasive, simple, and easy method to differentiated the AIT types, in order to establish the best therapy for these patients.
- The thyroid scan with Tc-99m MIBI may be used in differential diagnosis of benign/malignant nodules, especially with doubtful cytology. The malignant suspect nodules will present the same uptake in early and delayed images, while the benign ones will decrease their activity in the delayed images (Figs. 7.34 and 7.35).
- Recent articles present the usefulness of the method in the differential diagnosis of benign/malignant thyroid nodules, especially those with indeterminate cytology of FNAB.

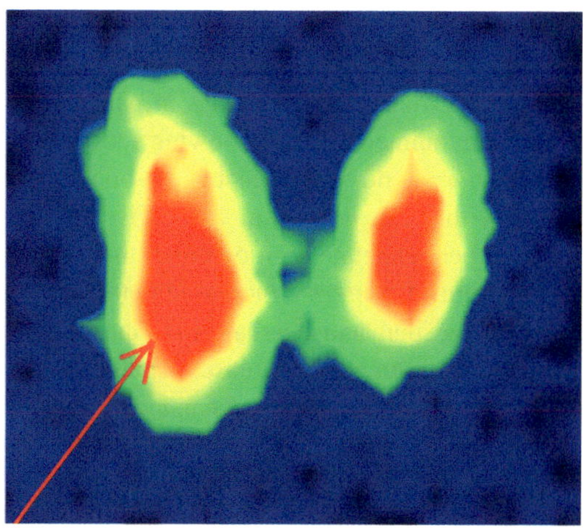

Fig. 7.34 Early image (15 min): nodule with intense uptake—highly probable benign

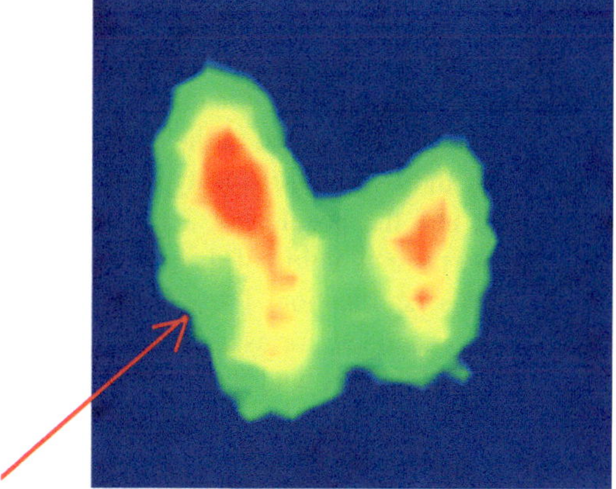

Fig. 7.35 Delayed image at 3 h: nodule with decreased uptake—highly probable benign

Giovanella et al. (2016) proposed a specific method for static thyroid scintigraphy where images were acquired 10 and 60 min after intravenous injection of 200 MBq of Tc-99m MIBI and visually assessed. Additionally, the MIBI washout index was calculated using a semiquantitative method. The team published that Tc-99m MIBI scintigraphy was superior to mutation analysis performed on patients with indeterminate cytology on FNAB, subsequently operated on to confirm or exclude a malignant lesion. Mutations for KRAS, HRAS, NRAS, and BRAF and translocations of PAX8/PPARγ, RET/PTC1, and RET/PTC3 were investigated.

The authors proposed a visual and a semiquantitative assessment of the nodules, in order to compare the risk of malignancy for the follicular neoplasm obtained at FNAB. The semiquantitative method consists of the following workflow: on each early image of MIBI thyroid scan, a region of interest (ROI) was drawn over the perimeter of the thyroid nodule and then moved to the opposite normal lobe; additionally, background ROIs were drawn above the inferior pole of thyroid lobe. These ROIs were then copied from the early to the delayed images. The mean count in each ROI was determined, and the early and delayed uptake results (EUR and DUR) were calculated by subtracting the count in the normal tissue (after correction for background activity) from the nodule count. The washout index (WOInd) was then calculated using the formula: WOInd = [(DUR/EUR × 100) − 100.

The visual assessment compares the Tc-99m pertechnetate and Tc-99m MIBI (early and delayed) thyroid images of a given patient. The authors recommended the following scoring system: *pattern 1* no increased uptake on Tc-99m MIBI within the nodule in comparison to the Tc-99m pertechnetate scan on either the early or delayed image, *pattern 2* increased uptake on the early image that had decreased on the delayed image, and *pattern 3* increased uptake on the early image that remained unchanged or had further increased on the delayed image. Giovanella et al. demonstrated that pattern 3 was considered suspicious for malignancy and patterns 1 and 2 were both considered negative for malignancy of the thyroid nodule concerned.

Reports:

- The reports respect the general format of the department with all the identification data of the patient, the institution, and the physician; the technical data related to the radiopharmaceutical, the used dose, the type of gamma camera; and the acquisition data; the report will note the estimation of the absorbed dose due to this examination. These data are available in predefined forms calculated for the majority of tracers and investigations. The report will include a description of the presence or absence of pathologic uptakes.

Normal image:

- Same features as other thyroid Tc-99m scans

Case 1: Severe Amiodarone-Induced Hyperthyroidism

History:

A 61-year-old male, without previous history of neck irradiation; no cases of familial thyroid cancer, with a history of 14 years of severe permanent atrial fibrillation submitted to radiofrequency ablation. After the first ablation in 2015, the patient has administered repeatedly large doses of amiodarone, between December 2015 and February 2016, a fact that leads to a very aggressive form of amiodarone-induced hyperthyroidism. It was decided to stop the intake of amiodarone, mainly because of the lack of cardiac response.

The patient developed an amiodarone-induced thyrotoxicosis type III (mixt), a very rare and confusing clinical situation, in a previously normal thyroid gland, with no nodules. The treatment consisted both of synthetic antithyroid drugs (carbimazole 65 mg/day) and large dose of prednisone (65–80 mg/day). The thyroiditis was with severe clinical expression and with massive thyroid hormones storm, very difficult to be controlled.

Clinical examination:

Symptoms: insomnia, sweating, and anxiety. No other clinical symptoms with relation to the thyroid.

The neck examination did not reveal any tumor mass in the anterior neck area; thyroid with elastic structure, ascending while patient has deglutition; no clinical evidence of lymph nodes. No signs of exophthalmia. The heart rate was 110–140/min.

Examinations:

The ultrasound revealed a diffuse destructive hypoechogenic thyroid structure, highly vascularized, with a microcyst of 3 mm in the left thyroid lobe. No pathologic lymph nodes (Fig. 7.36).

TSH < 0.001 mIU/L (N.V. 0.4–4.5 mIU/L), very low and undetectable.

Anti-TPO > 600 mIU/L (N.V. <34 mIU/L), very increased.

Anti-Tg—1280 kIU/L (N.V. <115 kIU/L), very increased.

FT4 > 100 pmol/L (N.V. 12–22 pmol/L),very increased.

EBR—12 mm/h, normal.

TRab negative.

Interleukin-6—6.3 (N.V. 5–15 pmol/L), normal; the value was against the type II AIT.

Iodemia—1762 (N.V. 46–71 μg/L), very increased.

Urinary iodine—10,464 (N.V 200–299 μg/L), very increased.

Findings:

The scintigraphy with Tc-99m Pt showed a very low uptake, without any thyroid tissue active in the neck area. There was very low Tc-99m Pt uptake (0.1%) while the normal values are 0.7–1.4% (Fig. 7.37). The scintigraphy with Tc-99m MIBI performed next day depicted the diagnosis between the types of AIT I, II, and III. Figure 7.38a shows the thyroid scan with very low uptake on

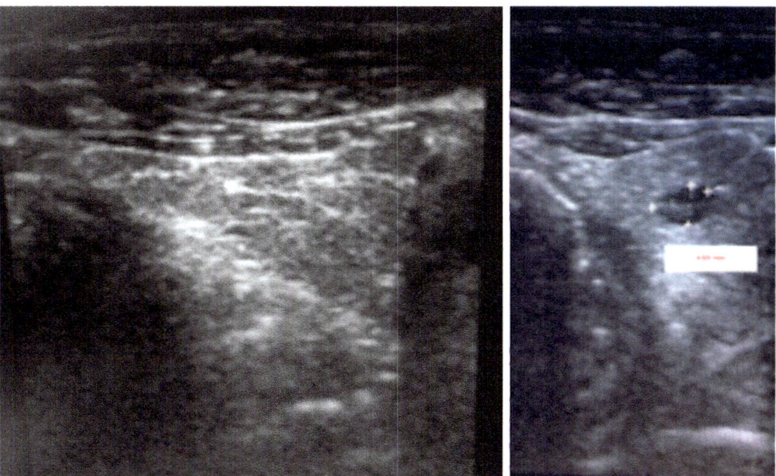

Fig. 7.36 Thyroid ultrasound gray-scale showing the important thyroid tissue destruction and microcyst in the left lobe; patient with AIT

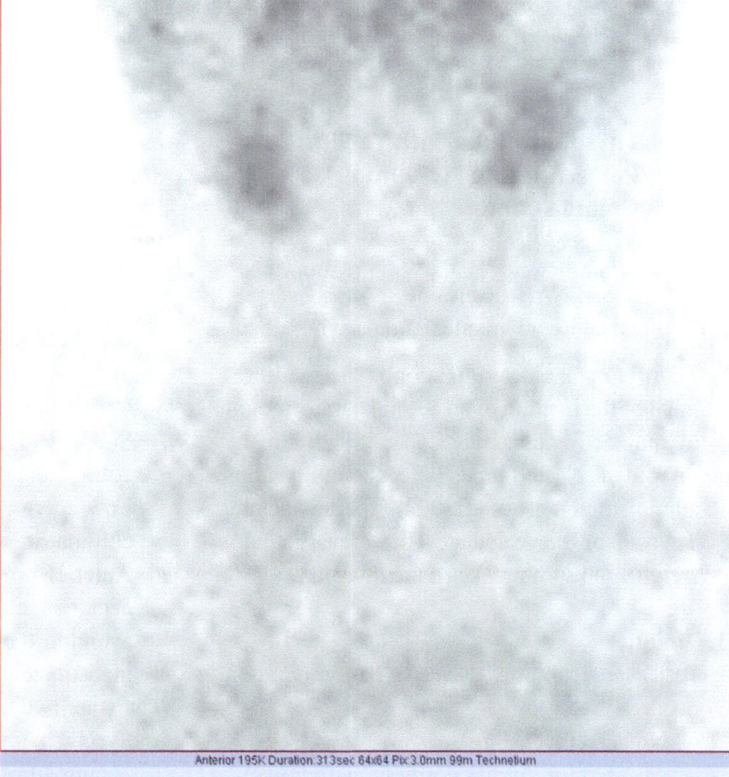

Fig. 7.37 Thyroid Tc-99m Pt scan showing the low uptake in the cervical area due to important thyroid tissue destruction; patient with AIT

early image and also low uptake in delayed images (Fig. 7.38b), suggestive for AIT type II/III, despite the lack of expression of serologic inflammatory factors. The results were crucial for the adequate selection of therapy.

Conclusion:

Amiodarone-induced hyperthyroidism. The Tc-99m MIBI scan is essential to differentiate AIT type I which needs antithyroid drugs from the AIT type II or III which needs corticotherapy.

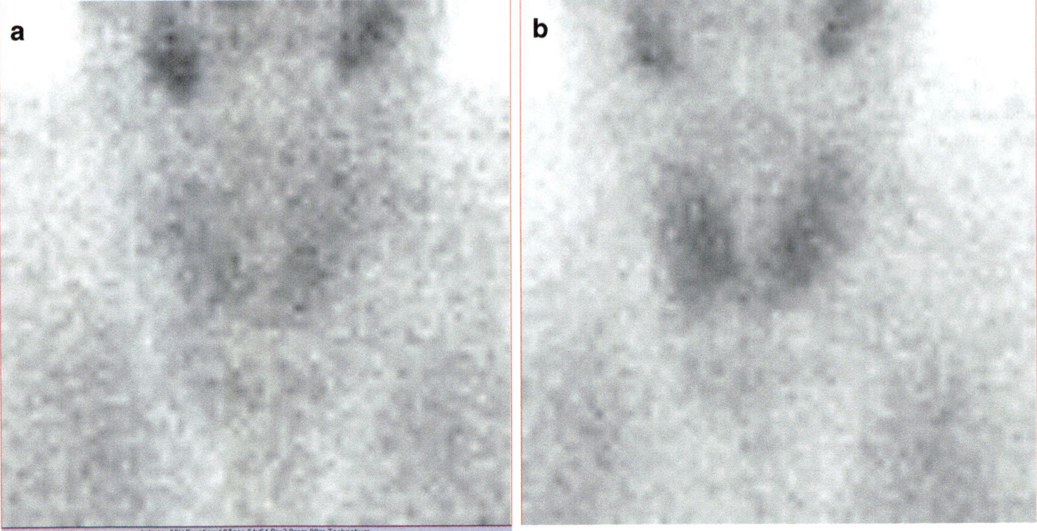

Fig. 7.38 Thyroid Tc-99m MIBI scan early image (**a**) and delayed image (**b**) showing the low uptake on both sequences, in the cervical area due to important thyroid tissue destruction; patient with AIT type II

7.3.5.4 Thyroid Uptake with Tc-99m Pertechnetate (Tc-99m Pt) Gamma Camera

Radiopharmaceutical:

- Technetium-99m pertechnetate (Tc-99m Pt)

Principle:

- Thyroid uptake determination is the measurement of the fraction of an administered amount of radioactive tracer that accumulates in the thyroid at selected times, after the intravenous administration of Tc-99m pertechnetate. Thyroid uptake calculates the area, volume, weight, and split uptake of the thyroid.

Technique:

- Patient preparation: No special preparation needed.
  - No need for fasting
  - No need for thyroid hormone withdrawal
  - No influence caused by other drugs
  - No influence caused by recent procedures with iodine contrast substances
  - Attention to breastfeeding patients, children, and potential fetal exposure (see chapter Radioprotection)
- Dose: 2–10 mCi (74–370) MBq/patient of Tc-99m Pt obtained from the generator of Tc-99m in the department, respecting the quality control requirements.
- Dose calibration.
- Injected I.V.
- 15–30 min are necessary for waiting, after the injection for the scan.
- Patient position: Supine, slight neck extension.
- Gamma camera:
  - Calibration and quality valid control tests
  - Small-field rectangular (optional pinhole collimator)
  - Low-energy high-resolution (LEHR) collimator
  - Anterior-posterior (AP) over the patient's neck, as close to the neck as possible, avoiding the influence of resolution by an inadequate distance
- There are two methods of acquisition:
  - Syringe images method—uses counts obtained from syringe images.

    Image containing a static view of the full syringe (Fig. 7.39)

    Image containing a static view of the empty syringe (Fig. 7.40)

    Image containing a static view of the injection site (optional)

    Image containing a static anterior view of the thyroid (Fig. 7.41)

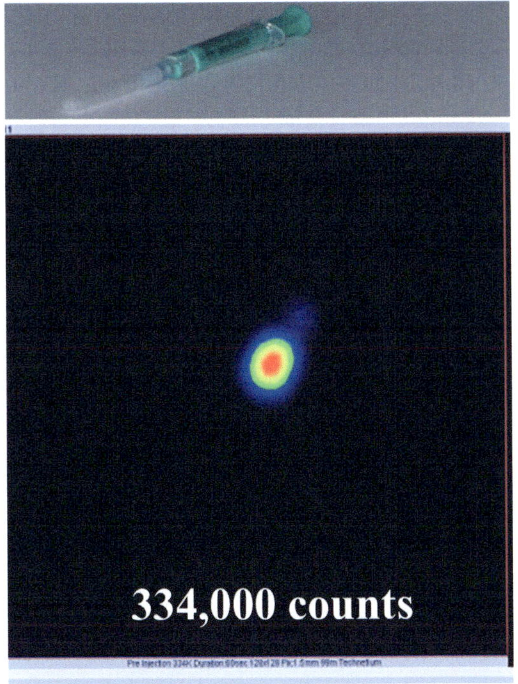

Fig. 7.39 Preinjection registered counts

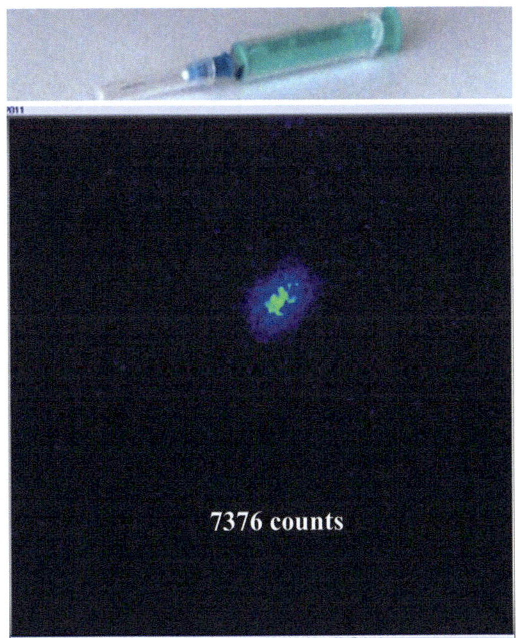

Fig. 7.40 Postinjection registered counts

- Dose calibrator and syringe images method
  Measures the activity of the full syringe.
  Measures the activity of the empty syringe following patient injection.

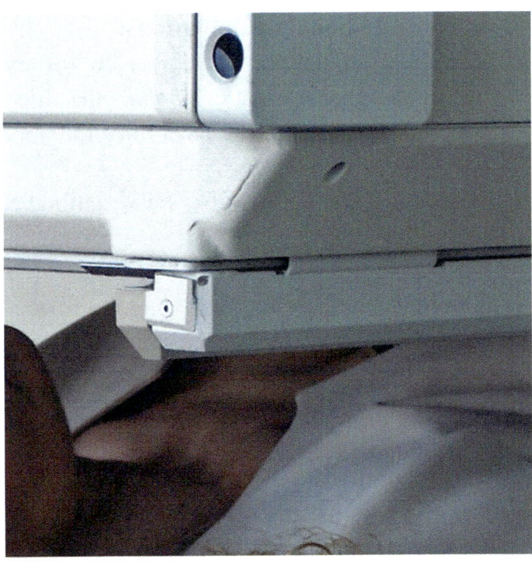

Fig. 7.41 Thyroid scan Tc-99m Pt uptake workflow

  Time and date when the full and empty syringe was measured.
  When using the dose calibrator method, a new calibration factor is needed each time.
- The camera parameters are:
  Anterior position using gamma camera
  Selected energy 140 keV
  Window 15–20%
  128 × 128 matrix or 256 × 256
  100,000–250,000 counts/image or 5 min

• Processing: There are special PC programs; the uptake values are obtained in workflow factory templates, present in the soft of the cameras.

Clinical applications:

• Assists in determining the amount of I-131 to be administered to patients for therapy of hyperthyroidism due to Graves' disease or toxic nodular goiter. The uptake should be performed as close as possible in time to the treatment.
• Differentiates subacute or painless thyroiditis and factitious hyperthyroidism from Graves' disease and other forms of hyperthyroidism.
• Assists in diagnosing and confirming the diagnosis of amiodarone-induced hyperthyroidism.

Necessary additional examinations:

- Clinical examination; remember to discuss and to examine the patient *before* the injection, in order to limit the hazardous radiation exposure.
- Serologic tests: TSH, FT4, FT3, antibodies TPO, TRab, etc.

Comments:

- The uptake also justifies the performance of the scan. In addition, with the same dose, we are able to obtain the structural information.

Reports:

- The reports respect the general format of the department with all the identification data of the patient, the institution, and the physician.
- The report will include the technical data related to the radiopharmaceutical, the used dose, the type of gamma camera, and the acquisition data. The report will note the estimation of the absorbed dose due to this examination. These data are available in predefined forms calculated for the majority of tracers and investigations. The report will include the value of the uptake and also the reference range of values, largely variable in different zones, areas, and countries (Fig. 7.42).

Most frequently, the normal thyroid uptake values determined by Tc-99m Pt uptake are reported to be between 0.5 and 1.6%.

Remember to ask from the nuclear medicine department the normal range established by the department standard. These values are set up according to some specific conditions: race, gender, age, geographical area, iodine-deficient region, etc.

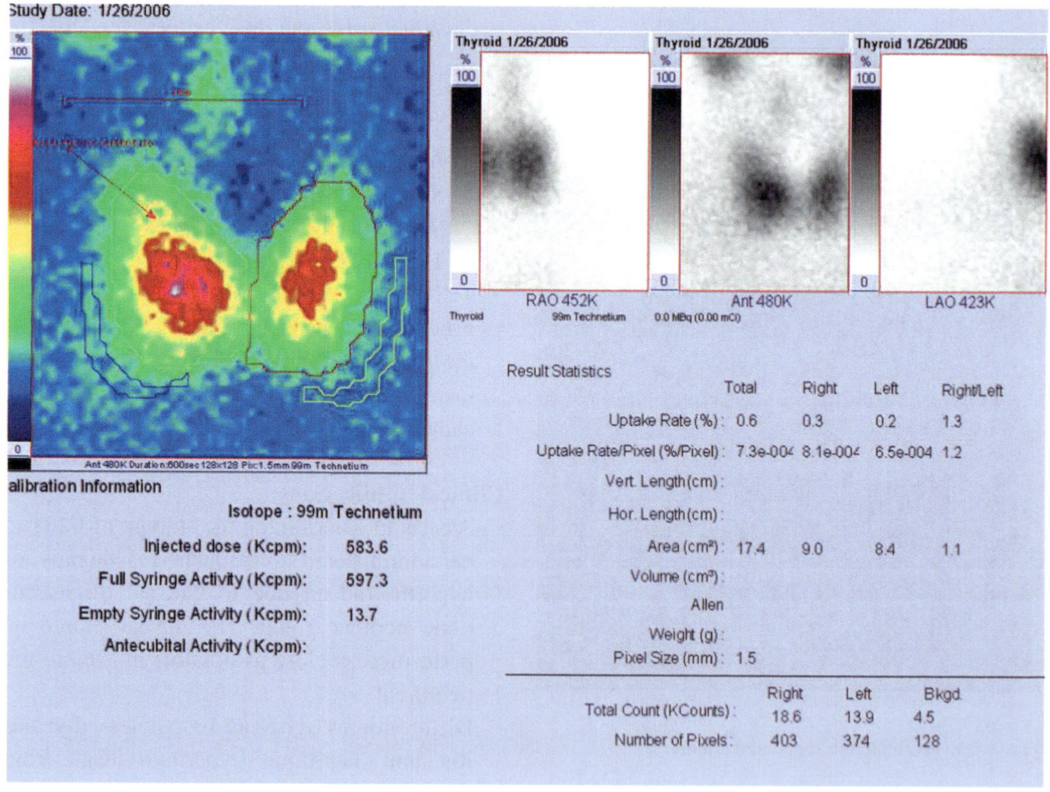

Fig. 7.42 Report of Tc-99m Pt thyroid uptake

7.3.5.5 Thyroid Uptake with I-131 or I-123 Sodium Iodide

Radiopharmaceutical:

- Radioiodine I-131 or I-123 sodium iodide capsules or liquid

Principle:

- Thyroid uptake determination is the measurement of the fraction of an administered amount of radioactive tracer that accumulates in the thyroid at selected times, after orally administered radioiodine. Radioiodine thyroid uptake (RAIU) calculates the uptake of the thyroid.

Technique:

- Patient preparation: Special preparation needed
  - It is necessary to have at least 4–6 h for fasting.
  - It is necessary to have a thyroid hormone withdrawal: for antithyroid drugs, 3–7 days, and for substitutive thyroid hormones, 14–20 days.
  - There can be an influence caused by other drugs.
  - Avoid or limit procedures with iodine contrast substances.
  - Low-iodine diet may be recommended at least 3–7 days before the test.
  - Attention to breastfeeding patients, children, and potential fetal exposure (see the chapter Radioprotection).
  - The amount of radioiodine is similar to daily intake of iodine, so the allergic side effects are very unusual and improbable.
- Dosage:
  - 50–100 μCi (1.85–3.7 MBq)/patient of I-131 NaI
  - 100–400 μCi (3.7–14.8 MBq)/patient of I-123 NaI
- Dose calibration.
- Orally administrated capsules or liquid.
- Measurements may be started at 2–5–6–24 h.
- Patient position: Supine, slight neck extension.
- Uptake system:
  - Calibration and valid quality control tests.
  - Immediate dose measurement, prior to patient administration, in a phantom model mimics the neck and the thyroid; the precise time and number of counts emitted by the dose are registered.
  - The capsules are swallowed with a little amount of water.
  - The measurement of counts emitted by the thyroid neck starts at 2 h for I-131 and at 6 h for I-123, and they are repeated in the same conditions after 24 h. There may be also other standard supplementary intervals created by the department.
- Processing: There are special PC programs; the uptake values are obtained in workflow factory templates present in the soft of uptake system or simply by calculating the ratio:

$$\text{RAIU} = \text{thyroid counts} / \text{capsule counts}$$

The details of the ratio are related to the measurement of the background and of the decay.

The formula is:

$$\text{RAIU} = \frac{\left(\begin{array}{l}\text{Thyroid counts} - \\ \text{background counts}\end{array}\right) \times \\ \text{decay correction factor}}{\begin{array}{l}\text{Iodine capsule counts} - \\ \text{background counts}\end{array}} \times 100\%$$

The decay correction factor is 0.918 for I-131 at 24 h, 0.730 for I-123 at 6 h, and 0.284 at 24 h (see Chap. 6).

Clinical applications:

- Assists in determining the amount of I-131 to be administered to patients for the therapy of hyperthyroidism due to Graves' disease or toxic nodular goiter. The uptake should be performed as close in time as possible to the treatment.
- Differentiates subacute or painless thyroiditis and factitious hyperthyroidism from Graves' disease and other forms of hyperthyroidism.

- Assists in diagnosing and confirming the diagnosis of amiodarone-induced hyperthyroidism.
- Tests of suppression.
- The measurement of the uptake is of limited value in the case of a hypothyroidism diagnosis.

Necessary additional examinations:
- Clinical examination; remember to discuss and to examine the patient before the administration of the capsule, in order to limit the hazardous radiation exposure.
- Serologic tests: TSH, FT4, FT3, antibodies TPO, TRab, etc.

Comments:
- The uptake also justifies the performance of the scan. In addition, the dose permits to obtain the structural information.

Reports:
- The reports respect the general format of the department with all the identification data of the patient, the institution, and the physician. The report will include the technical data related to the radiopharmaceutical, the used dose, the type of uptake system, and the acquisition data. The report will note the estimation of the absorbed dose due to this examination. These data are available in predefined forms calculated for the majority of tracers and investigations.
- The report will include the value of the uptake and also the reference range of values, largely variable in different zones, areas, and countries.

Normal values:
- At 2–6 h, the range is 3–8–15%.
- At 24 h, the range is between 5 and 35% in most regions of Northern America, and in many other parts of the world, the range is 15–50%.
- Some laboratories only measure RAIU at 24 h, which is the most accurate in many circumstances.
- Remember to ask the laboratory for the normal values set up for that specific region.

Increased RAIU:
- Hyperthyroidism (Graves' disease, Plummer's disease-toxic adenoma, trophoblastic disease, pituitary resistance to thyroid hormone, TSH-producing pituitary adenoma)
- Nontoxic goiter (endemic, inherited biosynthetic defects, generalized resistance to thyroid hormone, some cases of Hashimoto's thyroiditis)
- Excessive hormonal loss (nephrosis, chronic diarrhea, hypolipidemic resins, diet high in soybean)
- Decreased renal clearance of iodine (renal insufficiency, severe heart failure)
- Recovery of the suppressed thyroid (withdrawal of thyroid hormone and antithyroid drug administration, subacute thyroiditis, iodine-induced myxedema)
- Iodine deficiency (endemic or sporadic dietary deficiency, excessive iodine loss as in pregnancy or in the dehalogenase defect)
- TSH administration

Decreased RAIU:
- Hypothyroidism (primary or secondary); Hashimoto's thyroiditis
- Defect in iodide concentration (inherited "trapping" defect, early phase of subacute thyroiditis, transient hyperthyroidism)
- Suppressed thyroid gland caused by thyroid hormone (hormone replacement, thyrotoxicosis factitia, struma ovarii)
- Iodine excess (dietary, drugs, and other iodine contaminants)
- Miscellaneous drugs and chemicals (see Table 7.2)

Key Points
- All this blocking agents or situations must be analyzed according to the patient's special conditions. Even if it is well known, the blocking capability of contrast agents, the clinical presentation may decide the use of radioiodine despite the recent use of these substances. For example, in case of metastatic differentiated thyroid cancer, the recent CT with contrast media will not delay significantly the radioiodine therapy.

Table 7.2 Most frequent interfering drugs with the thyroid uptake

Interfering drug	Withhold	Study affected
Antithyroid medications	1 week	Decreases thyroid uptake
Thyroid hormones (T3, T4, or T3+T4)	2–3 weeks	Decreases thyroid uptake
Expectorants, vitamins	2 weeks	Decreases thyroid uptake
Phenylbutazone	1–2 weeks	Decreases thyroid uptake
Salicylates	1 week	Decreases thyroid uptake
Steroids	1 week	Decreases thyroid uptake
Sodium nitroprusside	1 week	Decreases thyroid uptake
Antihistamines	1 week	Decreases thyroid uptake
Antiparasitics	1 week	Decreases thyroid uptake
Penicillin	1 week	Decreases thyroid uptake
Sulfonamides	1 week	Decreases thyroid uptake
Tolbutamide	1 week	Decreases thyroid uptake
Thiopental	1 week	Decreases thyroid uptake
Benzodiazepines	4 weeks	Decreases thyroid uptake
I.V. contrast agents	1–2 months	Decreases thyroid uptake
Topical iodide agents	1–9 months	Decreases thyroid uptake
Oral cholecystographic agents	6–9 months	Decreases thyroid uptake
Bronchographic contrast oil-based iodinated agents	6–12 months	Decreases thyroid uptake
Mielographic contrast oil-based iodinated agents	2–10 years	Decreases thyroid uptake
Special attention to	Amiodarone—½–1–2 years	Blocks thyroid uptake
	Recent dose of radioiodine	Stunning effect
	Interferon alpha, interleukin-2	Blocking effect

7.3.5.6 Thyroid Scintigraphy with I-131 Sodium Iodide (I-131 NaI): Linear Scanner

Radiopharmaceutical:

- I-131 iodide (I-131 NaI)

Principle:

- I-131 NaI is absorbed from the gastrointestinal tract after per oral administration.
- The process of organification consists of I-131 trapped in the thyroid gland, undergoing the natural process of iodine metabolism. The active uptake of iodide (I−) by the follicular cells involves an active transport mechanism ATPase dependent, which allows I- to be taken up from capillary blood against both a concentration and an electrical gradient in exchange for Na+. This enables the thyroid gland to concentrate significantly the iodide and allows the very small quantities of radioactive isotopes to be used to investigate patients with thyroid disease.

Technique:

- Patient preparation:
  - Fasting for at least 6 h.
  - Thyroid hormone withdrawal (substitutive treatment between for 2–4–6 weeks and antithyroid drugs for 3–5–7 days).
  - Attention to the influence caused by other drugs.
  - Avoid or limit as much as possible the influence of recent procedures with iodine contrast substances.
  - Attention to breastfeeding patients.
  - The radioiodine is improbable to produce allergic effects; the allergic tests before this examination are recommended only in exceptional cases.
- Dose: 50–100 μCi (1.85–3.7 MBq)/patient of I-131 NaI.
- Administered P.O.
- Scan at 24 h after capsule administration.
- Patient position: Supine, slight neck extension.
- Linear scanner.

- Acquisition:
  - It has a single unchangeable head.
  - Anterior-posterior (AP) incidence over the patient's neck, as close to the neck as possible, avoiding the influence of resolution by an inadequate distance.
  - Static acquisition.
  - The counts acquisition, the speed of registering, and the subtract must be adjusted to each examination (the range of selected counts are 30, 102, 3 × 102, 103, 3 × 103, 104). The time constant is 5.
  - The energy selected is 364 keV.
  - Subtraction 20–40–60–80%; move in axe 2 mm.
  - Marks the suprasternal notch, with a point guided by a light marker.
  - Any palpable nodule should be marked on the images, during the acquisition, giving to the physician the facility to position the nodule.
- Processing: There is no need of special PC programs.

Clinical applications of the scan with or without uptake:

- Diagnosis of hyperthyroidism in:
  - Hyperfunctional nodular goiter
  - Autonomously hyperfunctional adenoma ("hot" nodule)
  - Hyperfunctional diffuse goiter (Basedow's disease)
- Diagnosis of hypothyroidism in:
  - Primary congenital (myxedema) and acquired hypothyroidism
  - Secondary hypothyroidism
- Thyroid cancer (cold nodule)
- Thyroiditis (de Quervain) and chronic thyroiditis (Hashimoto's disease)
- Thyroid cysts and other causes of nodules
- Thyroid anatomical variants: Retrosternal goiter, thyroid sublingual, left or right lateral-cervical thyroid, accessory lobe (Lalouette's pyramid), and agenesis of a lobe or of the entire gland

Necessary additional examinations:

- Thyroid ultrasound
- Serologic tests: TSH, FT4, FT3, TPO antibodies, calcitonin, thyroglobulin, TRab, etc.
- Fine needle aspiration biopsy (FNAB)

Comments:

- Scintigraphy is recommended according to the guidelines of thyroid disease diagnosis; its place is related to the national algorithm of evaluation of thyroid nodules.
- There are no allergic side effects that may be attributed to radioiodine; therefore, usually, there is no need for allergic tests before the nuclear tests with radioiodine. The amount of iodine is similar to the daily ingested iodine quantity, so it is very unlikely to determine allergic effects.

Reports:

- The reports respect the general format of the department with all the identification data of the patient, the institution, and the physician. The report will include the technical data related to the radiopharmaceutical, the used dose, the type of gamma camera, and the acquisition data. The report will note the estimation of the absorbed dose due to this examination. These data are available in predefined forms, calculated for the majority of tracers and investigations.
- The report will include a description of the:
  - Shape
  - Position
  - Size
  - Contour
  - Presence or absence of nodules in the thyroid area and the activity of the gland, of each lobe, and of the nodules
  - Presence of any special findings on the scintigraphy

Case 1: Autonomously Functioning Thyroid Nodule

History:

A 27-year-old female, without previous history of neck irradiation; no cases of familial thyroid cancer.

Clinical examination:

Symptoms: tremor, weight loss of 7 kg in 1 month, sweating, insomnia, and anxiety.

The neck examination revealed a tumor mass in the anterior neck area, not very firm, with elastic structure, ascending while patient has deglutition, developed quickly in the last

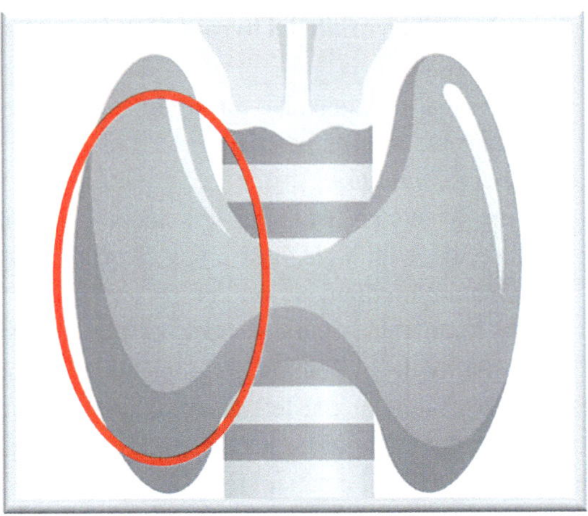

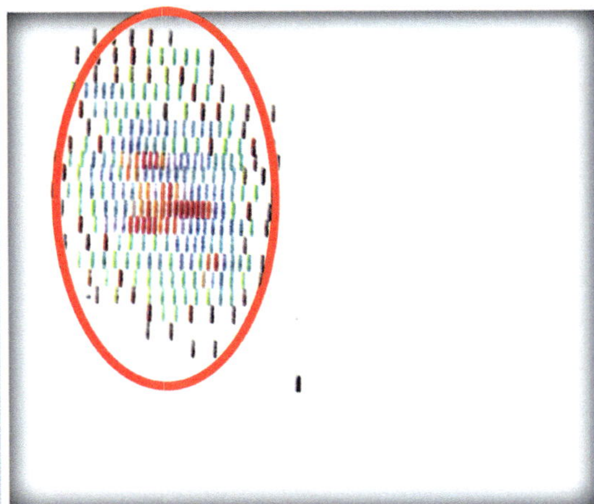

Fig. 7.43 Right thyroid lobe completely "hot" nodule

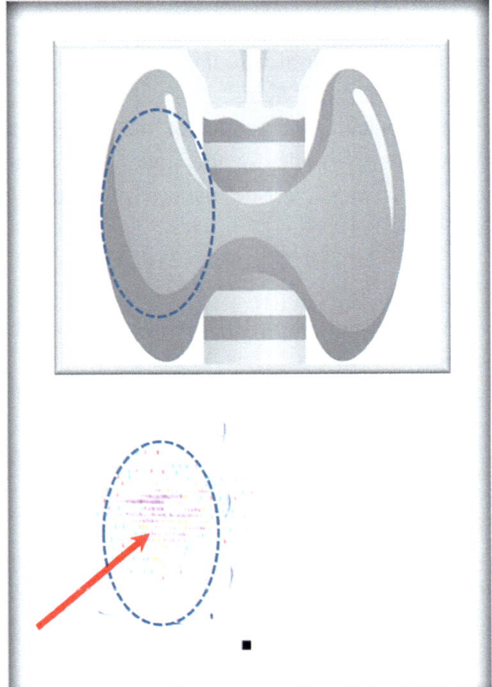

Fig. 7.44 Right thyroid lobe completely "hot" nodule

4 weeks. No clinical evidence of lymph nodes. The heart rate was 100–110/min. No signs of exophthalmia.

Examinations:

The ultrasound revealed a solid, hypoechogenic nodule involving almost entire right lobe of the thyroid. The nodule had regular contour and intense peripheral vascularity. No pathologic lymph nodes.

TSH <0.005 mIU/L (N.V. 0.4–4.5 mIU/L), undetectable

Findings:

The scintigraphy with I-131 NaI showed an intense uptake of the radiotracer in the entire right thyroid lobe ("hot" nodule), corresponding to the ultrasound finding.

The rest of the gland did not trap the tracer, due to the suppression of the tissue, by the dominant nodule; the rest of the gland did not appear on the image (Fig. 7.43).

Conclusion:

Autonomously hyperfunctioning right thyroid nodule (toxic adenoma)

Similar figures: Figs. 7.44 and 7.45

Key Points

- The radioiodine scintigraphy was largely used in the past due to the availability of the radiotracer, but today, its use is limited because of the radiation exposure.
- The stunning effect (blockage of radioiodine uptake after one previous dose of radioiodine) must be taken into consideration if there is an intention of applying a radioiodine therapy; the diagnostic dose must be as low as reasonable.

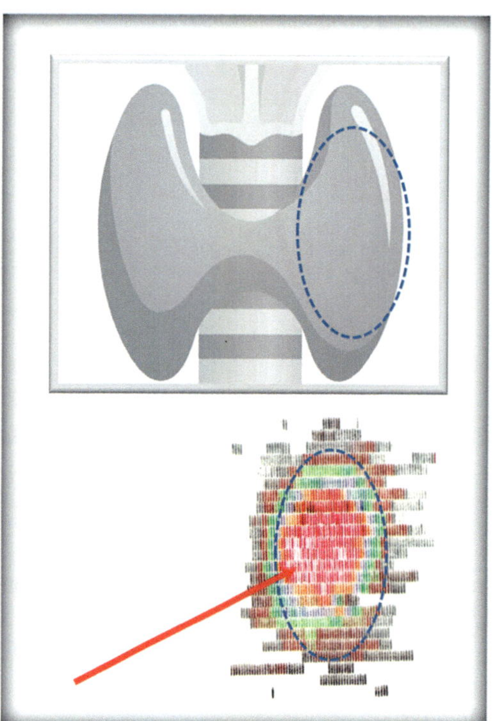

Fig. 7.45 Autonomously functioning left thyroid nodule

- The uptake associated to this scan may allow the calculation of the therapeutic dose.
- It is important to keep in mind that even in this situation, it is essential to rule out the cancer. Careful posttherapy follow-up of the patient and of the structure must be done. Increasing the volume or special patterns in ultrasound must lead to the indication of a FNAB.
- The initial FNAB is not recommended in this particular case. Thyroid cancer associated with toxic adenoma was rarely reported, but it is a clinical reality that should be in mind.

Case 2: Differentiated Thyroid Carcinoma

*History***:**

A 61-year-old male. No family history of thyroid cancers; no neck irradiation.

Clinical examination:

Clinical evidence of one left lateral-cervical lymph node, with high consistency, firm and having a maximum diameter of 3 cm.

No complaints; routine check of the thyroid gland during the evaluation of lymph node origin.

Enlargement of the left thyroid lobe, with a tumor in the left anterior neck area; the nodule is ascending while the patient is swallowing.

No other signs or symptoms to be mentioned.

Examinations:

The ultrasound revealed a nodule with intense hypoechogenicity in the interior, having multiple calcifications. It had irregular contour and abnormal, anarchic central vascularity, with the maximum diameter of 2.7 cm.

Pathological enlargement of the left lateral-cervical lymph nodes in the lower area of the neck, with characteristic pattern of metastatic disease.

TSH—4.6 mIU/L (N.V. 0.4–4.5 mIU/L), upper limit.

Anti-TPO < 34 mIU/L (N.V. <34 mIUL), normal.

FT4—13.2 pmol/L (N.V. 12–22 pmol/L), normal.

Calcitonin—2.1 pmol/L (N.V. <4 pmol/L), normal.

Findings:

The scintigraphy with I-131 NaI showed the distribution of a "cold" nodule in the 1/3 part of the left lobe of the thyroid gland. This metabolic feature was similar with the thyroid ultrasound, which concluded the diagnosis of probable thyroid carcinoma (Fig. 7.46).

Conclusion:

Left "cold" thyroid nodule. FNAB recommended.

The radical surgery was indicated and the final result was papillary thyroid carcinoma with left cervical lymph node metastasis.

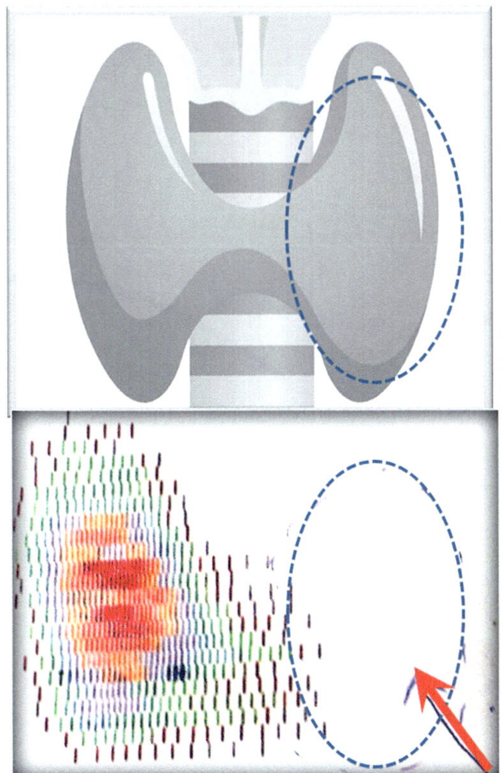

Fig. 7.46 "Cold" left thyroid nodule on radioiodine scan

Key Points

- The "cold" nodule in a radioiodine scintigraphy may be thyroid cancer in less than 10% of cases. In the majority of situations, this pathology is related to benign aspects.
- FNAB is the logic approach to establish the therapeutic sequence.
- In the image presented above, there is a risk of having a misinterpreted diagnosis without an inspection of the patient or without an ultrasound: "hot" nodule in the right lobe instead of "cold" nodule in the left lobe.

Case 3: Ectopic Thyroid Carcinoma

History:

A 58-year-old female. No family history of thyroid cancers or irradiation.

Clinical examination:

The inspection of the patient revealed an asymmetry in the central sternal area. No cutaneous changes in temperature or color, no pain symptoms. There was a deformation of the area highly probable due to the presence of a tumor.

No enlargement of the thyroid, no tumor in the anterior neck area; normally ascending thyroid while the patient is swallowing.

No other signs or symptoms to be mentioned. Patient referred for the sternal tumor.

Examinations:

The thorax CT described a solid mass of 5.4/9 cm lying in the posterior of the sternum, with minimum compression of the trachea, with sternum destruction. Mediastinum lymph nodes in the upper part.

TSH—0.61 mIU/L (N.V. 0.4–4.5 mIU/L), normal.

FT4—16.7 pmol/L (N.V. 12–22 pmol/L), normal.

Findings:

The scintigraphy with I-131 NaI showed a normal distribution of the radiotracer in the normal anterior cervical area.

Secondly, a second organ uptaking the radioiodine specifically situated in the sternum area was discovered; this image had a "cold" nodule in the 1/3 part of the right lobe of the thyroid gland.

The 24 h measured counts were almost equal (both in the normal situated thyroid and in the ectopic one) (Fig. 7.47).

Conclusion:

Ectopic thyroid gland with "cold" nodule is highly suggestive for neoplasm.

The radical surgery was indicated.

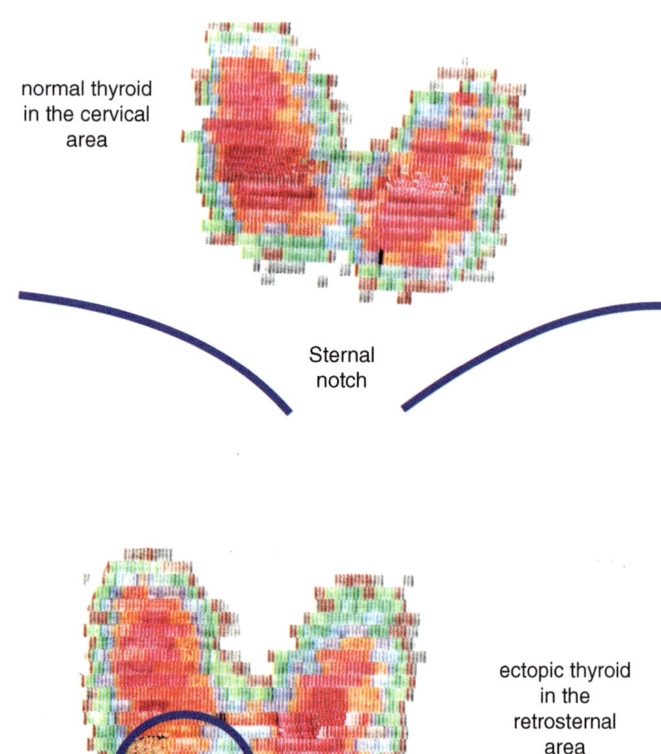

Fig. 7.47 Ectopic thyroid gland with right "cold" nodule situated in the retrosternal area

Key Points

- The radioiodine scintigraphy is the most specific imagistic test in the diagnosis of ectopic thyroid tissue.
- The ectopic tissues frequently evolve to malignancy.
- The particularity of this case is mainly due to the rare situation of the ectopic thyroid and to the method of scintigraphy; the linear scan is exceptionally used to scan large areas able to define the ectopy.
- In the intention to treat the neoplasm developed in an ectopic thyroid, it is also mandatory to ablate the normal thyroid gland.

Case 4: Hashimoto's Thyroiditis

History:

A 39-year-old female. No family history of irradiation or thyroid cancers. Recent menopause.

Clinical examination:

The inspection of the patient revealed a discrete enlargement of the thyroid gland; thyroid normally ascending while patient was swallowing.

No other signs or symptoms to be mentioned.

Examinations:

TSH—51.3 mIU/L (N.V. 0.4–4.5 mIU/L), high.

FT4—6.2 pmol/L (N.V. 12–22 pmol/L), low.

Anti-TPO > 600 mIU/L (N.V. <34 mIU/L), very high.

The thyroid ultrasound revealed an intense diffuse hypoechogenic structure in the thyroid gland, with multiple micronodules in both left

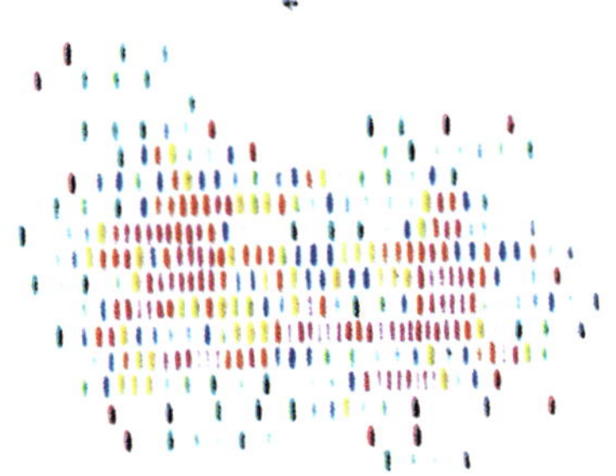

Fig. 7.48 Hashimoto's thyroiditis

RF 131I ; A 3,7 MBq ; S 20 % ; V 0,5 Imp. 10²

Thyroid uptake	2h 4 % (V.N. 10 – 12 %)
	24h 10,4 % (V.N. 35 – 48 %)

and right lobes; diffuse increasing of vascularity. No lymph nodes.

Findings:

The scintigraphy with I-131 NaI showed an abnormal distribution of the radiotracer in the anterior cervical area.

Diffuse reduced uptake in the entire gland;

The uptake is significantly reduced at the 2 h measurements and also after 24 h (Fig. 7.48).

Conclusion:

Hashimoto's thyroiditis

Case 5: Malignant Thyroid Tumor

History:

A 28-year-old female. No family history of irradiation or thyroid cancers.

Thyroid nodule discovered incidentally at the thyroid ultrasound.

Clinical examination:

The patient presented an enlargement of the left thyroid gland and a nodule of about 2 cm in the lower part of the left thyroid lobe; no lymph nodes clinically obvious.

Examinations:

Anti-TPO < 34 mIU/L (N.V. <34 mIU/L), normal.

TSH—1.63 mIU/L (N.V. 0.4–4.5 mIU/L), normal.

FT4—15.2 pmol/L (N.V. 12–22 pmol/L), normal.

The ultrasound revealed a solitary nodule with intense hypoechogenicity in the left lobe, with a maximum diameter of 1.7 cm, having an irregular contour; the existence of microcalcifications in the central area of the nodule; no other thyroid alterations.

Findings:

The Tc-99m Pt revealed a "hot" nodule corresponding to the ultrasound description of the left nodule (Fig. 7.49).

Because the patient refused FNAB, with the intention to improve the positive diagnostic, I-131 scan was recommended (there was no availability for I-123). This image was discordant to the previous Tc-99m scan presenting a "cold" nodule (Fig. 7.50).

Conclusion:

Left solitary nodule, highly probable to be malignant.

Key Points

- The discordant image: the "hot" nodule in Tc-99m Pt scan and the "cold" nodule in the I-131/I-123 scan are highly probable to be malignant.
- The FNAB is the first option in the morphological description, but there may be situation when the double-tracer scan may contribute to the improvement of the diagnosis.

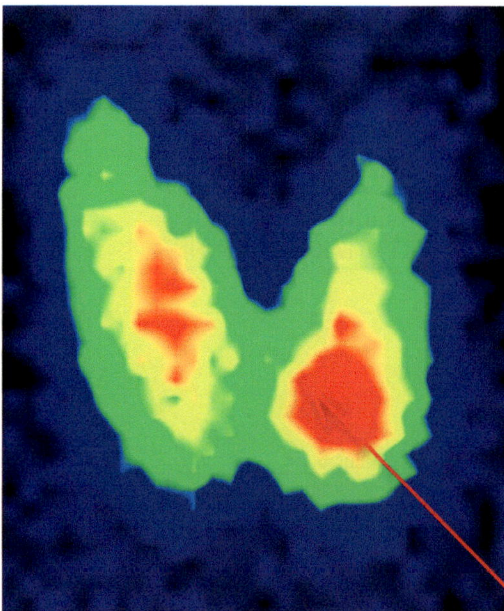

Fig. 7.49 Thyroid scan Tc-99m Pt: "hot" nodule in left inferior pole—discordant nodule highly probable to be malignant

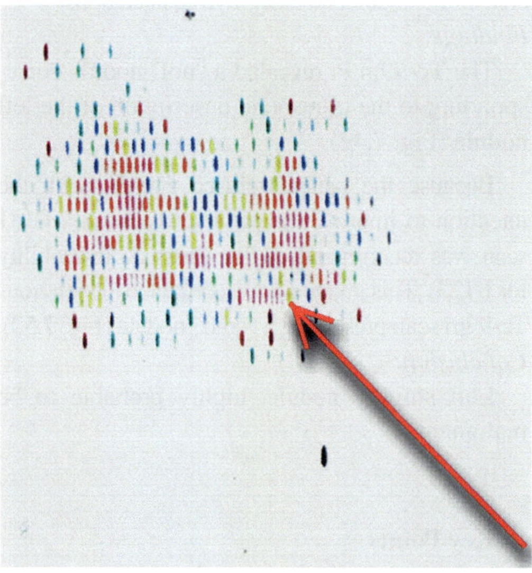

Fig. 7.50 Thyroid scan I-131: nodule "cold" in left inferior pole—discordant nodule highly probable to be malignant

7.3.5.7 Whole-Body Scan with I-131 Sodium Iodide (I-131 WBS): Gamma Camera

Radiopharmaceutical:

- I-131 iodide (I-131 NaI)

Principle:

- I-131 NaI is absorbed from the gastrointestinal tract after per oral administration.
- The process of organification consists in I-131 trapping in the thyroid gland and in all thyroid cells spread in the body from a differentiated thyroid carcinoma.
- The whole-body acquisition allows acquiring the data from a patient that is larger than the field of view of the gamma camera. Moving the patient's bed into or out of the gantry, while the image is acquired, realizes the acquisition.

Technique:

- Patient preparation:
  - Fasting for at least 6 h.
  - Thyroid hormone withdrawal (substitutive treatment) between 2, 4, and 6 weeks; thyrogen (recombinant TSH) administered in the situation of thyroid carcinoma without hormone withdrawal.
  - Avoid or limit the influence of the blocking drugs.
  - Avoid procedures with iodine contrast substances.
  - Attention to breastfeeding patient or potential fetal exposure (see chapter Radioprotection).
  - Unlikely to have allergic side effects, so the testing for allergic reactions is exceptional.
- Dose: 2–10 mCi (74–370 MBq)/patient of I-131 NaI in case of the diagnostic WBS, or after the radioiodine therapy, the dose is that of the administered activity (30–50–100–150–200 mCi) and is called post-therapeutic whole-body scan.
- The radioiodine is administered P.O. in case of the capsules or in liquid form.
- The scan may be performed at 24–48–72 h after the administration of the capsule; sometimes it can be performed after 5–7 days; the time is related to the activity of the radioiodine dose and the amount of the remnant tissue.
- Patient position: Supine, slight neck extension.
- Gamma camera (single head or dual head).
- Calibration and valid quality control tests.

- Large-field rectangular head.
- High-energy general-purpose (HEGP) collimator.
- Anterior-posterior (AP) and posterior-anterior (PA) over the patient's body, as close to the patient as possible, avoiding the influence of resolution by an inadequate distance.
- Acquisition:
  - Whole body.
  - Selected energy 364 keV.
  - Window 15–20%.
  - 1024 × 256 matrix.
  - 750,000–1000,000 counts/image.
  - Lateral or oblique-lateral images may be also obtained.
- It is possible to have also acquisition using single-photon emission computed tomography (SPECT) or SPECT/CT systems.
- Processing: There are special PC programs, which allow processing the images.

Clinical applications:
- Evaluation of remnant thyroid tissue postsurgery in differentiated thyroid cancer (DTC)
- Correct staging of DTC
- Assessment of the response to therapy in DTC

Necessary additional examinations:
- Thyroid ultrasound
- Serologic tests: TSH, Tg, and anti-Tg
- Fine needle aspiration biopsy (FNAB) of tumor or lymph nodes

Comments:
- Special attention to blocking drugs, mainly thyroid hormones and contrast media.
- Usually, there are no side effects related to allergy; therefore, there is no need for allergic tests.
- It is necessary to give a special attention to the stunning effect described as the blockage of trapping radioiodine; in case of targeted therapy for DTC, if previously it was done as a diagnostic I-131 WBS. This fact limits the pretherapeutic diagnostic WBS to some special situations: evaluation of large remnant tissues, in order to do another surgery, or when extensive metastasis is suspected.

Reports:
- The reports respect the general format of the department with all the identification data of the patient, institution, and physician. The report will include the technical data related to radiopharmaceutical, dose that was used, type of gamma camera, and acquisition data. The report will note the estimation of absorbed dose due to this examination. These are data available in predefined forms calculated for majority of tracers and investigations.
- The report will include a description of:
  - The presence of thyroid remnant in the thyroid area
  - The presence of uptake in the lymph nodes
  - The number and situation of metastasis
  - The normal sites of physiologic uptake of radioiodine
  - If there are areas of contamination that must be clarify and reported

Image description:
- Physiologic uptake (Figs. 7.51 and 7.52):
  - Radioiodine in central facial area (nose, mouth).
  - Uptake in the salivary glands (parotids, submandibular glands).
  - Stomach.
  - Bowel.
  - Sigma and rectum.
  - Urinary bladder.
  - There is a radioactive background of the entire body.
- Pathologic uptake (Figs. 7.53 and 7.54):
  - Thyroid remnant tissue in the neck area
  - Lymph nodes
  - Metastasis in the lungs
  - Metastasis in the brain
  - Metastasis in the bones
  - Any other sites that express radioiodine uptake, except the physiologic ones
- Contamination (Fig. 7.55):
  - Lack of contamination (no presence of uptake due to radioiodine in the surface of the skin, hair, or cloths of urinary, salivary, or swilling origin)

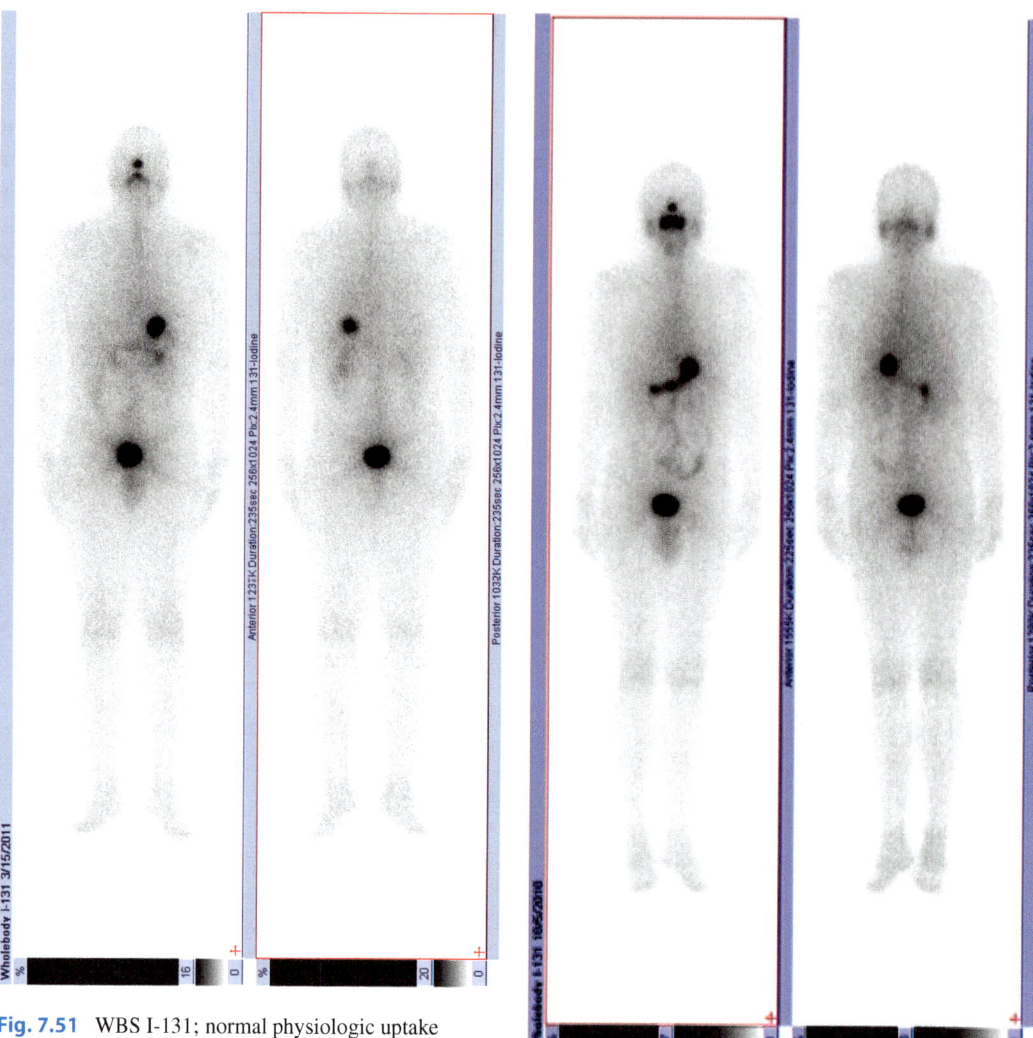

Fig. 7.51 WBS I-131; normal physiologic uptake

Fig. 7.52 WBS I-131; normal physiologic uptake

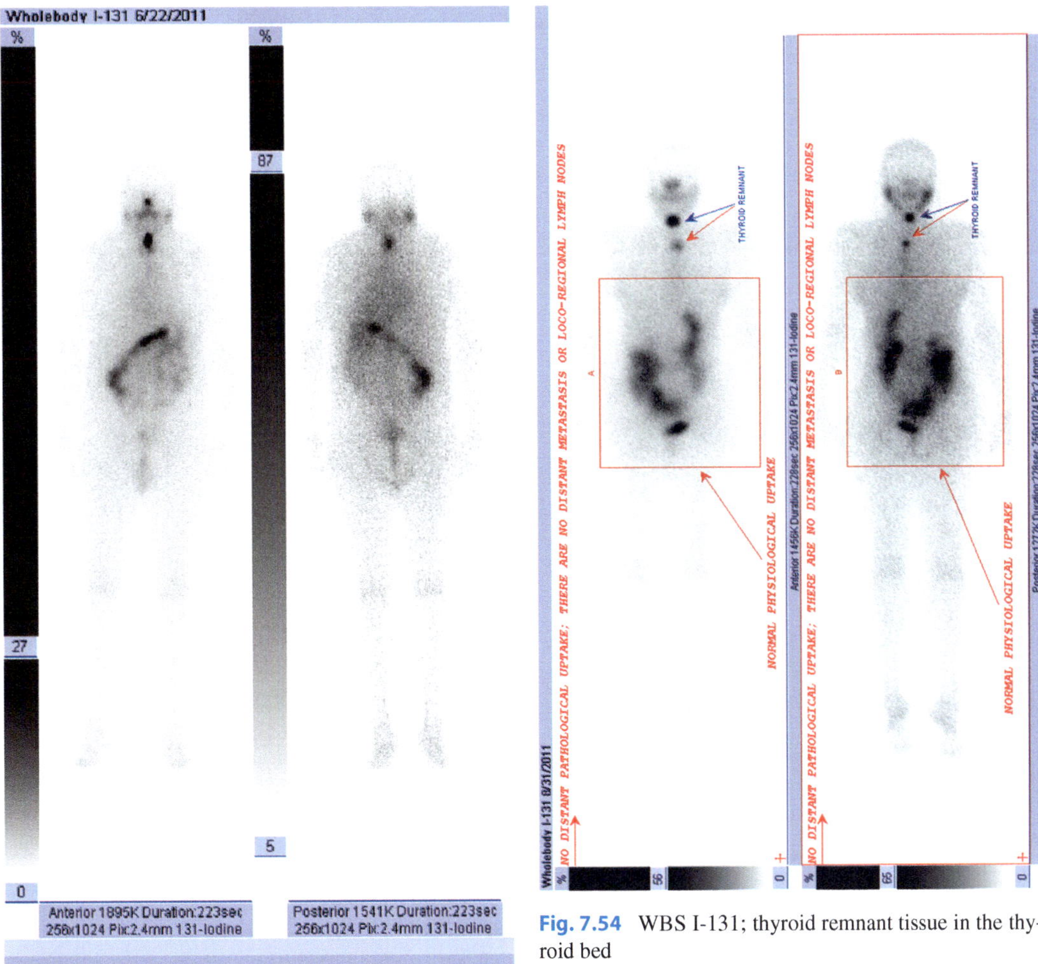

Fig. 7.53 WBS I-131; thyroid remnant tissue in the thyroid bed

Fig. 7.54 WBS I-131; thyroid remnant tissue in the thyroid bed

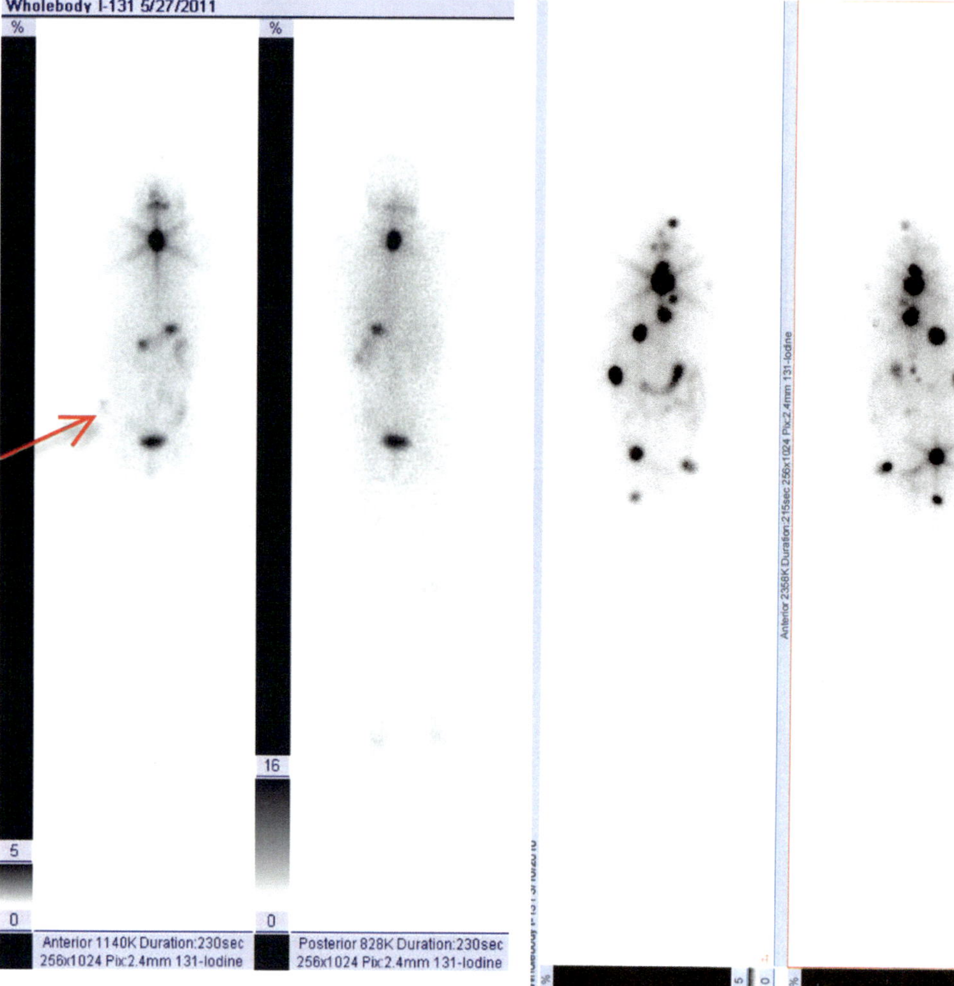

Fig. 7.55 WBS I-131 radioiodine contaminations on the clothes of the patient (handkerchief in the right pocket)

Fig. 7.56 WBS I-131—multiple radioiodine-avid metastases of papillary thyroid carcinoma

Case 1: Differentiated Thyroid Carcinoma

History:

A 52-year-old female. No family history of irradiation or thyroid cancers. In 2007 the patient suffered a total thyroidectomy for a multinodular goiter. She suffered a recent brain surgery for a tumor with the histology of papillary carcinoma.

Clinical examination:

She presented a surgical scar in the anterior neck area and in the left parietal bone due to craniotomy; minor speaking and equilibrium difficulties, with Parkinson-like symptoms.

Examinations:

- Brain MRI—no cerebral mass; defect of the cranium after craniotomy.
- Thorax CT—negative.
- Tg—42.724 μg/L (N.V. <0.1 μg/L), very high.
- Anti-Tg < 10 kIU/L (N.V. <115 kIU/L), normal.
- TSH < 0.001 mIU/L (N.V.—0.4–4.5 mIU/L), undetectable.
- FT4—27.2 pmol/L (N.V. 12–22 pmol/L), high. The values were obtained without any thyroid hormone replacement.

Findings:

The diagnostic whole-body scintigraphy with I-131 NaI (4 mCi) showed very important pathologic uptake of radioiodine in the patient's body (Fig. 7.56).

Conclusion:

Important thyroid remnant and multiple metastases in the brain, lungs, and bones due to papillary thyroid carcinoma

Key Points

- It is mandatory that the histology report be discussed and analyzed by a team who experimented in the evaluation of the thyroid pathology; any doubtful results must be clarified by additional tests (immunohistochemical analysis); if the borderline malignant/benign aspects persist, the patient must be followed up in a very careful manner.
- In the absence of thyroid hormone replacement after total thyroidectomy, the undetectable values of TSH with/without high serum levels of FT4 show the possible presence of extensive secreting thyroid tissue. In the particular case of thyroid cancer, this means multiple metastases or large thyroid remnant.
- If the histology report presents metastases of papillary carcinoma, do not forget the probability of thyroid or ovarian (struma ovarii) origins.
- Do not ask for the I-131 WBS for the complete assessment of the disease extent, when the thyroid gland is not yet ablated. The iodophilic character of normal thyroid cells is much higher than of the malignant cells; in this situation, the normal thyroid tissue will trap the radioiodine, and the metastatic sites will skip the examination test.
- When the extended metastases are suspected, the dose of radioiodine administered for WBS must be as low as possible with the intention to prevent a stunning effect; the therapy with I-131 will be performed as soon as possible after the diagnostic WBS.
- Avoid the examinations with contrast media.

Case 2: Differentiated Thyroid Carcinoma

History:

A 63-year-old male. No family history of irradiation or thyroid cancers. Nine years earlier suffered a total thyroidectomy for a compressive goiter and thyroid adenoma without further evaluation and follow-up, with inconstant hormone replacement. He suffered a pathologic fracture of the left femur, 1 month before being referred to the thyroid center; the report from the surgery suggested the diagnosis of metastatic follicular carcinoma.

Clinical examination:

The patient expressed very important mobility limitation with severe pain; he presented a surgical scar in the anterior neck area and a recent left femoral scar after the prosthesis surgery. No clinical evidence of lymph nodes.

Examinations:

Brain MRI—no cerebral mass.

Thorax CT—multiple metastases in the lungs.

Tg—150.552 μg/L (N.V. <0.1 μg/L), very high.

Anti-Tg < 10 kIU/L (N.V. <115 kIU/L), normal.

TSH—0.77 mIU/L (N.V. 0.4–4.5 mIU/L), normal.

FT4—9.2 pmol/L (N.V. 12–22 pmol/L), low.

The values were obtained without any thyroid hormone replacement.

Findings:

The diagnostic whole-body scintigraphy with I-131 NaI (4 mCi) showed very important pathologic uptake of radioiodine in the patient's body (Fig. 7.57).

Conclusion:

Important thyroid remnant and multiple metastases in the lungs and bones due to the follicular thyroid carcinoma.

Key Points

- The histology of follicular adenoma must be careful reported, in order to be sure about the exclusion of follicular thyroid carcinoma.
- The differential diagnosis between follicular adenoma and follicular carcinoma is set mainly depending on the

vascular invasion; due to this behavior, this type of tumors spread firstly into the body not via the lymphatic system; therefore, the sites of the metastases are frequently the bones, not the lymph nodes.

- The thyroid pathology occurring in male patients is by far less frequent than in the case of female patients, but the natural history of the tumor is definitely more aggressive; this is the reason why special attention must be granted to this category of patients.

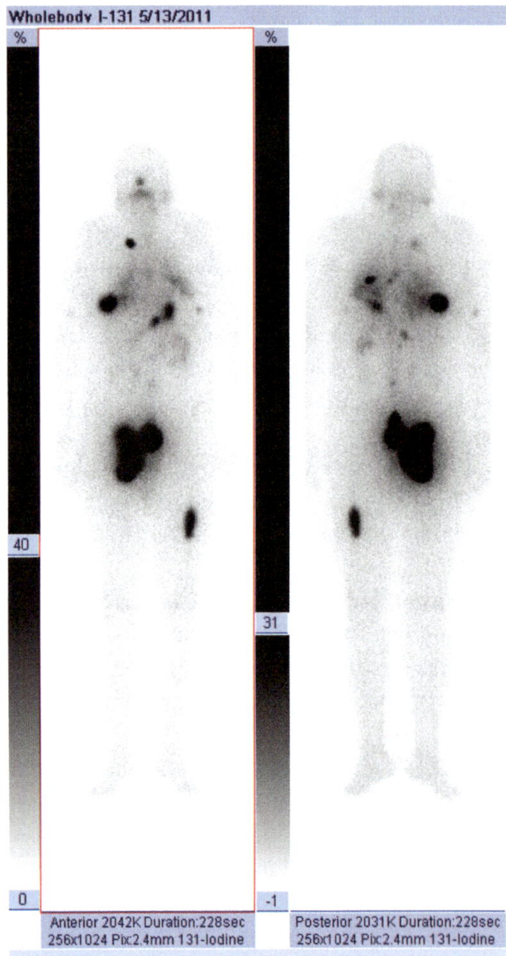

Fig. 7.57 I-131 WBS—multiple metastases of follicular thyroid carcinoma

Case 3: Hiatal Hernia

History:

A 64-year-old female patient was referred to the Institute of Oncology under "Prof. Dr. I. Chiricuță" Cluj–Napoca with the diagnosis of papillary thyroid carcinoma. Besides thyroid pathology, she complained of headache and cardiac symptoms such as chest pain and tachycardia, every time after the meals. She was investigated in order to treat a cardiac pathology associated with these symptoms but without a significant improvement. After the total thyroidectomy for thyroid carcinoma, the patient underwent the radioiodine therapy.

Clinical examination:

The patient presented minimal side effects of myxedema because of a 3-week hormone withdrawal; anterior neck post-thyroidectomy scar; no clinical lymph nodes or tumor detected; no other significant complaints. After having a meal, the symptoms became dramatic, with severe chest pain and tachycardia.

Examinations:

Thorax CT—negative

Tg < 0.1 μg/L (N.V. <0.1 μg/L), normal.

Anti-Tg < 10 kIU/L (N.V. <115 kIU/L), normal.

TSH—76.2 mIU/L (N.V. 0.4–4.5 mIU/L), significantly elevated on hormone withdrawal.

Negative ultrasound for thyroid recurrence or lymph nodes metastases.

Findings:

The diagnostic whole-body scintigraphy with I-131 NaI (4 mCi) showed very important pathologic uptake of radioiodine in the thorax of the patient.

The images obtained at 24 h post-radioiodine therapy revealed an unusual radioiodine uptake in the left hemithorax (Fig. 7.58).

This aspect was interpreted as a benign uptake produced by the presence of an isotope in the herniated stomach and because of the poor drainage.

At 48 h after administration, in fasting conditions, the images revealed a drained aspect (Fig. 7.59).

The hiatal hernia was confirmed by planar posterior-anterior and lateral chest radiography, which revealed the presence of the stomach in the

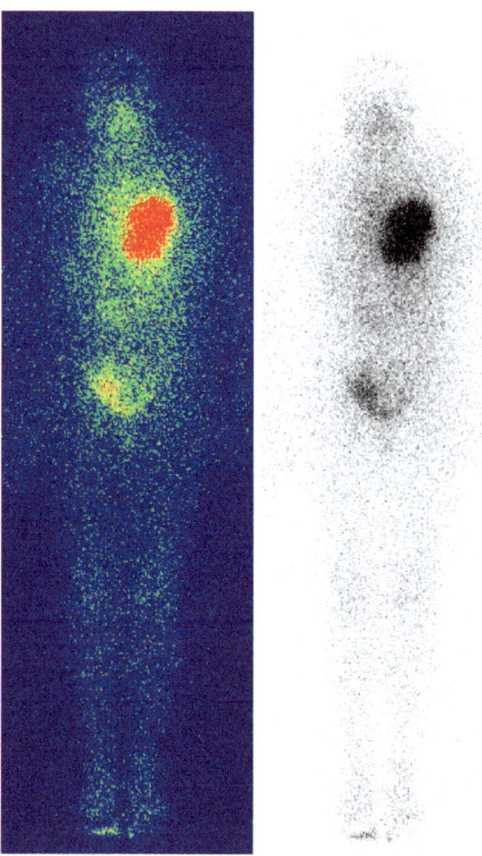

Fig. 7.58 WBS I-131 at 24 h; hiatal hernia

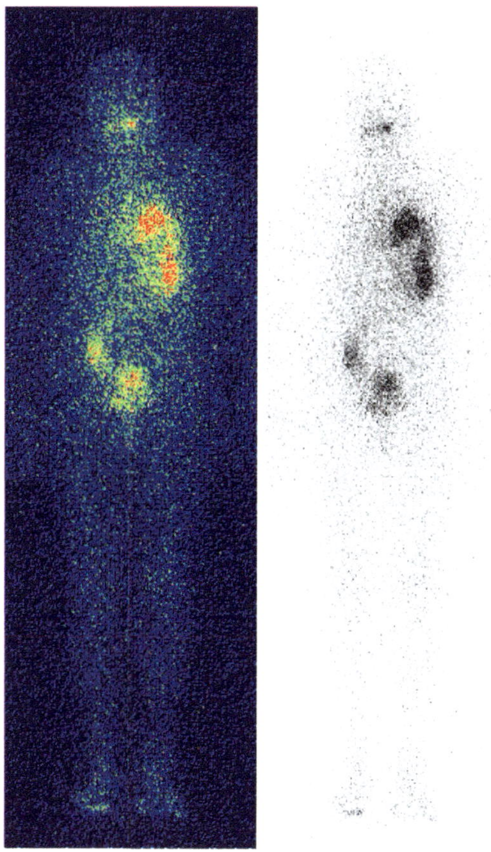

Fig. 7.59 WBS I-131 at 48 h; hiatal hernia and drainage of I-131

thorax. After an appropriate surgical treatment, the patient had complete remission of symptoms.

Conclusion:

Important radioiodine uptake in the left hemithorax because of hiatal hernia

Key Points

- The presence of radioiodine in the digestive system allows obtaining images about the transit and may suggest important information regarding the motility and obstruction at this level.
- The early images of WBS obtained at 24 h posttherapy are potentially inadequate; these may mask distant metastases because of the high level of radioactivity from the digestive system.

7.3.5.8 Thyroid Scintigraphy with I-123 Iodide (I-123 NaI): Gamma Camera

Radiopharmaceutical:

- Iodide I-123 sodium (I-123 NaI) capsules; the capsules are available with activities of 3.7 and 7.4 MBq (100 and 200 μCi) I-123 at time of calibration.

Principle:

- Sodium iodide is absorbed from the gastrointestinal tract. Following the absorption, the iodide is primarily distributed within the extracellular fluids of the body.
- It is trapped and organically bound by the thyroid gland and concentrated in the stomach, choroid plexus, and salivary glands and excreted by the kidneys.

Technique:

- Patient preparation: Special preparation.
  - At least 4–6 h is needed for fasting.
  - Thyroid hormone withdrawal is necessary.
  - There can be an influence caused by other drugs.
  - Avoid or limit procedures with iodine contrast substances.
  - Low-iodine diet may be recommended at least 3–7 days before the test.
  - Attention to breastfeeding patients, children, and potential fetal exposure (see chapter Radioprotection).
  - Unlikely to produce allergic effects.
- Dose: 100–500 μCi (3.7–18.5 MBq)/patient of I-123; higher doses up to 74 MBq (2 mCi) in case of WBS.
- Oral administration of capsules.
- The scan and also the uptake may be performed 6 h after the ingestion of the capsule.
- Patient position: Supine, slight neck extension.
- Gamma camera:
  - The low-energy high-resolution or general-purpose (LEHR or LEGP) collimator
  - Detector position: Anterior-posterior (AP) over the patient's neck, as close to the neck as possible, avoiding the influence of resolution by an inadequate distance
- Acquisition:
  - Static acquisition.
  - 128 × 128 matrix; if is acquired WBS 1024 × 256 matrix.
  - 50,000–100,000 counts/image.
  - Energy—159 keV.
  - Mark the suprasternal notch, with a point source of Tc-99m or Cobalt-57; this mark will be registered on the images.
  - Lateral or oblique-lateral images may also be obtained.
  - Any palpable nodule should be marked on the images, during the acquisition, giving to the physician the facility for positioning the nodule.
- Processing: There is no need of special PC programs; additional analysis of counts in different regions of interest (ROI) may be used; image interpretation.

Clinical applications:

- Same indication as I-131, but due to the less aggressive proprieties (no beta emitter, short half-life of 13.2 h, and low energy of 159 keV), it is more suitable.

Necessary additional examinations:

- Thyroid ultrasound
- Serologic tests: TSH, FT4, FT3, TPO antibodies, calcitonin, thyroglobulin, TRab, etc.
- Fine needle aspiration biopsy (FNAB)

Comments:

- The assessment of thyroid nodules is correlated with ultrasound diagnosis and the national algorithm of thyroid nodule evaluation.
- It may be safely used for children.

Reports:

- Same reports as in I-131 scintigraphy

Normal image and uptake:

- Same as in I-131

Key Points

- I-123 has ideal proprieties regarding the physiologic testing of the thyroid, following the same patterns of organic iodine.
- The short half-life of 13 h is perfect for the thyroid evaluation, allowing performing the uptake and the scan earlier than with I-131.
- The main advantage of I-123 in diagnosis is the absence of beta particles, and in consequence, the irradiation and cell damage are considerably lower than that due to I-131.
- Unfortunately, I-123 has a worldwide limited availability and considerable high costs.
- WBS with I-123 has the advantage of avoiding the stunning effect in a patient with thyroid carcinoma who will receive the therapeutic dose of I-131.

7.3.5.9 Thyroid Scintigraphy with I-125 Iodide (I-125 NaI) Gamma Camera

Radiopharmaceutical:

- Iodide I-125 sodium (I-125 NaI) capsules or liquid.

Principle:

- Sodium iodide is absorbed from the gastrointestinal tract. Following the absorption, the iodide is primarily distributed within the extracellular fluids of the body.
- It is trapped and organically bound by the thyroid gland and concentrated in the stomach, choroid plexus, and salivary glands and excreted by the kidneys.

Technique:

- Patient preparation: Special preparation
  - At least 4–6 h is needed for fasting.
  - Thyroid hormone withdrawal is necessary.
  - There can be an influence caused by other drugs. Avoid or limit procedures with iodine contrast substances.
  - Low-iodine diet may be recommended at least 3–7 days before the test.
  - Attention to breastfeeding patients, children, and potential fetal exposure (see chapter Radioprotection).
- Dose: 100–400 μCi MBq/patient of I-125
- Oral administration
- The scan and also uptake may be performed 6 h after the ingestion of the capsule.
- Patient position: Supine, slight neck extension.
- Gamma camera.
- The low-energy high-resolution or general-purpose (LEHR or LEGP) collimator
- Acquisition:
  - Static acquisition.
  - 128 × 128 matrix.
  - Minimum 100,000 counts/image.
  - Energy: 35 keV.
  - Mark the suprasternal notch, with a point source of Tc-99m or Cobalt-57; this mark will be registered on the images.
  - Lateral or oblique-lateral images may also be obtained.
  - Any palpable nodule should be marked on the images, during the acquisition, giving to the physician the facility for positioning the nodule.
- Processing: There is no need of special PC programs; additional analysis of counts in different regions of interest (ROI) may be used; image interpretation.

Clinical applications:

- Same indication as I-131; has less aggressive proprieties (no beta emitter and low energy of 35 keV). Long half-life of 59.4 days.
- Rarely used

Necessary additional examinations:

- Thyroid ultrasound
- Serologic tests: TSH, FT4, FT3, antibodies TPO, calcitonin, thyroglobulin, TRab, etc.
- Fine needle aspiration biopsy (FNAB)

Comments:

- The tracer is no longer used in clinical practice.
- Because of its relatively long half-life and emission of low-energy photons, I-125 is the preferred isotope for tagging antibodies in radioimmunoassay and other gamma-counting procedures involving proteins outside the body. The same properties of the isotope make it useful for brachytherapy (as noted) and for certain nuclear medicine scanning procedures, in which it is attached to proteins (albumin or fibrinogen) and where a longer half-life than provided by I-123 is required, in order to follow the isotope during the several days of test.
- Iodine-125 is sometimes used in imaging the thyroid, but iodine-123 is preferred for this purpose, due to better radiation penetration and shorter half-life.

Reports:

- Same reports as in I-131 scintigraphy

Normal image and uptake:

- Same as for I-131

7.3.5.10 Thyroid Scintigraphy with Thallium 201 Chloride (Tl-201 Chloride) Gamma Camera

Radiopharmaceutical:

- Thallium chloride (Tl-201chloride)

Principle:

- Tl-201 is trapped from the bloodstream by malignant thyroid cells, after the intravenous injection.

Technique:

- Patient preparation: No special preparation needed.
  - No need for fasting
  - No need for thyroid hormone withdrawal
  - No influence caused by other drugs
  - No influence of recent procedures with iodine contrast substances
  - Attention to breastfeeding female and potential fetal exposure
- Dose: 1.5–2 mCi (55–74 MBq)/patient of Tl-201.
- Injected I.V.
- After the injection, it is necessary to wait 5–15 min, in order to have early images, and 3–5 h for delayed images.
- Patient position: Supine, slight neck extension.
- Parallel collimator for low-energy 80 keV (LEGP or LEHR).
- Window width 20%.
- Acquisition:
  - Static acquisition.
  - Anterior position using gamma camera.
  - 128 × 128 matrix.
  - 250,000–500,000 counts/image.
  - Mark the suprasternal notch, with a point source of Tc-99m or Cobalt-57; this mark will be registered on the images.
  - Lateral or oblique-lateral images may also be obtained.
  - Any palpable nodule should be marked on the images, during the acquisition, giving to the physician the facility for positioning the nodule.
- Processing: There is no need of special PC programs; additional analysis of counts in different regions of interest (ROI) may be used; image interpretation.

Clinical applications:

- Differential diagnosis of malignant and benign thyroid nodules
- Complementary in the diagnosis of medullar thyroid cancer
- In non-avid iodine differentiated thyroid cancers

Necessary additional examinations:

- Thyroid ultrasound
- Serologic tests: TSH, FT4, FT3, antibodies TPO, calcitonin, thyroglobulin, TRab, etc.
- Fine needle aspiration biopsy (FNAB)

Comments:

- Method of scintigraphy complementary to FNAB, in some special situations (Thy 3—undetermined cytology?)
- Method mainly used in the evaluation of myocardial perfusion

Reports:

- The reports respect the general format of the department with all the identification data of the patient, the institution, and the physician. The report will include the technical data related to the radiopharmaceutical, the used dose, the type of gamma camera, and the acquisition data. The report will note the estimation of the absorbed dose due to this examination. These data are available in predefined forms calculated for the majority of tracers and investigations.
- The report will include a description of the:
  - Shape
  - Position
  - Size
  - Contour
  - Presence or absence of nodules in the thyroid area and the activity of the gland, each lobe, and the nodules
  - Presence of any special findings on the scintigraphy

Key Points
- There are controversial studies regarding the usefulness of Tl-201 thyroid scintigraphy using early/delayed images for increasing the accuracy of differential diagnosis between malignant and benign nodules.
- Until nowadays the method has been used only as a complementary one.

7.3.5.11 Thyroid Scintigraphy with Ga-67 Citrate Gamma Camera

Radiopharmaceutical:
- Gallium-67 (Ga-67) citrate

Principle:
- Accumulation mainly due to increased capillary permeability occurring during the inflammation processes.

Technique:
- Patient preparation: No special preparation needed.
  - Attention to breastfeeding and childbearing-age patients (see chapter of Radioprotection).
- Dose: 5 mCi (185 MBq)/patient of Ga-67 citrate.
- Injected I.V. 24 h is necessary for waiting, after the injection for the first images. Delayed images may be registered at 48 h.
- Patient position: Supine.
- Gamma camera:
  - Medium-energy general-purpose (MEGP) collimator at 300 keV
- Acquisition:
  - Spot planar acquisition.
  - First image at 24 h and the next image at 48–72 h.
  - Anterior and posterior position using gamma camera.
  - 128 × 128 matrix.
  - Min 500,000 counts/image.
  - Spot images on the region of interest may also be obtained.
  - SPECT is usually recorded with 360° acquisition of 20–30 s/image, for a total collection time of 20 min, along with the cross-sectional presentation.
- Processing: There are special PC programs for image processing; additional analysis of counts in different regions of interest (ROI) may be used; image interpretation.

Clinical applications:
- Diagnosis of inflammatory process involving the thyroid gland

Necessary additional examinations:
- Thyroid ultrasound
- Serologic inflammatory tests
- Fine needle aspiration biopsy (FNAB)

Comments:
- It is a rarely used method.
- Evaluation of the thyroid may occur during other investigations of the organs.

Reports:
- The report will include a description of the normal distribution and pathologic uptakes.

7.3.5.12 Thyroid Scintigraphy with I-123/131 MIBG: Gamma Camera

Radiopharmaceutical:
- Metaiodobenzylguanidine (MIBG) or iobenguane is a combination of an iodinated benzyl and a guanidine group. It may be labeled with I-131 for imaging and for treatment or with I-123 only for diagnosis.

Principle:
- MIBG enters the neuroendocrine cells by an active uptake mechanism via the epinephrine transporter and is stored in the neurosecretory granules, resulting in a specific concentration in contrast to the cells of other tissues.
- Theoretical considerations and clinical experience indicate that the I-123-labeled agent is to be considered the radiopharmaceutical of choice as it has a more favorable dosimetry

and provides better image quality allowing an accurate anatomical localization by the use of SPECT/CT hybrid systems. Nonetheless, I-131-MIBG is widely employed for most routine applications mainly in adult patients because of its ready availability and the possibility of obtaining delayed scans.

Technique:

- Patient preparation: A special topic in MIBG scans is the blocking of the thyroid gland if the target organ is not the thyroid.
- If the scan is performed for the diagnosis of a neuroendocrine pathology involving the thyroid gland, the blocking protocol should not be used; but if the scan is performed for the diagnosis of other sites, the protocol must be applied in order to avoid the trapping of the substance, mainly by the highly receptive thyroid tissue.
- Tracer injection, dosage, and injected activity MIBG, diluted in compliance with the manufacturer's instructions, are administered by slow intravenous injection (at least 5 min) in a peripheral vein. The preparation should have a high specific activity.
- The activity administered to adults should be:
  - I-131-MIBG, 20–40–80 MBq (0.6–1.2–2.2 mCi).
  - I-123-MIBG, 200–400 MBq (5.4–10.8 mCi).
  - The activity administered to children should be calculated on the basis of a reference dose for an adult, scaled to body weight according to the schedule proposed by special preparation.
- Patient position: Supine.
- Gamma camera:
  - A single (or multiple) head gamma camera with a large field of view is necessary to acquire planar and/or tomographic (SPECT) images. Fusion images with SPET/CT hybrid systems can improve diagnosis accuracy. The use of modern SPECT/CT systems is highly recommended.
  - Low-energy high-resolution or general-purpose (LEHR or LEGP) collimators for I-123 MIBG. Medium-energy collimators may improve image quality, by reducing scatter while preserving acceptable sensitivity (i.e., without increasing acquisition time).
  - I-131-MIBG: High-energy, parallel hole.
- Acquisition:
  - The timing of imaging: Scanning with I-131-MIBG is performed 1 and 2 days after the injection and can be repeated the third day or later.
  - Scanning with I-123-MIBG is performed between 4, 20, and 24 h. Selected delayed images (never later than day 2) may be useful in case of equivocal findings in day 1.
  - The patient should be placed in the supine position.
  - Views: WBS with additional limited field images or spot images.
  - Imaging field I-131-MIBG: WBS (speed 4 cm/s) or both anterior and posterior limited field or static spot views (>150K counts) of the head, neck, chest, abdomen, pelvis, and upper and lower extremities.
  - Imaging filed I-123-MIBG: WBS (speed 5 cm/s) or both anterior and posterior limited field or static spot views (about 500K counts or 10 min acquisition) of the head, neck, chest, abdomen, pelvis, and upper and lower extremities. In neuroblastoma patients, for head imaging, both anteroposterior and lateral views are recommended. Spot views are often superior to whole-body scans in contrast and resolution, especially in low-count regions, and therefore, they are preferable in the case of young children (who may bear much easier this exam, longer in total time, but with interruptions in between).
  - A pixel size of about 2 mm requires a 256 × 256 matrix or a 128 × 128 matrix with zoom. For quantification, different levels of approximation can be adopted for attenuation correction. The basic method of geometric mean between conjugate views can be improved using a standard source phantom-based method. For the whole body, 256 × 1024 matrix should be used.
  - SPECT protocol consists of 120 projections, in 3° steps, in continuous or

step-and-shoot mode, with 25–35 s per step. The data are acquired on a 128 × 128 matrix. In case of noncooperative patients, it is possible to reduce acquisition time using 6° steps or a 64 × 64 matrix with shorter time per frame.
  - In SPECT/CT imaging, the CT image should be taken with high resolution in order to have a better characterization of the anatomical surroundings. These images are also important for dosimetry calculations (uptake and size of the tumor).
  - SPECT/CT is performed at the region of interest 4 and 24 h p.i. Suitable acquisition parameters for SPECT are 25 s per view using 64 views, 180-degree rotation, and a matrix of 128 × 128. Low-dose CT may be acquired, for example, using 17 mA, 130 keV, slice thickness of 5 mm and reconstructed FOV 500 mm, and slice width of 5 mm.
- Processing: No particular processing procedure is needed for planar images. In case of SPECT, one should take into account the different types of gamma camera and software available. Careful choice of processing parameters should be adopted in order to optimize image quality. Iterative reconstruction with a low-pass post-filter often provides better images than filtered back projection. Any reporting should clearly state the methodology adopted for image processing and quantification.

Necessary additional examinations:
- Thyroid ultrasound
- Fine needle aspiration biopsy (FNAB)
- Laboratory test results: plasma and urinary catecholamine dosage, CEA, 5-HIAA (5-hydroxyindoleacetic acid), NSE (neuron-specific enolase), chromogranin A, calcitonin, etc.
- Results of any other imaging studies (CT, MRI, US, X-ray)
- History of recent biopsy, surgery, chemotherapy, hormone therapy, and radiation therapy

Clinical applications:
- MIBG scintigraphy is used to image tumors of neuroendocrine origin, particularly those of the neuroectodermal (sympathoadrenal) system (pheochromocytomas, paragangliomas, and neuroblastomas).
- Although other neuroendocrine tumors (e.g., carcinoids, medullary thyroid carcinoma) can also be visualized.
- In addition, MIBG can be employed to study disorders of sympathetic innervation, for example, in ischemic and nonischemic cardiomyopathy, as well as in the differentiation between idiopathic Parkinson's syndrome and multisystem atrophy.

Comments:
- I-123 MIBG avoids hazardous irradiation due to beta emitters.
- I-131 MIBG scan may have prognostic value in perspective therapy with I-131 MIBG.

Reports:
- The nuclear medicine physician should record all information regarding the patient, the type of examination, the date, the radiopharmaceutical, the dose, concise patient history, all correlated data from previous diagnostic studies, and the clinical questions.
- The report to the referring physician should describe whether the distribution of MIBG is physiological or not, all abnormal areas of uptake (intensity, number, and site; if necessary, retention of MIBG over time), and comparative analysis: the findings should be related to any previous information or results from other clinical or instrumental examinations.
- Interpretation: A clear diagnosis of malignant lesion should be made if possible, accompanied by a differential diagnosis when appropriate; comments on factors that may limit the accuracy of scintigraphy are sometimes important (lesion size, artifacts, interfering drugs, etc.).
- Same requirements as in other scintigraphies.

Normal image and uptake:
- *Physiological* distribution *of MIBG*
  - The uptake of radiolabeled MIBG in different organs depends on catecholamine

excretion and/or adrenergic innervation. Since MIBG is excreted in the urine, the bladder and urinary tract show intense activity.
  - Mainly the liver normally takes up MIBG; smaller uptake is described in the spleen, lungs, salivary glands, skeletal muscles, and myocardium.
  - Normal adrenal glands are usually not seen, but faint uptake may be visible 48–72 h after injection in up to 15% of cases when using MIBG I-131.
  - Free iodine in the bloodstream may cause some uptake in the digestive system and in the thyroid (if not properly blocked). No skeletal uptake should be seen. Extremities show only slight muscular activity.
- *Pathological* MIBG soft tissue uptake is observed in primary tumor and in metastatic sites including the lymph nodes, liver, bone, and bone marrow. The increased uptake in the skeleton (focal or diffuse) is indicative of bone marrow involvement and/or skeletal metastases (Fig. 7.60).
- *Sources of error*:
  - Clinical and biochemical findings that are unknown or have not been considered.
  - Insufficient knowledge of physiological MIBG biodistribution and kinetics.
  - Small lesions, below the resolution power of scintigraphy.
  - Incorrect patient preparation (e.g., pelvic) views cannot be correctly interpreted if the patient has not voided before the acquisition.
  - Lesions close to the areas of high physiologic or pathologic uptake; tumor lesions that do not uptake MIBG (e.g., changes in differentiation, necrosis, interfering drugs, etc.).
  - Patient motion (mainly in children).
  - Increased diffuse physiologic uptake (hyperplastic adrenal gland after contralateral adrenalectomy); increased focal physiologic uptakes (mainly in the urinary tract or bowel); thyroid activity (if no adequate thyroid blockade is performed).
  - Urine contamination or any other external contamination (salivary secretion).

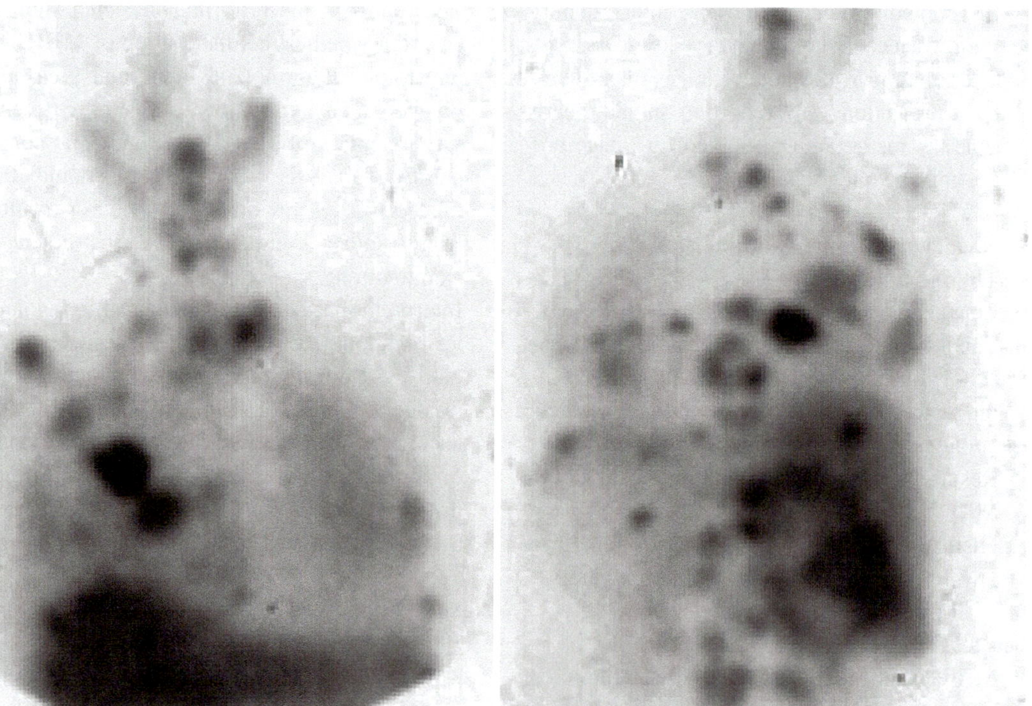

Fig. 7.60 I-123 MIBG—AP and PA incidence scans of metastatic medullary thyroid carcinoma

7.3.5.13 Thyroid Single-Photon Emission Computed Tomography and SPECT/CT

Radiopharmaceutical:

- All anterior described radiopharmaceuticals might be used also in SPECT and SPECT/CT techniques; most suitable are I-123 or I-131, Tc-99m MIBI, I-123-MIBG, and Tl-201 chloride.

Principle:

- This technique offers better localization of the lesions.

Technique:

- Patient preparation: According to the radiotracer used
- Patient position: Supine
- Acquisition:
  - SPECT is usually recorded with 360° acquisition for 30 s/image, for a total of 64 images "step and shoot."
  - 128 × 128 matrix.
  - CT spiral low dose, tube voltage 130 keV, pitch 1.5, rotation time 1 s. The recommendation is to use low-dose diagnostic parameters for CT.
  - Processing: There are special PC programs for image reconstruction and processing; filtered back projection; attenuation correction.
  - The most frequent application of the method is the diagnosis and follow-up of thyroid cancer. Depending on the therapeutic activity applied, whole-body scintigraphy is performed 24–48 h to 8 days after application of I-131. A dual-headed camera with a high-energy collimator is recommended, and acquisition should be performed with a scan speed of at most 20 cm/min. SPECT/CT is added if anatomical correlation of an iodine-positive finding is necessary. It is also mandatory to exclude/resolve a projection of a thyroid remnant onto a metastasis. SPECT/CT may be performed without the use of iodinated contrast agent and in low-dose technique, as the CT is used for anatomical correlation only. Suitable acquisition parameters for SPECT are 25 s per view using 64 views, 2 × 180° rotation, and a matrix of 128 × 128. Low-dose CT may be acquired using 17 mAs, 130 keV, slice thickness of 5 mm, FOV 500 mm, and slice width of 5 mm (parameters depending on the applied device).

Clinical applications:

- Diagnosis mainly of malignant tumors and distant metastasis.

Necessary additional examinations:

- Thyroid ultrasound
- Serologic tests
- Fine needle aspiration biopsy (FNAB)

Comments:

- It is not a frequently used method in the algorithm of thyroid nodule diagnosis but may be used in selected situations, like multinodular goiter (Fig. 7.61).
- The evaluation of the thyroid may occur during the investigation of other organs.
- In the latest years, SPECT/CT has a special attention in the evaluation protocol of thyroid cancer during follow-up, increasing significantly its importance.

Reports:

- The report will include a description of the normal distribution and pathologic uptakes.

In the protocol of thyroid carcinoma, the use of I-131 SPECT/CT has been reported to change clinical management in significant numbers of patients, both when used routinely or on selected patients with inconclusive planar images. Avram (2014) proposed the following changes in the thyroid carcinoma strategy according to SPECT/CT findings: deciding whether to give or withhold radioiodine treatment, indicating and guiding the extent of surgery, selecting patients for external beam radiation therapy, and indicating the need for alternative imaging strategies such as 18F-FDG PET. The information obtained with planar imaging and SPECT/CT impacts management in a significant number of patients. An example about the specific impact of SPECT/CT

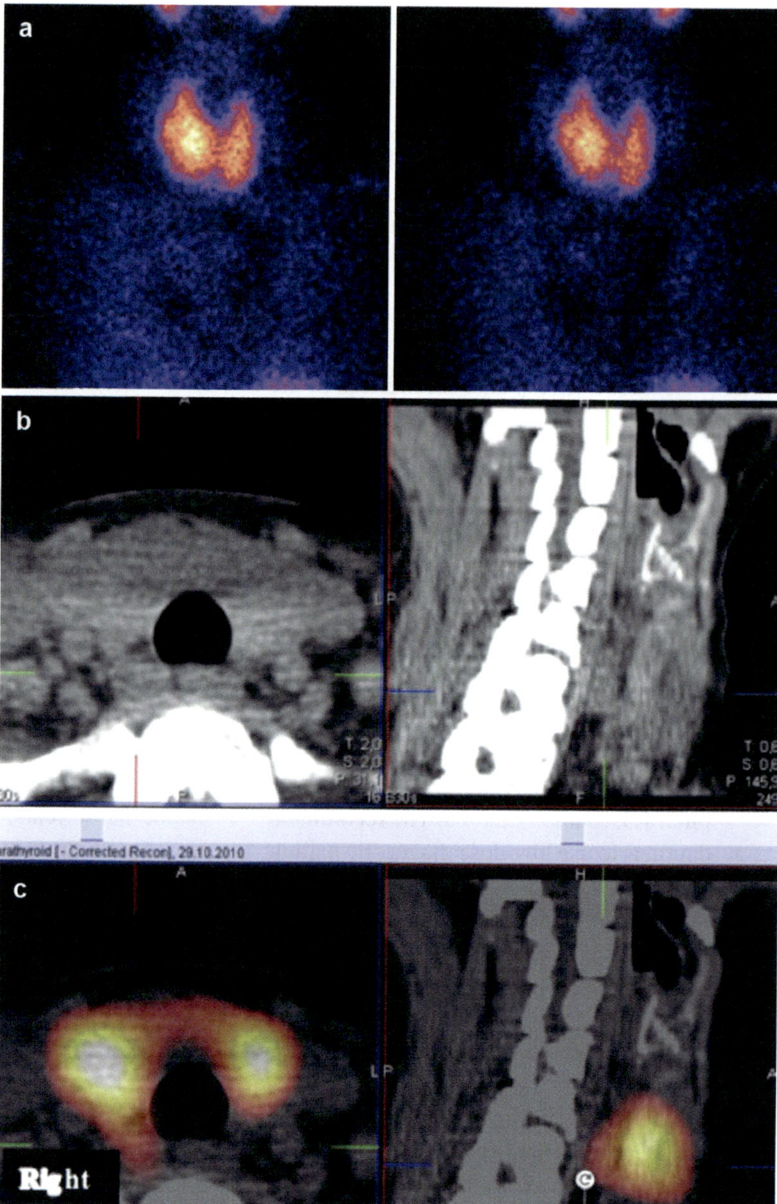

Fig. 7.61 Thyroid scan Tc-99m Pt of a multinodular goiter on planar gamma camera (**a**), CT (**b**), and hybrid imaging, SPECT/CT (**c**)

in the management of patients with DTC submitted for radioiodine therapy is presented in Fig. 7.62. Image A shows a planar whole-body scan (WBS) after therapeutical dose of I-131 for ablation in differentiated thyroid cancer and reveals pathologic uptake in the right lateral-cervical area (metastatic lymph node?) and minimal residual tissue in the left thyroid bed. The hybrid image SPECT/CT (B) shows clearly that the right lateral-cervical uptake is due to retention in the right salivary gland, without any further oncological impact. Depending on patients' clinical context, the timing of the radioiodine scan (preablation or posttherapy), and the therapeutic protocols at each institution, change in management has been reported in 11–58% of patients, by decreasing the rate of equivocal findings.

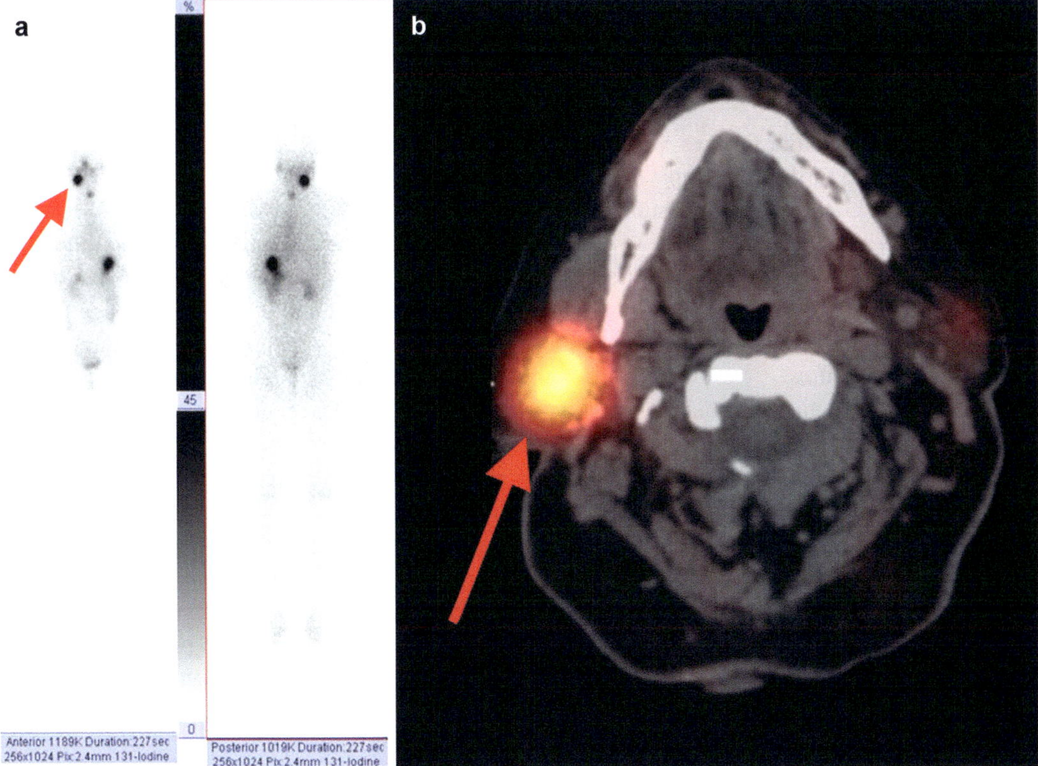

Fig. 7.62 Whole-body scan (WBS) after therapeutical dose of I-131 for ablation in differentiated thyroid cancer. The planar WBS image (**a**) reveals pathologic uptake in the right lateral-cervical area (metastatic lymph node?) and minimal residual tissue in the thyroid bed. The hybrid image SPECT/CT (**b**) shows clearly that the uptake is due to retention in the right salivary gland, without any further oncological impact

The new technology of SPECT/CT has changed the field and led to reassessment of current management protocols and guidelines in thyroid cancer. In this light, the American Thyroid Association (ATA) 2015 guideline underlines the role of SPECT/CT in the treatment decision and follow-up of differentiated thyroid carcinoma: "whole-body SPECT/CT performed after the administration of a diagnostic or a therapeutic activity (30 mCi or more) of I-131 is associated with an increased number of patients with a diagnosis of metastatic lymph node and a decreased frequency of equivocal findings. Furthermore, the CT portion of the SPECT/CT provides additional information on non-iodine-avid lesions; SPECT-CT changed tumor risk classifications in 25% of the patients according to the International Union Against Cancer classification and in 6% of the patients according to the ATA risk of recurrence classification. Finally, SPECT-CT avoids the need for further cross-sectional imaging studies such as contrast CT or MRI. Neoplastic lesions with low uptake of RAI or without any uptake may be a cause of false negative SPECT-CT."

Searching the literature, 31 systematic review studies are available, and these underline that SPECT/CT imaging has improved the ability to localize disease and distinguish benign and otherwise normal, anatomical variants from thyroid cancer in the neck and elsewhere.

The addition of anatomical maps that can be directly combined with the distribution of radioiodine in multi-planar orthogonal projections has changed the approach to diagnosis, staging, therapy, and prognostic assessment of well-differentiated thyroid cancer.

The impact of SPECT/CT on management of DTC is summarized below, adapted from Belhocine et al. (2008):

- Physiologic or benign uptakes vs pathologic uptakes with no further work-up:
  - Head: hair contamination, mastoiditis, dental works
  - Neck: thyroid bed, thyroglossal tract, salivary glands
  - Mediastinum: esophagus, thymus, gastroesophageal reflux
  - Lung: diaphragmatic hernia
  - Abdominal: colon
  - Pelvis: rectum, uterus
- Accurate localization of I-131 avid metastases:
  - Brain
  - Lung
  - Bone
  - Cervical and supraclavicular lymph nodes

7.3.5.14 Orbital Single-Photon Emission Computed Tomography with Tc-99m DTPA for the Evaluation of Graves' Ophthalmopathy

Radiopharmaceutical

- Tc-99m DTPA—Tc-99m diethylenetriamine pentaacetic acid

Principle:

- Tc-99m DTPA is a chelate, primarily excreted by glomerular filtration. It is uniformly distributed throughout the extracellular space and does not normally cross the blood-tissue barriers. The uptake has been reported as related to the inflammatory process, disappearing with resolution of the infection/inflammation.
- The theoretical basis of the method is that the high capillarisation and edema in the orbit may be reflected on Tc-99m DTPA images in GO.

Technique:

- Patient preparation: No special preparations.
- Patient position: Supine.
- 7 MBq/kg patient (370–500 MBq) Tc-99m DTPA intravenously.
- Acquisition starts at 20 min after the injection.
- Acquisition:
  - 128 projections by a four-headed SPECT (a double-headed camera may also be used).
  - On the sum of six transversal slices containing the entire bulbar region of the skull, a triangle-like region of interest (ROI) is drawn (orbital ROI-OR).
  - This ROI is "slipped" to the right temporal region of the brain as reference site (brain ROI-B). The count ratios of OR/B must be calculated.
  - SPECT is usually recorded with 360° acquisition for 30 s/image, for a total of 64 images "step and shoot."
  - 128 × 128 matrix.
- Processing: There are special PC programs for image reconstruction and processing; filtered back projection; attenuation correction.

Clinical applications:

- Differential diagnosis of Graves' ophthalmopathy sensitive or resistant to the immune suppressive therapy.

Necessary additional examinations:

- Orbital ultrasound
- Ophthalmic measurements of the ocular globes
- Serologic tests
- MRI T2 time of relaxation

Comments:

- Even if this method is minimally aggressive, safe, easy, and cheap, it is not a frequently used method in the algorithm of GO diagnosis.
- Comparing with MRI, this nuclear medicine test has a better physiologic response to the therapy definition requested by the endocrinologist.
- The orbital uptake of the radionuclide (activity uptake, AU) is calculated (references values 4.7–12.2 MBq/cm3).
- The most frequent AU higher than 12.2 MBq/cm^3 is the value considered that

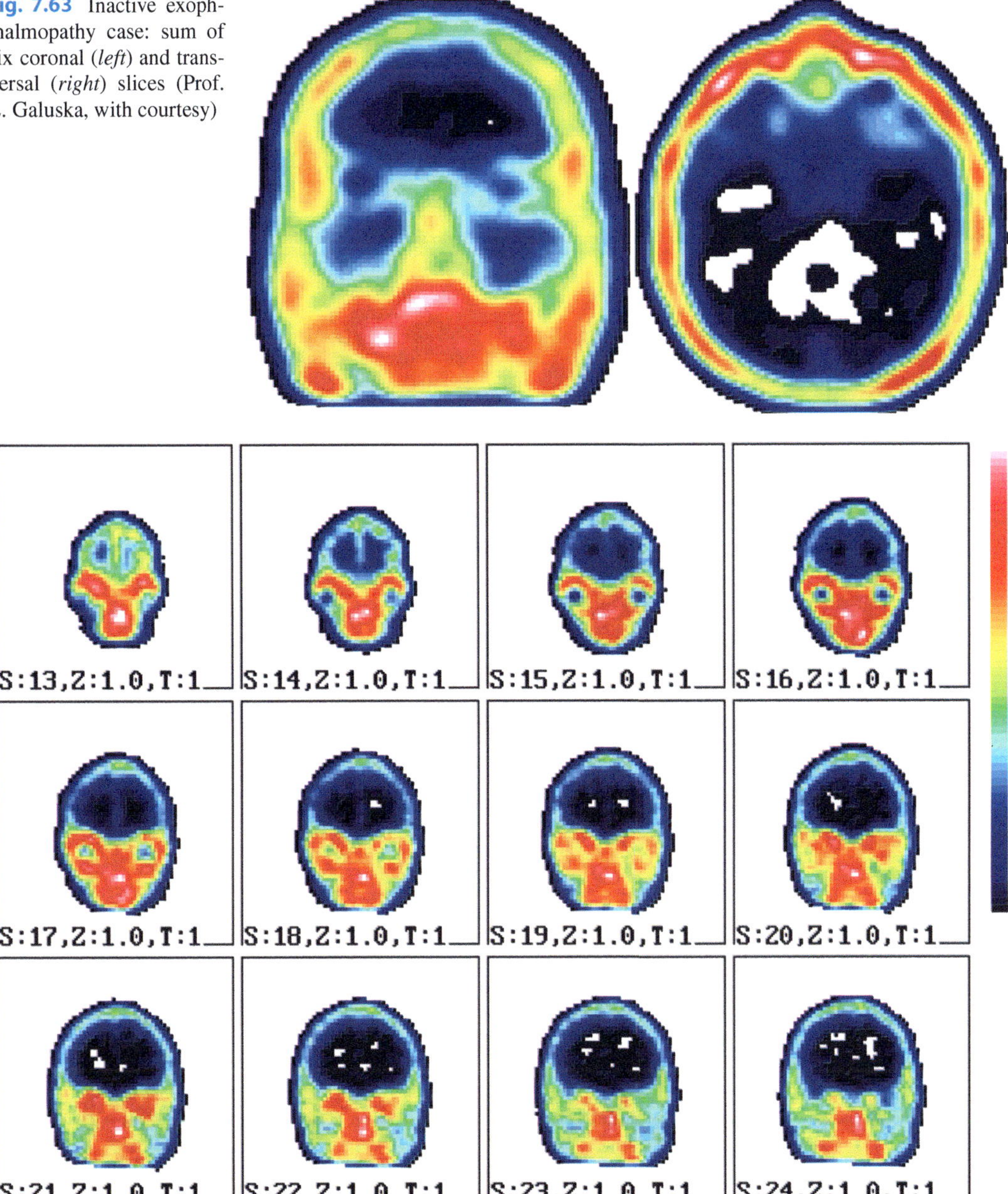

Fig. 7.63 Inactive exophthalmopathy case: sum of six coronal (*left*) and transversal (*right*) slices (Prof. L. Galuska, with courtesy)

Fig. 7.64 Active exophthalmopathy: original coronal (4 mm) slices (from 13 to 24) (Prof. L. Galuska, with courtesy)

GO is active and sensitive to immunosuppressive therapy.

The technique described above and the following images (Figs. 7.63, 7.64, 7.65, 7.66, and 7.67) were obtained with the courtesy of Prof. Galuska Laszlo from the Department of Nuclear Medicine of the University of Debrecen, Hungary.

Key Points

- The technique may improve significantly the treatment choice and the outcome of the patient with GO.
- The results obtained in the classic dual-headed camera are very similar to those obtained in the quadruple-headed camera, far less common than the first one.

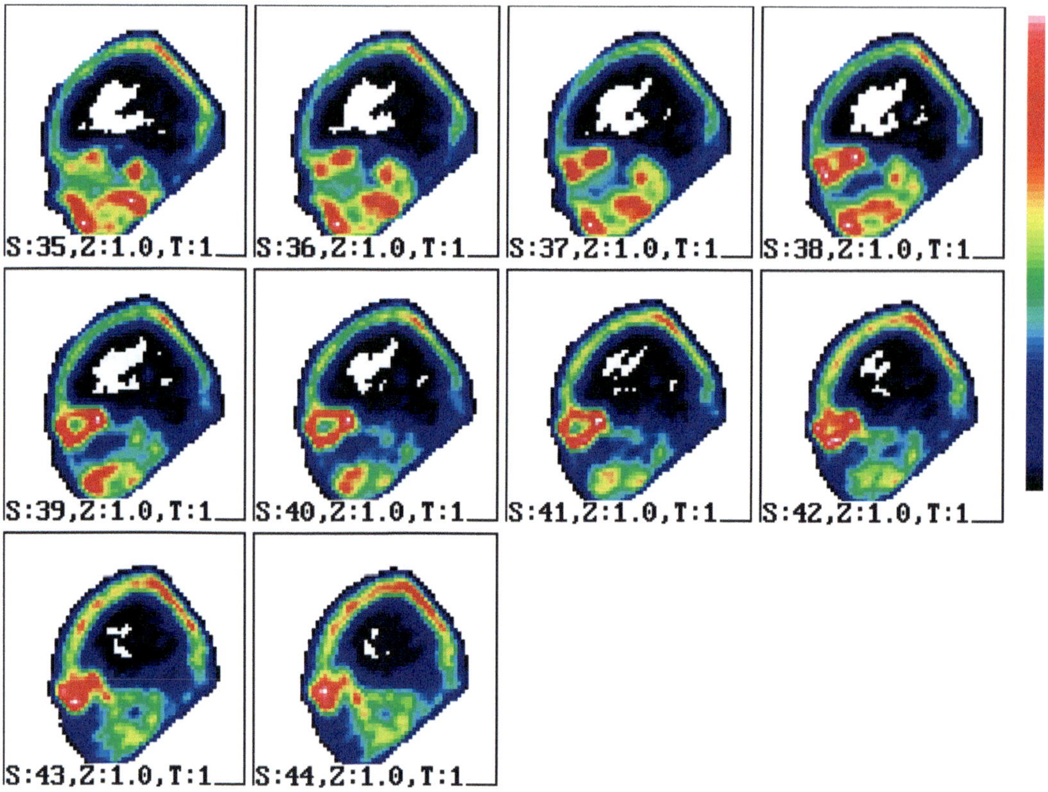

Fig. 7.65 Active exophthalmopathy: original left eye sagittal (4 mm) slices (from 35 to 44), (Prof. L. Galuska, with courtesy)

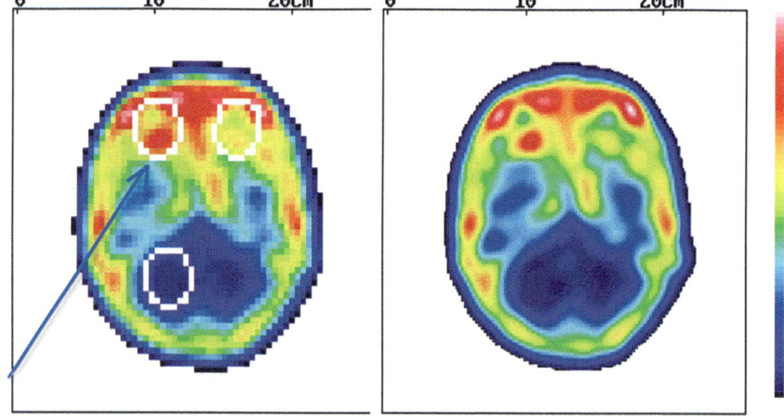

Fig. 7.66 Right-sided active exophthalmopathy case (*arrow*). ROI selection on the sum of six transversal slices to calculate the uptake value (*UV*) (Prof. L. Galuska, with courtesy)

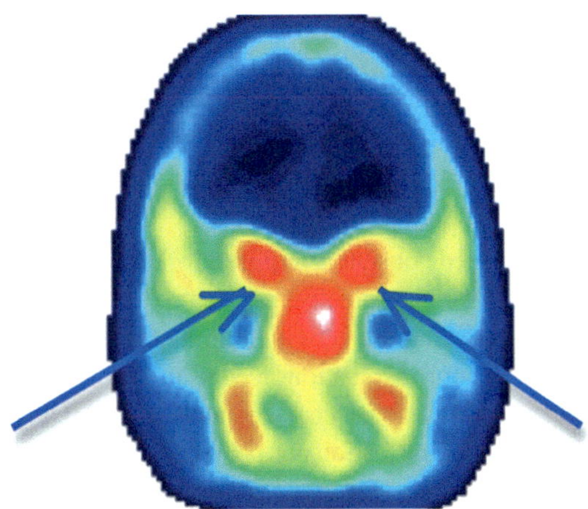

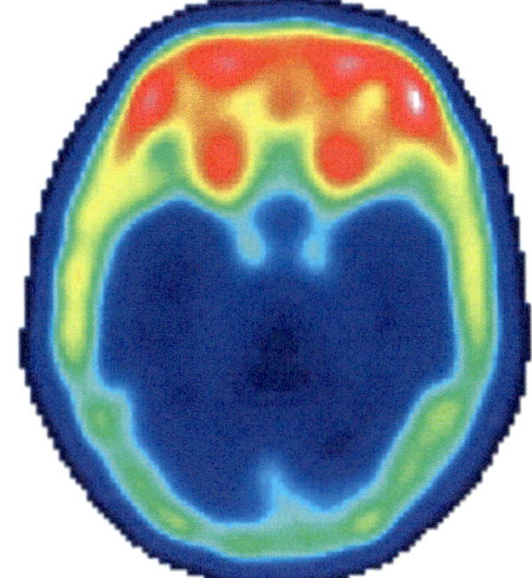

Fig. 7.67 Active exophthalmopathy case: sum of six coronal (*up*) and transversal (*below*) slices (Prof. L. Galuska, with courtesy)

7.4 Radioiodine Therapy in Benign Thyroid Diseases

Radioiodine (*I-131*) has been used to treat benign conditions of the thyroid gland since the 1940s. This therapy may be used for patients with hyperthyroidism, which is a consequence of excessive thyroid hormone action (ATA/AACE 2011 and ATA 2016; Ross et al. 2016):

- Autoimmune hyperthyroidism (Graves' disease)
- Solitary hyperfunctioning thyroid nodule
- Toxic multinodular goiter

Also patients with a large nontoxic goiter who are euthyroid may benefit from a reduction in thyroid volume after radioiodine therapy.

In patients with hyperthyroidism, the aim of the treatment with I-131 is to achieve a nonhyperthyroid status, which can be euthyroid or hypothyroid, consequently treated by LT4 (levothyroxine) medication. In patients with nontoxic large goiter, the aim of the treatment with I-131 is to diminish the size of the goiter and, consequently, to reduce the symptoms related to gland enlargement and nodule formation.

According to different pathophysiological conditions, the treatment options of hyperthyroidism are:

- Antithyroid drugs
- Radioiodine
- Surgery

Indications of I-131 therapy:

- Graves' disease
- Toxic multinodular goiter
- Solitary hyperfunctioning nodule
- Nontoxic multinodular goiter
- Goiter recurrence
- Ablation of residual thyroid tissue in case of malignant ophthalmopathy after surgery but during an inactive state of the orbitopathy

Contraindications of I-131 therapy:

Absolute

- Pregnancy
- Breastfeeding

Relative

- Uncontrolled hyperthyroidism
- Active thyroid orbitopathy (especially at smokers)

Procedure

The national regulations may request the therapy being done only in inpatient conditions even though the doses are not high; there are also countries that allow the treatment in ambulatory conditions.

The facility requirements for the unit performing therapy for thyroid disease according to national legislation must be a nuclear unit, with appropriate authorization for using therapy doses of radioiodine. The facility in which treatment is performed has appropriate personnel, radiation safety equipment, and procedures for waste handling and disposal, handling of incidental contamination, and monitoring of personnel for accidental contamination and controlling/limiting its spread. This facility may be easily achieved either in an endocrinology department or nuclear medicine unit.

Patient Preparation

Patient evaluation before radioiodine therapy should include (Stokkel et al. 2010):

- Patient history with special emphasis on previous treatments (e.g., use of ATS, contrast media, amiodarone, other iodine-containing medication, and iodine-containing food).
- Laboratory testing, including FT4, FT3, TSH, anti-TPO, and TRab.
- Thyroid Tc-99m scintigraphy or radioiodine scan + radioiodine 24 h uptake (RAIU), according to the availability in the department. The RAIU at 24 should be >20%, and if lower, other treatment modalities should be considered. Uptake measurements are not absolutely required when fixed activities are used.
- Assessment of thyroid target volume (ultrasonography) and intrathoracic extension in those with a large goiter (magnetic resonance imaging/computed tomography). However, we have to note that assessment of the target volume by computed tomography using contrast agents impairs the radioiodine uptake for weeks to months, making therapy with I-131 impossible during that time.
- Fine needle aspiration biopsy (FNAB) of nodules larger than 1–1.5 cm with a suspicious ultrasound appearance and hypo-/iso-functioning on scan. In autonomously functioning nodules, as the risk of malignancy is very low, FNAB should only be considered in those with suspicious ultrasound features.
- In female patients of childbearing potential, a routine testing for pregnancy is performed within 72 h before the administration of I-131. When the patient history clearly indicates that pregnancy is excluded, a pregnancy test may be omitted at the discretion of the treating physician. In case of suspicious situation, a serologic analysis of beta HCG may be requested.
- In patients with Graves' ophthalmopathy, establishment of the status of thyroid eye disease activity should be done by an experienced ophthalmologist.
- Informed consent is required for every patient.
- All documents including identity data, medical information, activity administered, indication about medication needed to be restarted, radioprotection aspects, contact data, and physician identification are provided to patients.

Special Considerations

- If the antithyroid drugs (ATS) are used in the initial treatment of patients with hyperthyroidism, the procedure is to be stopped 5–7 days before radioiodine and the beta-blockers within 24 h before. Propylthiouracil is stopped at least 2 weeks before therapy.
- ATS are restarted after I-131 only if a previous treatment was applied before therapy and there were no side effects on ATS.
- In patients with Graves' ophthalmopathy, if they are already on steroid therapy, orally, prednisolone is administered. It is not a routine to start the corticotherapy.
- In patients with thyrotoxicosis induced by amiodarone or in those receiving compounds that contain iodine (e.g., radiographic contrast agents), radioiodine can be administered as definitive therapy, if the drug has been stopped sufficiently long enough. In amiodarone-induced thyrotoxicosis, the excess of iodine is eliminated during at least 3–6 months, after withdrawal of the drug. In this respect, the assay of urinary iodine excretion can be used as an indicator of normalization of iodine upload.
- The use of other drugs in preparing the therapy, such as lithium, is not a routine and is reserved to the specific conditions of some patients.

Patient Information and Instruction

Patients receive both written and verbal information about the procedure before receiving therapy. A written informed consent from the patient is obtained. Radiation protection measures are detailed in the leaflets given to the patient in order to reduce radiation doses to children, family members, and other people in the general population, according to national rules. Contraception for 4 months after I-131 therapy is also recommended. As the result is evaluated 6 months after therapy, this interval is necessary in clinical practice to avoid interference with retreatment in the event of recurrent disease (The American Thyroid Association Taskforce on Radioiodine Safety 2011.

Radiopharmaceutical and Administration

Radioiodine is orally administered. Patients should be encouraged to drink a large volume of fluids (1.5–2 L) for a 24 h period following radioiodine therapy to lower the radiation dose to the bladder.

Two procedures are in use:

- Empirically established doses
- Calculated doses, especially in young patients and with less severe symptoms

Currently, an absorbed radiation dose of 100–150 Gy is recommended, requiring about 3.7–5.5 MBq (0.1–0.15 mCi) per gram of thyroid tissue corrected for the 24-h I-131 uptake. In patients with autonomously functioning nodules, the recommended dose is of 300–400 Gy.

In patients with Graves' disease, the dose with the aim of restoring a euthyroid status is approximately 150 Gy, whereas the dose to achieve complete ablation is in the range of 200–300 Gy.

The fixed-dose approaches are usually based on an estimation of the size of the gland realized by palpation or by the measurement on ultrasonography or scintigraphy.

The range of activities currently prescribed vary in the range of 200–800 MBq (5–21 mCi), with the majority of patients receiving 200–500 MBq (5–15 mCi). The amount of activity is prescribed according to clinical features, volume of gland, and disease.

Radioiodine therapy for children younger than 5 years old is done only in exceptional cases.

For children between 5 and 15 years of age, radioiodine therapy may be considered. The side effects should be clearly discussed by all the staff involved in the treatment of a young patient with Graves' disease.

The calculated doses are decided according to the following formula by Marinelli (Eq. 7.1):

$$\text{MBq} = \frac{V \times 25 \times (100 - 300\ \text{Gy})}{\text{RAIU 24 h} \times T_{\text{ef}}} \tag{7.1}$$

MBq—the calculated activity in MBq
V—the gland volume estimated at ultrasound in mL (cm^3)
100–300 Gy—estimated required dose at thyroid level, between 100 and 300 Gy
RAIU 24 h—% of thyroid uptake at 24 h
T_{ef}—effective half-time, estimated in hyperthyroidism at 4.5 days and in euthyroidism at 6 days
25—constant

Example (Eq. 7.2):

Thyroid gland volume—30 mL
Constant—25
Estimated dose—200 Gy
RAIU 24 h—67%
T_{ef}—4.5

$$\text{MBq} = \frac{30 \times 25 \times 200}{67 \times 4.5} = \frac{150{,}000}{301.5} = 497.5 \tag{7.2}$$

37 MBq = 1 mCi
497.5 MBq = 13.44 mCi

Result: the necessary dose for therapy is of 13.5 mCi.

Side Effects of I-131 Therapy

Acute patients with a large goiter may notice transient edema of the goiter and dyspnea. This symptom may last several days following therapy, and some discomfort or dyspnea may be associated with it. Slight discomfort of the salivary glands may be present. In some patients, a thyroid storm may develop. This rare condition must be treated with intravenous infusion of ATS, corticosteroids, and beta-blockers. This situation is extremely rare and does not represent a reason to not recommend the therapy.

Hypothyroidism is the main side effect of radioiodine treatment. Its rate varies, and its incidence continues to increase over time, so that lifelong follow-up is essential. According to all published data in the literature, the rate of hypothyroidism at 1 year after radioiodine therapy is very similar to the rate from the surgery approach.

The administration of prednisone helps prevent exacerbation of ophthalmopathy, and this is now the standard approach in patients who have clinically active ophthalmopathy at the time of treatment. The determination of periorbital inflammation tissue by nuclear test with Tc-99m DTPA may identify the cases that will benefit from steroid treatment.

Follow-up After Radioiodine Treatment

Regular review of thyroid function tests in patients who have undergone radioiodine treatment for thyroid disease is essential to assess the efficacy of the treatment and for timely detection of developing hypothyroidism or posttreatment immunogenic hyperthyroidism. First, TSH and FT4 examination is performed not longer than 4–6 weeks after radioiodine therapy. Shorter intervals of about 2–3 weeks are recommended for patients who have received ATS or who have an increased risk of endocrine ophthalmopathy because of hypothyroidism.

The level of TSH serum is slowly increasing so the determination of TSH is less useful in the monitoring in the first 3–6 months, than FT4 is. If the treatment was performed for (overt) hyperthyroidism, ATS is restarted, about 3–5 days after the radioiodine administration. In those with persistent hyperthyroidism, the radioiodine treatment can be repeated after 6–12 months. In those with posttherapy immunogenic hyperthyroidism, ATS for some months appears to be adequate, and a second radioiodine treatment is not necessary in most patients. Annual laboratory tests (at least including TSH) are necessary for life even in patients with euthyroidism after I-131 therapy.

7.5 Radioiodine Therapy in Malignant Thyroid Diseases

Overview

The thyroid cancer is a possible aggressive thyroid condition, which continues to be the most frequent endocrine tumor. The incidence of thyroid cancer, mainly differentiated, is one of the most rapidly increasing human cancers, especially in the last decade (ATA 2015; Gaengler et al. 2017; Hodgson et al. 2004; Pacini et al. 1999, 2004, 2010, 2016; Perros 2014, 2016; Piciu et al. 2014; Sassolas et al. 2009). Despite this situation, it is still considered to be one of the rare cancers. According to the European surveillance of rare cancers project (rare cancers list), a rare cancer is defined as a tumor with an annual incidence lower than 6 cases per 100,000 persons.

Thyroid cancer can be identified as a thyroid nodule detected by palpation and, more frequently nowadays, by neck ultrasound. Thyroid ultrasound is a widespread technique that is used as a first-line diagnostic procedure for detecting and characterizing nodular thyroid disease. There are some special patterns of ultrasound image, which may suggest the malign transformation. These features relate to a previous neck irradiation or a family history of thyroid cancer, and the presence of cervical lymph nodes leads to the cytology evaluation of the nodule despite its size. Otherwise, the limit of 1 cm in maximum diameter of the highly suspicious thyroid nodule is the one recommending as routine the fine needle aspiration biopsy (FNAB) (Braga et al. 2001; Goldstein et al. 2002; Pacini et al. 2010; ATA 2015; Haugen 2017). The FNAB sensitivity may be of 83%, and its specificity could be 72–100%.

According to the latest studies, the use of various immunohistochemical markers in cytological samples (such as BRAF, RAS, RET/PTC, etc.) might increase the accuracy of the positive diagnosis (Bongiovanni et al. 2010; ATA 2015).

The serum hormonal tests and scan images will be indicated according to the protocols of thyroid nodule diagnosis (AACE/AME/ETA 2010; AACE 2002; Hegedus 2001; Guarino et al. 2005; Frates et al. 2005; Marqusee et al. 2000; Dunn 1994; Pacini et al. 2004; ATA guidelines 2015; BTA 2014); all investigations are made with the aim of limiting the unjustified surgery and improving the positive diagnosis of malignancy prior surgery.

The papillary type is the most frequent form (Hay et al. 1993, 2002; AACE/AME/ETA 2010; Leger et al. 2005; Machens et al. 2005; Shah et al. 1992; ATA 2015) (nearly 80%), and its microscopic presentation (thyroid microcarcinoma) is by far the most challenging problem regarding the increasing frequency.

There is a need for a uniform diagnosis and treatment strategies for thyroid nodules and differentiated thyroid cancer (DTC), since the disease requires a multidisciplinary approach. Thyroid cancer comprises 0.5–1.5% of all childhood tumors and represents the most common head and neck malignant tumor in young people (Robbins 1992; Zimmermann et al. 1988; Piciu et al. 2012; Francis et al. 2015).

An accurate treatment strategy can cure this disease, can minimize recurrence risks, and can give an excellent prognosis to these patients (Mazzaferri et al. 1994).

7.5.1 Classification of Thyroid Tumors

WHO classification of carcinoma of the thyroid (DeLellis 2004)

Papillary carcinoma

Variants (in alphabetical order):

- Classical (usual)
- Clear cell variant
- Columnar cell variant
- Cribriform-morular variant
- Diffuse sclerosing variant
- Follicular variant
- Macrofollicular variant
- Microcarcinoma (occult, latent, small, papillary microtumor)
- Oncocytic or oxyphilic variant (follicular variant, non-follicular variant)
- Solid variant
- Tall cell variant
- Warthin-like variant
- Hobnail variant of papillary thyroid cancer
- Cribriform-morular variant of papillary thyroid cancer

Follicular carcinoma

Variants:

- Clear cell variant
- Oncocytic (Hürthle cell) variant
- Poorly differentiated thyroid carcinomas including insular carcinoma

Medullary carcinoma

Undifferentiated (anaplastic) carcinoma

Carcinoma, type cannot be determined

Others:

- Squamous cell carcinoma
- Mucoepidermoid carcinoma
- Sclerosing mucoepidermoid carcinoma with eosinophilia
- Mucinous carcinoma
- Mixed medullary and follicular cell carcinoma
- Spindle cell tumor with thymus-like differentiation (SETTLE)
- Carcinoma showing thymus-like differentiation (CASTLE)

Other thyroid tumors:

- Teratoma
- Primary lymphoma and plasmacytoma
- Ectopic thymoma
- Angiosarcoma
- Smooth muscle tumors
- Peripheral nerve sheath tumors
- Paraganglioma
- Solitary fibrous tumor
- Follicular dendritic cell tumor
- Langerhans' cell histiocytosis
- Secondary tumors of the thyroid

Well-differentiated malignant neoplasms (85% of the thyroid cancers):

- Papillary thyroid carcinoma (PTC) (Figs. 7.68, 7.69, 7.70, and 7.71)
- Follicular thyroid carcinoma (FTC) (Figs. 7.72 and 7.73)

Poorly differentiated malignant neoplasms:

- Medullary thyroid carcinoma (MTC) (Figs. 7.74 and 7.75)
- Anaplastic thyroid carcinoma (ATC) (Figs. 7.76 and 7.77)

These images were obtained with the courtesy of the colleagues from the pathology department of the Institute of Oncology "Prof. Dr. I. Chiricuță" Cluj-Napoca.

From a clinical perspective, molecular studies are being used to guide management of thyroid nodules with indeterminate FNAB and to better define prognosis. Also, the genetic profile aids to more rationale selection of novel therapeutic agents that are able to target the aggressive and advanced disease. A summary of most common genotypes found in DTC is presented in Table 7.3.

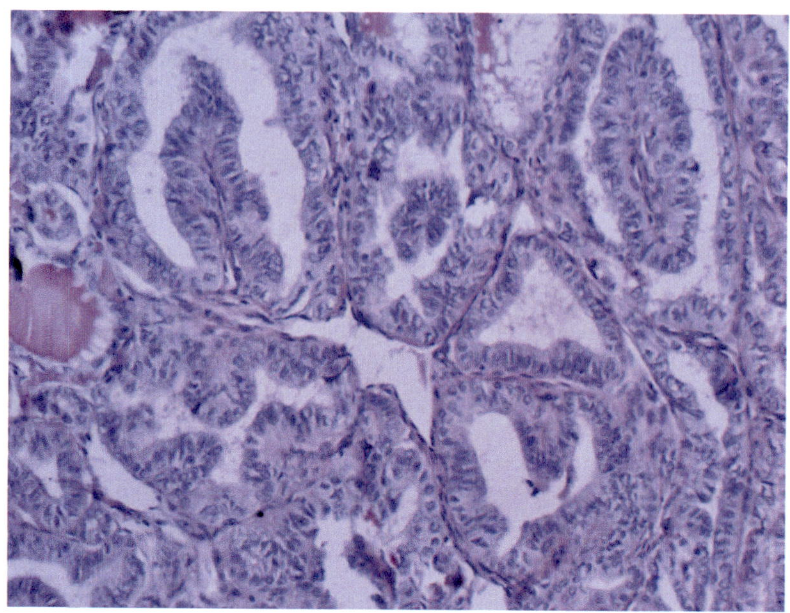

Fig. 7.68 Papillary thyroid carcinoma tall cell variant HE ×100

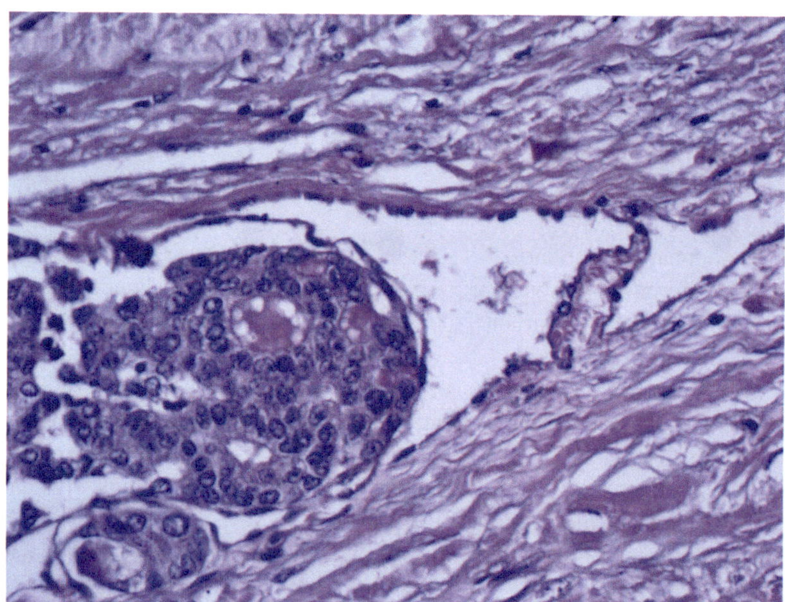

Fig. 7.69 Papillary thyroid carcinoma with vascular invasion HE ×200

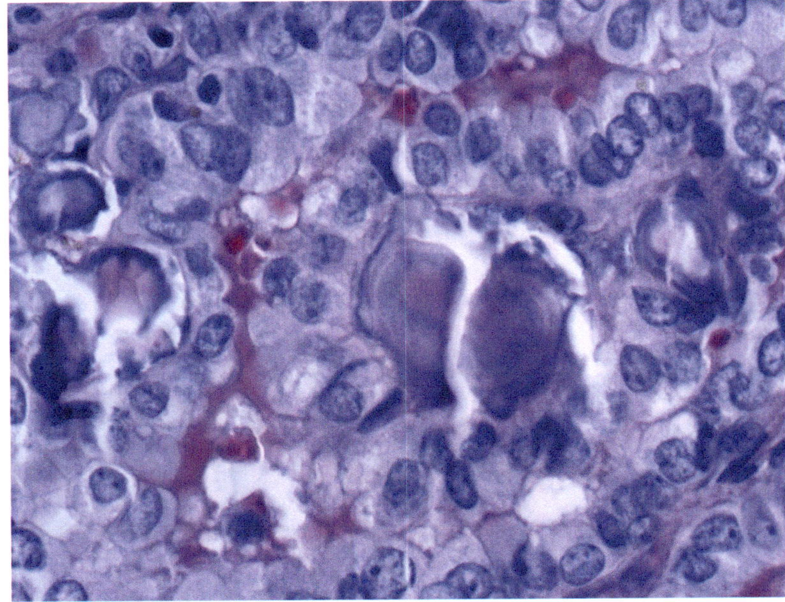

Fig. 7.70 Papillary thyroid carcinoma calcospherite HE ×400

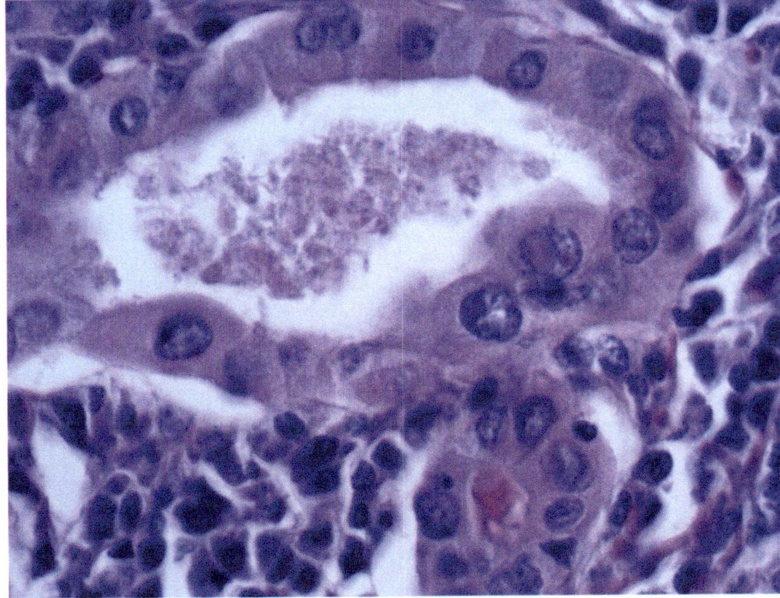

Fig. 7.71 Papillary thyroid carcinoma Warthin like HE ×400

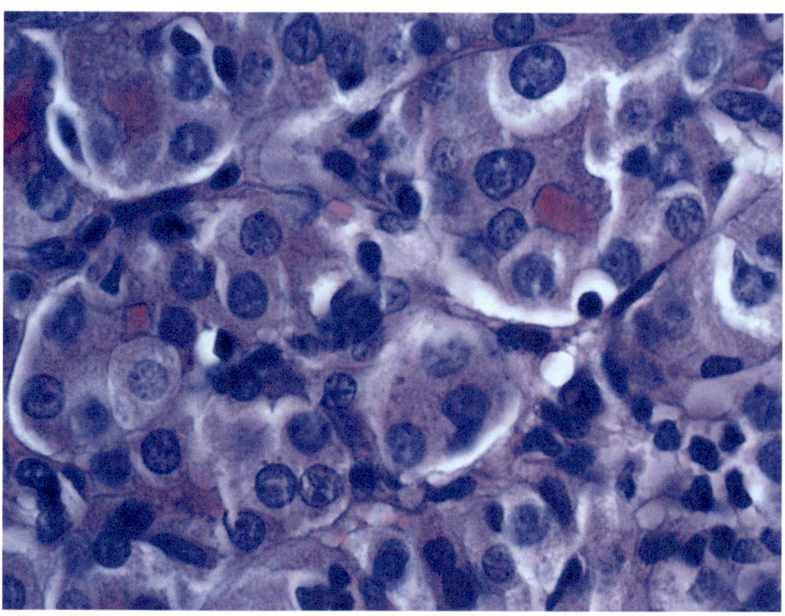

Fig. 7.72 Follicular thyroid carcinoma HE ×400

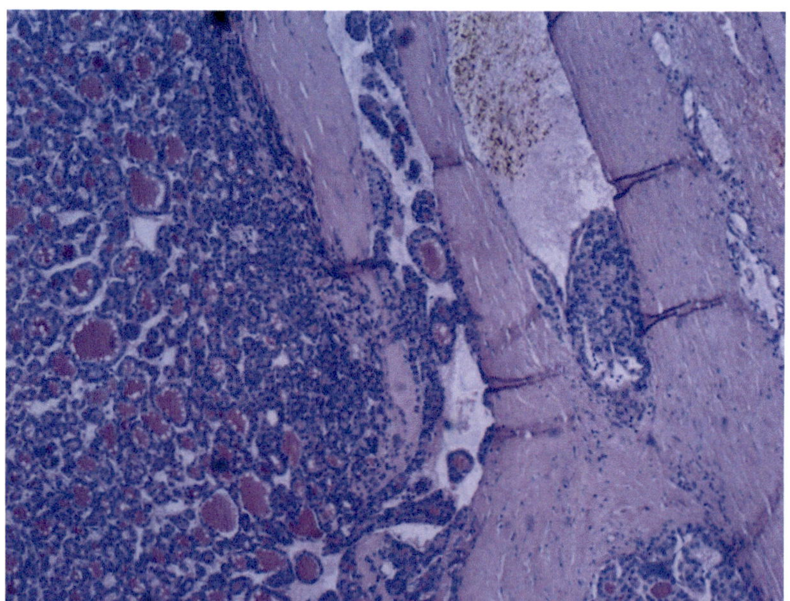

Fig. 7.73 Follicular thyroid carcinoma with invasion HE ×100

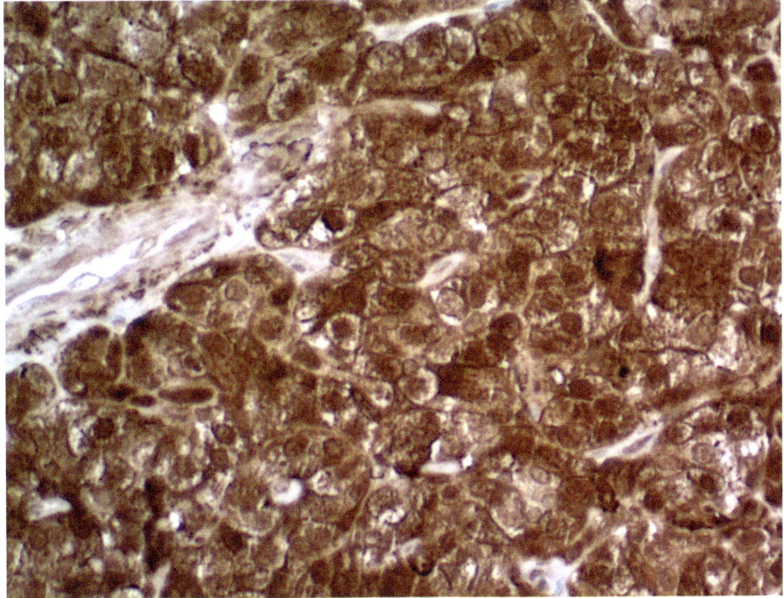

Fig. 7.74 Medullary thyroid carcinoma calcitonin ×200

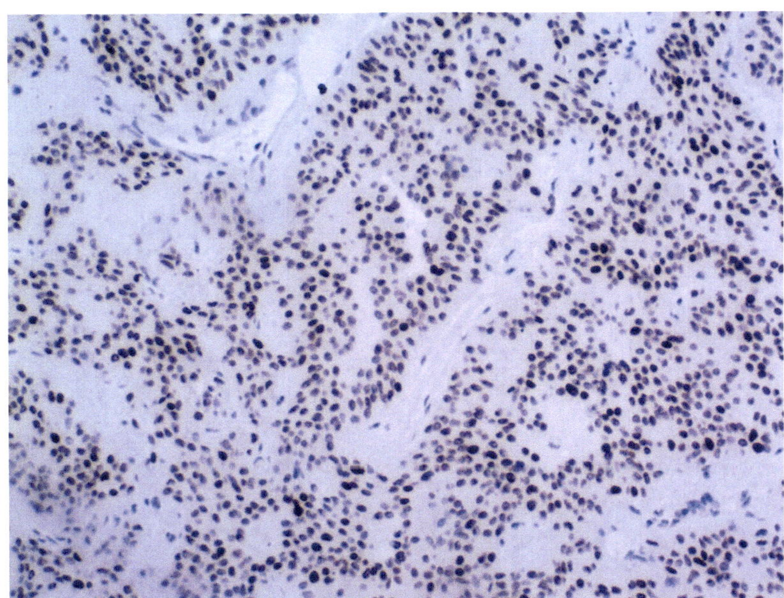

Fig. 7.75 Medullary thyroid carcinoma TTF1 ×100

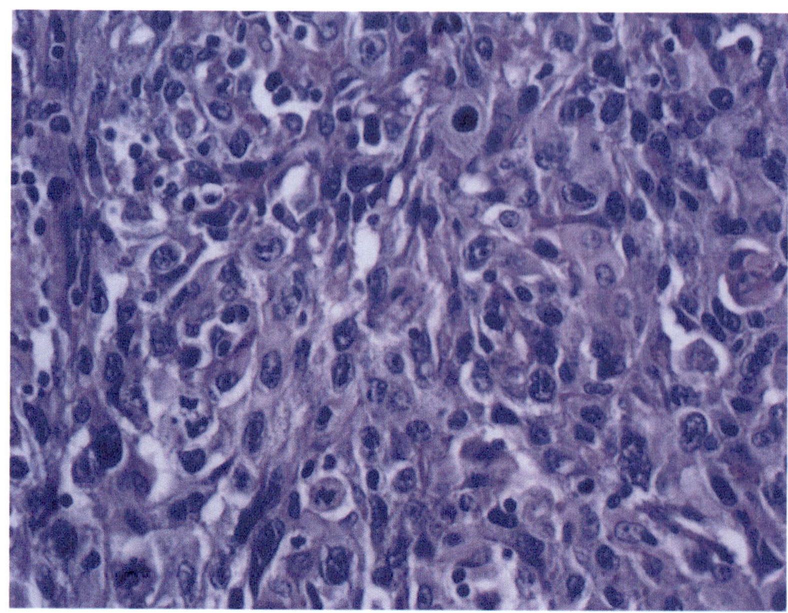

Fig. 7.76 Anaplazic thyroid carcinoma HE ×200

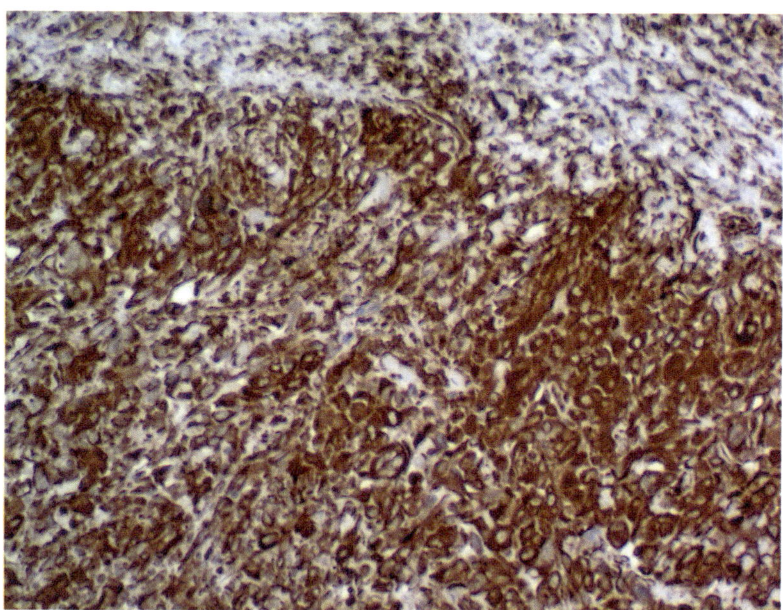

Fig. 7.77 Anaplazic thyroid carcinoma vimentine

Table 7.3 Genotype in differentiated thyroid carcinoma (DTC) (Adapted from Schulmberger et al. 2016)

Genotype	DTC histological variant
RET/PTC1, RET/PTC 3	PTC, PTC solid variant
TRK	PTC, radiation induced
ALK	ATC, poorly DTC
BRAF V600E	PTC, tall cell PTC
RAS	FTC, ATC, poorly DTC, follicular variant of PTC, follicular adenoma
PAX8-PPARγ	FTC, follicular variant of PTC, follicular adenoma
PI3K/AKT	FTC, ATC, poorly DTC
PTEN	ATC, poorly DTC
TERT	ATC, PTC, poorly DTC

7.5.2 The TNM Staging System

The majority of thyroid cancer forms is not aggressive and has an excellent prognosis. In order to select the best therapeutic options, many scientific committees proposed during the years the prognostic factors for thyroid cancer.

Prognostic factors:

- Age
- Sex
- Tumor size
- Extrathyroidal extension
- Distant metastases
- Lymph node involvement
- Histological grade
- Histological type
- Multicentricity
- Incomplete resection

According to these factors, some prognostic scores were proposed as follows:

- *AGES*: Patient age, histologic grade of tumor, and extent and size of primary tumor
- *AMES*: Patient age, presence of distant metastases, and extent and size of primary tumor
- *EORTC*: European Organization for Research and Treatment of Cancer; age, sex, extrathyroidal extension, distant metastases, and histological type
- *MACIS*: Metastasis, patient age, completeness of resection, local invasion, and tumor size
- *MSKCC*: Memorial Sloan-Kettering Cancer Center; age, tumor size, extrathyroidal extension, distant metastases, lymph node involvement, histologic grade, and histological type
- *NTCTCS*: National Thyroid Cancer Treatment Cooperative Study; age, tumor size, extrathyroidal extension, distant metastases, lymph node involvement, histological type, and multicentricity
- *OSU*: Ohio State University; tumor size, extrathyroidal extension, distant metastases, lymph node involvement, and multicentricity
- *TNM*: Tumor-node-metastasis (American Joint Committee on Cancer staging system)

The most common system used to describe the stages of thyroid cancer is the American Joint Committee on Cancer (AJCC) TNM system (American Joint Committee on Cancer (AJCC) TNM Staging for Thyroid Cancer (7th ed. 2010), Tuttle et al. (2017))

T indicates the size of the main (primary) *tumor* and whether it has grown into nearby areas.

N describes the extent of spread to nearby (regional) lymph *nodes*.

M indicates whether the cancer has spread (*metastasized*) to other organs of the body. (The most common sites of spread of thyroid cancer are the lungs, the liver, and the bones.)

T categories for thyroid cancer (other than anaplastic thyroid cancer)

Primary tumor (T)

Note: All categories may be subdivided.

- (s) Solitary tumor
- (m) Multifocal tumor (the largest determines the classification):

TX: Primary tumor cannot be assessed.

T0: No evidence of primary tumor.

T1: The tumor is 2 cm or smaller and has not grown out of the thyroid.

T1a: The tumor is 1 cm or smaller and has not grown outside the thyroid.

T1b: The tumor is larger than 1 cm but not larger than 2 cm across and has not grown outside of the thyroid.

T2: The tumor is between 2 and 4 cm across and has not grown out of the thyroid.

T3: The 8th edition of AJCC/TNM cancer staging has divided in T3a and T3b. The tumor is larger than 4 cm, or it has begun to grow into nearby tissues outside the thyroid. Tumor more than 4 cm in greatest dimension limited to the thyroid (T3a) or any tumor with minimal extrathyroidal extension (T3b), limited to strap muscles (e.g., extension to the sternothyroid muscle).

T4a: The tumor is of any size and has grown extensively beyond the thyroid gland into the nearby tissues of the neck, such as the larynx, trachea, esophagus, or the nerve to the larynx. This is also called moderately advanced disease.

T4b: A tumor of any size that has grown either back toward the spine or into nearby large blood vessels. This is also called very advanced disease.

T categories for anaplastic thyroid cancer

All anaplastic thyroid cancers are considered T4 tumors at the time of diagnosis.

T4a: Tumor is still within the thyroid.

T4b: Tumor has grown outside of the thyroid.

Unlike previous edition where all anaplastic thyroid cancers were classified as T4 disease, the 8th edition AJCC/TNM has modified also this classification. Anaplastic cancers will use same T definition as differentiated thyroid cancer (T1a,b;T2;T3a,b;T4a,b).

N categories for thyroid cancer:

NX: Regional (nearby) lymph nodes cannot be assessed.

N0: No spread to nearby lymph nodes.

N0a: Cytological and histologically proven as benign lymph nodes.

N0b: Radiological or clinical negative.

N1: The cancer has spread to nearby lymph nodes.

N1a: Spread to lymph nodes pretracheal, paratracheal, and prelaryngeal.

N1b: Spread to other cervical lymph nodes or to lymph nodes behind the throat (retropharyngeal) or in the upper mediastinum.

M categories for thyroid cancer:

M0: No distant metastasis.

M1: Spread to other parts of the body, such as the distant lymph nodes, brain, internal organs, bones, etc.

7.5.3 Thyroid Cancer Staging

Papillary or follicular (differentiated) thyroid cancer in patients younger than 45 years old

The 8th edition of AJCC/TNM cancer staging has modified the age at 55 years old.

All people younger than 55 years old having these types of cancers are considered to have a *stage I* cancer if they have no distant spread and a *stage II* cancer if they have distant spread.

Stage I (*any T, any N, M0*):

The tumor can be of any size (any T) and may or may not have spread to nearby lymph nodes (any N). It has not spread to distant sites (M0).

Stage II (*any T, any N, M1*):

The tumor can be of any size (any T) and may or may not have spread to nearby lymph nodes (any N). It has spread to distant sites (M1).

Papillary or follicular (differentiated) thyroid cancer in patients of 55 years old and older (the 8th edition of AJCC/TNM cancer staging); in the previous edition, the cut-off age was 45 years old and the staging was different

Stage I (*T1–2, N0, M0*):

The tumor is of 2–4 cm (T1-2) and has not grown outside the thyroid. It has not spread to nearby lymph nodes (N0) or distant sites (M0).

Stage II: One of the following applies:

T1-2, N1, M0: The tumor is 2–4 cm across and has not grown outside the thyroid (T1–2) and it has spread to nearby lymph nodes (N1), but it has no distant metastases (M0).

T3*a/3b any N, M0*: The tumor is larger than 4 cm limited to thyroid (T3a) or has grown slightly outside the thyroid, invading only strap muscles (T3b), might involve or not the nearby lymph nodes (N0/N1), but it has not spread to distant sites (M0).

Stage III: *T4a, any N, M0*:

The tumor is of any size and has grown gross beyond the thyroid gland and into nearby tissues of the neck (T4a). It may or may not have spread to nearby lymph nodes (any N). It has not spread to distant sites (M0).

Stage IVA (*T4b, any N, M0*):

The tumor is of any size and has grown either back to the spine, invading prevertebral fascia or into nearby large blood vessels (T4b). It may or may not have spread to nearby lymph nodes (any N), but it has not spread to distant sites (M0).

Stage IVB (*any T, any N, M1*):

The tumor is any of size and may or may not have grown outside the thyroid (any T). It may or may not have spread to nearby lymph nodes (any N). It has spread to distant sites (M1).

Medullary thyroid cancer

Age is not a factor in the stage of medullary thyroid cancer.

Stage I (*T1, N0, M0*):

The tumor is of 2 cm or less across and has not grown outside the thyroid (T1). It has not spread to nearby lymph nodes (N0) or distant sites (M0).

Stage II—one of the following applies:

T2, N0, M0: The tumor is more than 2 cm but not larger than 4 cm across and has not grown outside the thyroid (T2). It has not spread to nearby lymph nodes (N0) or distant sites (M0).

T3, N0, M0: The tumor is larger than 4 cm or has grown slightly outside the thyroid (T3), but it has not spread to nearby lymph nodes (N0) or distant sites (M0)

Stage III (*T1 to T3, N1a, M0*):

The tumor is of any size and may have grown slightly outside the thyroid (T1 to T3). It has spread to lymph nodes around the thyroid in the neck (N1a) but not to distant sites (M0).

Stage IVA—one of the following applies:

T4a, any N, M0: The tumor is of any size and has grown beyond the thyroid gland and into nearby tissues of the neck (T4a). It may or may not have spread to nearby lymph nodes (any N). It has not spread to distant sites (M0).

T1 to T3, N1b, M0: The tumor is of any size and may have grown slightly outside the thyroid gland (T1 to T3). It has spread to certain lymph nodes in the neck (cervical nodes) or to lymph nodes in the upper chest or behind the throat (retropharyngeal nodes) (N1b) but not to distant sites (M0).

Stage IVB (*T4b, any N, M0*):

The tumor is of any size and has grown either back toward the spine or into nearby large blood vessels (T4b). It may or may not have spread to nearby lymph nodes (any N), but it has not spread to distant sites (M0).

Stage IVC (*any T, any N, M1*):

The tumor is of any size and may or may not have grown outside the thyroid (any T). It may or may not have spread to nearby lymph nodes (any N). It has spread to distant sites (M1).

Anaplastic (undifferentiated) thyroid cancer

All anaplastic thyroid cancers are considered to be a stage IV, reflecting the poor prognosis of this type of cancer.

Stage IVA (*T1–3a, any N, M0*):

The tumor is still within the thyroid T1–T3a. It may or may not have spread to nearby lymph nodes (any N), but it has not spread to distant sites (M0).

Stage IVB

T1–T3a, N1, Mo

T3b, any N, M0

T4, any N, M0

The tumor is T1–T4. It may or may not have spread to nearby lymph nodes (any N), but it has not spread to distant sites (M0).

Stage IVC (any T, any N, M1):

The tumor is of any size and may or may not have grown outside of the thyroid (any T). It may or may not have spread to nearby lymph nodes (any N). It has spread to distant sites (M1).

The last years brought a more conservative approach of the non-aggressive histologies of thyroid cancer. In this light, some guidelines were revised and endorsed their recommendations. An example is ATA 2015 guidelines that redefined in 2017 (Haugen 2017) the histopathologic nomenclature for encapsulated follicular variant papillary thyroid carcinoma (EFVPTC) without invasion as a NIFTP, given the excellent prognosis of this neoplastic variant. Nevertheless, it is recommended to validate the observed patient outcomes (and test performance in predicting thyroid cancer outcomes), as well as implications on patients' psychosocial health and economics.

Nikiforov et al. in 2016 published the results of an international, multidisciplinary, retrospective study of patients with thyroid tumors currently diagnosed as noninvasive EFVPTC; the authors concluded that EFVPTC has a very low risk of adverse outcome and should be termed NIFTP. This reclassification will affect a large population of patients worldwide and result in a significant reduction in psychological and clinical consequences associated with the diagnosis of cancer.

According to histology and the stage, thyroid carcinoma has different therapy approaches. There are multiple guidelines of diagnosis and therapy, many of them published by national and international committees of experts in endocrinology, endocrine surgery, nuclear medicine, and oncology. All these algorithms were frequently reviewed with the intention to minimize the inadequate diagnosis and surgery and to provide the best option for surgery and complementary therapies.

The European Thyroid Association (ETA), the American Thyroid Association (ATA 2009 and 2015), the American Association of Clinical Endocrinologists (AACE/AME/ETA 2010), the American Association of Endocrine Surgeons (AAES), the Associazione Medici Endocrinologi (AME), the British Thyroid Association (BTA 2007, 2014), and the National Cancer Comprehensive Network (NCCN 2016) have produced the most comprehensive guidelines of diagnosis and treatment of thyroid cancer; many completed and renewed in the last 2 years.

7.5.4 Treatment Recommendations

Stage I and II Papillary and Follicular Thyroid Cancer

- Surgery is the therapy of choice for all primary lesions. Surgical options include total thyroidectomy or lobectomy. The choice of procedure is influenced mainly by the age of the patient and the size of the nodule.
- Total thyroidectomy: Preferred due to the high incidence of multicentric involvement of both lobes of the gland and the possibility of dedifferentiation of any residual tumor to the anaplastic cell type.
- Lobectomy: This term represents the total ablation of one lobe including the isthmus.
  - I-131: A therapeutic ablative dose of I-131 results in a decreased recurrence rate among high-risk patients with papillary and follicular carcinomas (NCCN 2016; ATA 2015; Pacini et al. 2006a, 2010, Schulmberger et al. 2016; Chianelli et al. 2009; Franzius et al. 2007). Patients presenting with papillary thyroid microcarcinomas (tumors <10 mm) have an excellent prognosis when treated surgically, and additional therapy with I-131 is limited (Verburg et al. 2010).
  - Following surgery and radioiodine therapy procedure, patients should receive postoperative treatment with exogenous thyroid hormone in doses sufficient to suppress the thyroid-stimulating hormone (TSH); the suppression is not lifelong, except the group of persistent/aggressive disease (Biondi et al. 2005; ATA 2015; BTA 2014; Mitchell et al. 2016).

Stage III Papillary and Follicular Thyroid Cancer

- Total thyroidectomy including removal of involved lymph nodes or other sites of extrathyroidal disease

- I-131 ablation following total thyroidectomy if the tumor demonstrates uptake of this isotope
- External beam radiation therapy if I-131 uptake is minimal (Clark and Duh 1990; Braverman and Utiger 2000; ATA 2015)

Stage IV Papillary and Follicular Thyroid Cancer

The most common sites of metastases are the lymph nodes, the lung, and the bone. The treatment of lymph node metastases alone is often curative. Treatment of distant metastases is usually not curative but may produce significant palliation (DeVita et al. 2001; Pacini et al. 2006b).

Standard treatment options:

- I-131: Metastases that demonstrate uptake of this isotope may be ablated by therapeutic doses of I-131.
- External beam radiation therapy for patients with localized lesions which are unresponsive to I-131.
- Resection of limited metastases, especially symptomatic metastases, should be considered when the tumor has no uptake of I-131.
- Thyroid-stimulating hormone suppression with thyroxin is also effective in many lesions not sensitive to I-131.

Patients unresponsive to I-131 should also be considered candidates for systemic therapies and clinical trials testing new approaches to this disease (Haugen 2017; ATA 2015; NCCN 2016; Pacini et al. 2010).

According to actual knowledge, 1/3 of metastatic DTC are definitely cured by radioiodine, the others being difficult to be managed regarding tumor progression. In France, 350 cases/year of refractory differentiated thyroid carcinoma (RDTC) (Sassolas et al. 2009) and metastatic RDTC refractory about 200 cases/year were reported.

Radiosensitivity to classic therapy with radioiodine is related to the following factors:

- Young patient
- Small foci
- Low FDG uptake at PET
- Well differentiation of tumor

Differentiated thyroid carcinoma is generally indolent in nature, and even though it metastasizes to distant organs, the prognosis is frequently excellent. In contrast, the overall survival of patients with radioactive iodine refractory and progressive metastases is unpredictable. Until recently, treatment options for patients with progressive, radioactive iodine-resistant differentiated thyroid cancer (DTC) have been limited. However, the last years demonstrated consistent data about the administration of tyrosine kinase inhibitors (TKIs) (Cabanillas et al. 2010); the drug has become a new line of therapy for RAI-refractory and progressive metastases. Previous studies have reported significant improvement regarding the progression-free survival rates of patients with metastatic lesions. However, TKIs cause various severe adverse effects that damage patients' quality of life and can even be life-threatening. Additionally, metastatic lesions may progress significantly after stopping TKI therapy. Therefore, it is difficult to determine who is a candidate for TKI therapy, as well as how and when physicians start and stop the therapy. Among other professionals, the committee of pharmacological therapy for thyroid cancer of the Japanese Society of Thyroid Surgery (JSTS) and the Japan Association of Endocrine Surgeons (JAES) summarized in the review published in 2016 (Ito et al. 2016) how to appropriately use TKIs by describing what they recommend to do and not in the treatment using TKIs.

The molecular pathogenesis of thyroid cancer has led to the discovery of driving somatic genetic alterations and suggested better methods to risk-stratify patients prior to surgery and also identification of patients at risk for recurrence and dedifferentiation, into a more aggressive thyroid cancer (Nikiforov 2015). Molecular profiling offers tremendous benefit in the refractory metastatic disease, and identification of targetable pathogenic lesions may select for more precise therapeutic options, such as the molecular kinase inhibitors. Figure 7.78 summarizes the most important molecular pathways that might be targeted by these therapies.

Selection criteria (Brose et al. 2014):

- L-T4: TSH <0.1 mUI/L
- Radical treatment of DTC

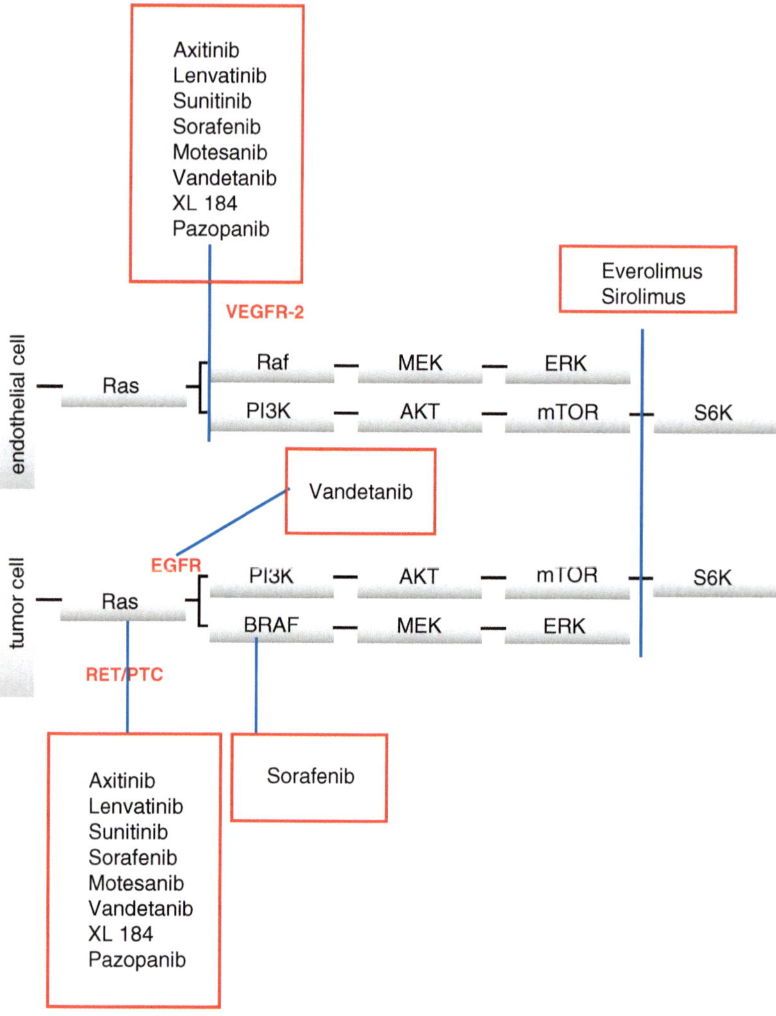

Fig. 7.78 Systemic therapy in radioactive iodine-refractory DTC

- WBS I-131 negative, no I-131 uptake in the lesions
- No resectability of the tumor
- No indication for external irradiation
- Significant progression of the disease in the last 6–12 months, according to RECIST criteria

Radiological evaluation at 6 months:

- Stable disease monitoring
- Progression of the disease—systemic therapy

Rates of response:

- 0–35% motesanib, axitinib, sunitinib, vandetanib, and vemurafenib
- ≥50% lenvatinib, pazopanib, and cabozantinib

Progression-free survival (PFS) vs placebo

- Vandetanib—phase II random (11.1 vs 5.9 months)
- Sorafenib—phase III-DECISION trial (10.8 vs 5.8 months)
- Lenvatinib—phase III-SELECT trial (18.3 vs 3.6 months)

Brose et al. published in 2014 the results of the trial DECISION. This multicenter, randomized (1:1), double-blind, placebo-controlled, phase III study investigated sorafenib (400 mg orally twice daily) in patients with RAI-refractory locally advanced or metastatic DTC progressing within the past 14 months. The primary endpoint was progression-free survival (PFS) by central independent review. Patients receiving placebo could cross over to open-label sorafenib upon progression. Archival tumor tissue was examined for BRAF and RAS mutations. Serum thyroglobulin was measured at baseline and each visit. Sorafenib significantly improved PFS compared with placebo in patients with progressive RAI-refractory DTC. Adverse events were consistent with the known sorafenib safety profile. These results suggest that sorafenib represents a new treatment option for patients with progressive RAI-refractory DTC.

A novel area of development is usage of TKIs as radioiodine resensitizing agents. A pilot study evaluated the role of selumetinib, a MEK inhibitor. Selumetinib increased iodine uptake in 12 patients, and 8 were retreated with RAI (Ho et al. 2013), suggesting that MEK inhibition therapy can lead to resensitization. The use of dabrafenib, a selective BRAF inhibitor, was also evaluated; the study demonstrated new radioiodine uptake following treatment (Schulmberger et al. 2016).

Medullary Thyroid Cancer

Medullary thyroid cancer (MTC) comprises less than 5% of all the thyroid cancers. MTC may be diagnosed through screening family members, determining serum calcitonin in basal or stimulated conditions, or determining RET proto-oncogene mutation (Dunn 1994; Mayr et al. 1999; Elisei et al. 2004; Schulmberger et al. 2016). MTC may be also diagnosed by evaluation of thyroid nodule or lymph nodes. Approximately 25% of the reported cases of MTC are familial, others being sporadic MTC. Familial MTC syndromes include MEN 2A and MEN 2B and familial non-MEN syndromes. Any patient with a familial variant should be screened for other associated endocrine tumors, particularly parathyroid hyperplasia and pheochromocytoma (Sipple 1961). MTC can secrete calcitonin and other peptide substances. Family members who are gene carriers should undergo prophylactic thyroidectomy at an early age.

Treatment options (AACE 2002; Pacini et al. 2006b, 2010; ATA 2009):

- Thyroidectomy: Patients with medullary thyroid cancer should be treated by total thyroidectomy, unless there is evidence of distant metastasis. In patients with clinically palpable medullary carcinoma of the thyroid, the incidence of microscopically positive nodes is more than 75%; routine central and bilateral modified neck dissections have been recommended. When cancer is confined to the thyroid gland, the prognosis is excellent.
- External radiation therapy: External radiation therapy has been used for palliation of locally recurrent tumors, without evidence that it provides any survival advantage.
- Radioactive iodine has no place in the treatment of patients with MTC.
- Chemotherapy: Palliative chemotherapy has been reported to produce occasional responses in patients with metastatic disease. No single-drug regimen can be considered standard. Some patients with distant metastases will experience prolonged survival and can be managed expectantly until they become symptomatic.

Anaplastic Thyroid Cancer

Standard treatment options (Braverman and Utiger 2000; NCCN 2016):

- Surgery: Frequently surgery is resumed to biopsy because of the aggressive extent of the tumor. If the disease is confined to the local area, which is rare, total thyroidectomy is warranted to reduce symptoms caused by the tumor mass.
- Radiation therapy: External beam radiation therapy may be used in patients who are not surgical candidates or whose tumor cannot be surgically excised.
- Chemotherapy: Anaplastic thyroid cancer as MTC is not responsive to I-131 therapy; the treatment with individual anticancer drugs has been reported to produce partial remissions in some patients. Single or in combination with other drugs, the doxorubicin appears to be active and has been reported to produce an improvement of the disease.

7.5.5 European Thyroid Association and American Thyroid Association: Indications for Postsurgical Radioiodine Thyroid Ablation, Procedure, and Follow-up

As the trend in thyroid cancer management continues to move toward a personalized therapy and monitoring, it is even more important that the professionals involved in this pathology be able to accurately assess the risk of recurrence and risk of disease-specific mortality in order to ensure that the recommendations are specifically tailored for each patient and the quality of life is appropriate.

In this light, the former guidelines referring to the therapy and follow-up of thyroid cancer, presented in the first edition of this book, are still available, but there are new tendencies worldwide to improve quality of life and to adjust every single recommendation to specific particularities of each patient, having a more conservative approach for the indolent forms and a clearer defined systemic approach in the aggressive forms.

The next paragraphs will cover both the former and the newest guidelines, in order to have an overview about the changes that were made. From the personal point of view, the authors' opinion is that one of the major attention in this new approach was focused on patients' perspective and quality of life, considering that this pathology is in the majority of cases a curable and life-threatening and monitoring disease, completely different compared with other cancers.

As in the previous edition, we will focus on the recommendations made by the most important opinion leaders which continue to be the European Thyroid Association (ETA), American Thyroid Association (ATA), and American Association of Clinical Endocrinologists (AACE). The latest guidelines will be also summarized from ETA (2010) and ATA (2015) and completed with the endorsements from other professional associations involved in this pathology: European Association of Nuclear Medicine (EANM 2010; Luster et al. 2008), UK National Multidisciplinary Guidelines (2016), British Thyroid Association (2014), Italian Thyroid Association (2016), South Korean Thyroid Association (Lee et al. 2017; Yi et al. 2016), Japanese Thyroid Association (Koizumi et al. 2004; Takami et al. 2014), and Latin-American Thyroid Society (LATS, 2009) revised guidelines.

European Thyroid Association (ETA) (Pacini et al. 2006b, 2010)

Very low-risk group, no indication for *postoperative* I-131

- Unifocal microcarcinoma (≤1 cm)
- No extension beyond the thyroid capsule
- No lymph node metastases
- Complete surgery

Low-risk group, probable indication for I-131: no concensus

- Less than total thyroidectomy, no lymph node dissection
- Age <18 years
- Unfavorable histology, T1 > 1 cm, T2, N0, M0

High-risk group, definite indication for I-131

- T3, T4, N1, M1
- Incomplete surgery
- High risk of recurrence

American Thyroid Association (ATA 2009)

The American guidelines have a classification of recommendations in six groups: A, B, C, D, E, F, and I related to the strength of medical evidence-based studies.

A. *Strongly recommends*. The recommendation is based on good evidence and includes consistent results from well-designed, well-conducted studies in representative populations.
B. *Recommends*. The recommendation is based on fair evidence that the service or intervention can improve important health outcomes. The evidence is sufficient to determine effects on health outcomes, but the strength of the evidence is limited.
C. *Recommends*. The recommendation is based on expert opinion.
D. *Recommends against*. The recommendation is based on expert opinion.
E. *Recommends against*. The recommendation is based on fair evidence that the service or

intervention does not improve important health outcomes or that harms outweigh benefits.

F. *Strongly recommends against.* The recommendation is based on good evidence that the service or intervention does not improve important health outcomes or that harms outweigh benefits.

G. *Recommends neither for nor against.*

Recommendation R 32—radioiodine ablation is recommended for:

- Patients with stage III and IV (AJCC 7th edition, TNM classification)
- All patients with stage II younger than 45 years old
- Most patients with stage II 45 years old or older
- Selected patients with stage I, with multifocal (>2 foci) disease, nodal metastases, extrathyroidal and vascular invasion, and/or aggressive histology. Recommendation B

ETA—staging and recommendations after thyroidectomy and radioiodine therapy (Pacini et al. 2006b)

Very low risk

- Unifocal T1a (≤1 cm) N0M0 and no extension beyond thyroid capsule
- LT4 replacement: TSH −0.5–1 mIU/L

Low risk

- T1b (>1 cm, but less 2 cm) N0M0 or T2N0M0 or multifocal T1aN0M0
- LT4 replacement: TSH—0.5–1 mIU/L for 6–12 months

High risk

- Any T3 and T4 or any T, N1, or M1
- LT4 suppressive dose TSH < 0.1 mIU/L for 3–5 years

ATA—staging and recommendations after thyroidectomy and radioiodine therapy (2009)

Low risk

- No local or distant metastases
- All macroscopic tumor removed
- No tumor invasion of locoregional tissues or structures
- No aggressive histology (e.g., tall cell, insular, columnar carcinoma)
- TSH must be between 0.3 and 2 mIU/L. Recommendation C

Intermediate risk

- Microscopic invasion in perithyroidal soft tissues
- Aggressive histology or vascular invasion

High risk

- Macroscopic tumor invasion
- Incomplete tumor resection
- Distant metastases
- I-131 uptake outside the thyroid bed after the posttreatment WBS scan.
- TSH must be between 0.1 and 0.5 mIU/L for 5–10 years. Recommendation C

LATS (Pitoia et al. 2009) proposed a disease staging system based on three categories:

Very low risk

- Unifocal T1a (<1 cm) N0M0 and no extension beyond thyroid capsule

Low risk

- T multifocal 1–4 cm N0M0

High risk

- T > 4 cm (>45 years)
- Macroscopic extrathyroidal extension (>45 years)
- N1
- M1
- Residual disease
- Aggressive histology

According to BTA 2014**,** the following algorithm of disease staging should be used:

No indications of I-131 therapy

All criteria below should be met:

- Tumor <1 cm unifocal or multifocal
- Histology classical papillary or follicular variant of papillary carcinoma or follicular carcinoma
- Minimally invasive without angioinvasion
- No invasion of thyroid capsule (extra thyroidal extension)

Definite indications of I-131 therapy

Any one of the criteria below should be met:

- Tumor >4 cm
- Any tumor size with gross extra-thyroidal extension
- Distant metastases present

Uncertain indications; selective use of I-131

All other cases

One or more of the following risk factors may identify patients at higher risk of recurrence who may benefit from RRA:

- Large tumor size
- Extra-thyroidal extension
- Unfavorable cell type (tall cell, columnar or diffuse sclerosing papillary cancer, poorly differentiated elements)
- Widely invasive histology
- Multiple lymph node involvement, large size of involved lymph nodes, high ratio of positive to negative nodes, and extracapsular nodal involvement
- WBS posttherapy at 3–5 days

ETA/ATA—management of metastatic and recurrent disease (Pacini et al. 2006b, 2010)

Local and regional recurrence:

- Surgery and I-131
- External beam therapy of 40–45 Gy in 25–30 sessions only if surgery is not possible and there is no I-131 uptake

Distant metastases:

- Lungs: 100–200 mCi every 4–8 months during the first 2 years
- Bones: Surgery and I-131 and external beam therapy
- Brain: Surgery and external beam therapy and I-131 only after external radiotherapy

Second malignancies:

- ETA—over 600 mCi I-131, the risk is significantly higher for second malignancy (Canchola et al. 2006; Pacini et al. 2006a; Rubino et al. 2003).
- ATA—the risk of second malignancy is dose related; long-term follow-up studies demonstrate a very low risk. There appears to be an increased risk of breast cancer; it is unclear whether this is a result of screening basis, radioiodine therapy, or other factors (recommendation C).

We strongly suggest having cancer screening programs to all the patients with thyroid malignancy, most of them women, who have the opportunity of regular breast examination and genital control.

In order to do our best for this disease, there has to exist a close relation between all the specialists involved in the diagnostic and treatment of this pathology.

The prognosis of these patients strongly depends on some presurgical, intraoperative, and postoperative criteria, as synthetized by Schulmberger et al. (2016) and presented in Fig. 7.79.

The new ATA 2015 guidelines proposed a new risk stratification, summarized in Table 7.4; to be noted, compare to the previous guideline the introduction of genotype criteria and of number and/or sizes of metastatic vessels or lymph nodes.

Recommendations for radioiodine ablation according to **ATA 2015** are summarized in Table 7.5.

A novelty proposed by the new guidelines was the response classification to therapy. The response to therapy restaging system was designed and specifically developed to guide specific therapeutic decisions after primary therapy is completed. Prospective studies of the value of this system for guiding extent of primary treatment, including adjuvant treatment decisions, are needed. However, given that there is emerging evidence that such a reclassification system has potential to be of great importance in the management of DTC patients after primary treatment, there will be presentation of the systems proposed by BTA 2014 (Table 7.6) and ATA 2015 (Table 7.7).

BTA proposed the following terminology:

ATA proposed the following terminologies, for the assessment of therapy response:

1. **Excellent response**: no clinical, biochemical, or structural evidence of disease after initial therapy; <1% disease-specific death
2. **Biochemical incomplete response**: abnormal Tg/anti-Tg values in the absence of localizable disease; <1% disease-specific death
3. **Structural incomplete response**: persistent or newly identified locoregional or distant metastases; 11% disease-specific death (locoregional metastases) and 50% disease-specific death (distant metastases)

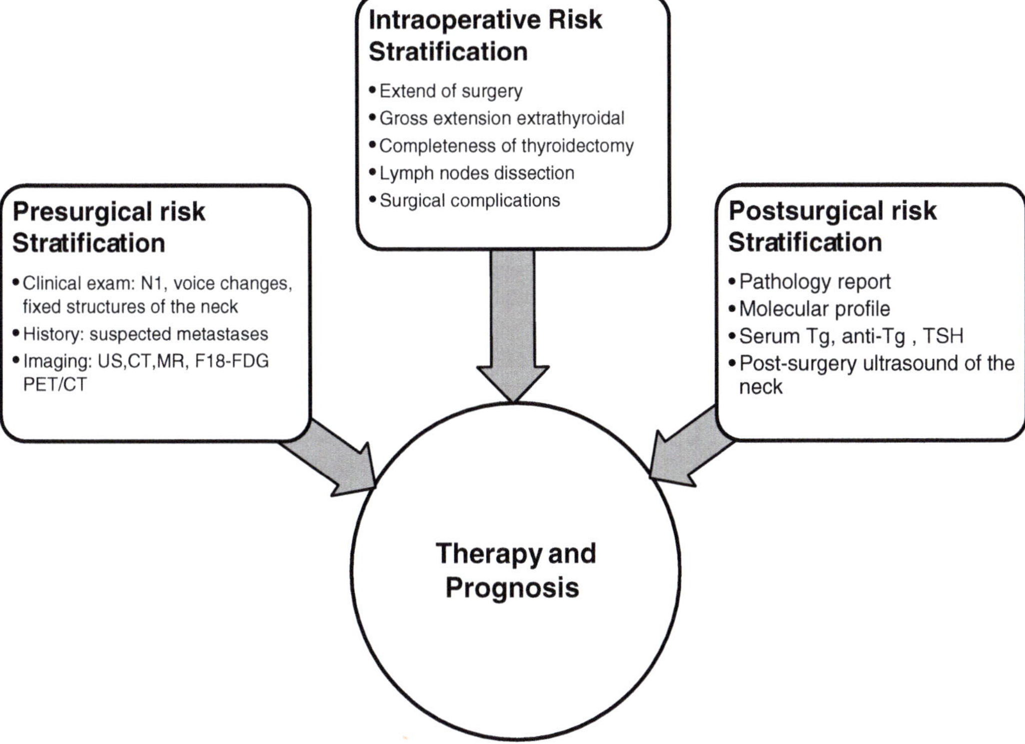

Fig. 7.79 Initial risk stratification factors (Adapted from Schulmberger et al. 2016)

Table 7.4 Risk stratification system ATA 2015

Low risk	Intermediate risk	High risk
1. Papillary thyroid cancer, with all of the following: • No local or distant metastases • All macroscopic tumor has been resected • No tumor invasion of locoregional tissues or structures • The tumor does not have aggressive histology (e.g., tall cell, hobnail variant, columnar cell carcinoma) • If I-131 is given, there are no I-31-avid metastatic foci outside the thyroid bed on the first posttreatment whole-body RAI scan • No vascular invasion • Clinical N0 or ≤5 pathologic N1 micrometastases (<0.2 cm in largest dimension) 2. Intrathyroidal papillary microcarcinoma, unifocal or multifocal, including BRAF^{V600E} mutated (if known) 3. Intrathyroidal, encapsulated follicular variant of papillary thyroid cancer 4. Intrathyroidal, well-differentiated follicular thyroid cancer with capsular invasion and no or minimal (<4 foci) vascular invasion	1. Microscopic invasion of tumor into the perithyroidal soft tissues 2. I-131-avid metastatic foci in the neck on the first posttreatment whole-body RAI scan 3. Aggressive histology (e.g., tall cell, hobnail variant, columnar cell carcinoma) 4. Papillary thyroid cancer with vascular invasion 5. Clinical N1 or >5 pathologic N1 with all involved lymph nodes <3 cm in largest dimension 6. Multifocal papillary microcarcinoma with extrathyroidal extension and BRAF^{V600E} mutated (if known)	1. Macroscopic invasion of tumor into the perithyroidal soft tissues (gross extension) 2. Incomplete tumor resection 3. Distant metastases 4. Postoperative serum thyroglobulin suggestive of distant metastases 5. Pathologic N1 with any metastatic lymph node ≥3 cm in largest dimension 6. Follicular thyroid cancer with extensive vascular invasion (>4 foci of vascular invasion)

Table 7.5 Characteristics according to the ATA risk stratification system and AJCC/TNM staging system with postoperative radioiodine decision-making

Risk staging ATA, 2015	Features	Radioiodine indication (RAI)
ATA low risk T1a, N0/Nx, M0/Mx	Tumor size ≥1 cm (uni- or multifocal)	No
ATA low risk T1b, T2, N0/Nx, M0/Mx	Tumor size >1–4 cm	Not routine—may be considered for patients with aggressive histology or vascular invasion
ATA low to intermediate risk T3, N0/Nx, M0/Mx	Tumor size >4 cm	Consider—need to consider presence of other adverse features. Advancing age may favor RAI use in some cases, but specific age and tumor size cutoffs subject to some uncertainty
ATA low to intermediate risk T3, N0/Nx, M0/Mx	Microscopic ETE, any T	Consider—generally favored based on risk of recurrent disease. Smaller tumors with microscopic extension may not require RAI
ATA low to intermediate risk T1-3, N1a, M0/Mx	Central compartment neck lymph node metastases	Consider—generally favored, due to somewhat higher risk of persistent or recurrent disease, especially with increasing number of large (>2–3 cm) or clinically evident lymph nodes or presence of extranodal extension. Advancing age may also favor RAI use. However, there is insufficient data to mandate RAI use in patients with few (<5) microscopic nodal metastases in central compartment in absence of other adverse features
ATA low to intermediate risk T1-3, N1b, M0/Mx	Lateral neck or mediastinal lymph node metastases	Consider—generally favored, due to higher risk of persistent or recurrent disease, especially with increasing number of macroscopic or clinically evident lymph nodes or presence of extranodal extension. Advancing age may also favor RAI use
ATA high risk T4 Any N, Any M	Any size, gross ETE	Yes
ATA high risk M1, Any T, Any N	Distant metastases	Yes

Table 7.6 Dynamic risk stratification: definitions of response to initial therapy of DTC (9–12 months after total thyroidectomy with subsequent radioiodine therapy, adapted BTA 2014)

Excellent response	*All the following:* • Suppressed and stimulated Tg <1 ng/mL (anti-Tg negative) • Neck US without evidence of disease • Cross-sectional and/or nuclear medicine imaging negative (if performed)	*Low risk*
Indeterminate response	*Any of the following:* • Suppressed Tg < 1 ng/L and stimulated Tg ≥1 and <10 ng/L (anti-Tg negative) • Neck US with nonspecific changes or stable <1 cm lymph nodes • Cross-sectional and/or nuclear medicine imaging with nonspecific changes, although not completely normal	*Intermediate risk*
Incomplete response	*Any of the following:* • Suppressed Tg≥1 ng/mL or stimulated Tg ≥ 10 ng/L (anti-Tg negative) • Rising Tg values • Persistent or newly identified disease on cross-sectional and/or nuclear medicine imaging	*High risk*

Table 7.7 Proposed terminology to classify response to therapy and clinical implications (Adapted from ATA 2015)

Excellent response	*Negative imaging* and either • Suppressed Tg <0.2 ng/mL or • TSH-stimulated Tg <1 ng/mL	An excellent response to therapy should lead to: • An early decrease in the intensity and frequency of *follow-up* • And the *degree of TSH suppression*
Biochemical incomplete response	*Negative imaging* and • Suppressed Tg ≥1 ng/mL or • Stimulated Tg ≥10 ng/mL or • Rising anti-Tg antibody levels	A biochemical incomplete response should lead to: • If associated with *stable or declining serum Tg values*, continued observation with ongoing TSH suppression in most patients • *Rising Tg or anti-Tg antibody values* should prompt additional investigations and potentially additional therapies
Structural incomplete response	*Structural or functional evidence of disease* with any Tg level, with or without anti-Tg antibodies	A structural incomplete response may lead to • Additional treatments or ongoing observation depending on multiple clinicopathologic factors including the size, location, rate of growth, RAI avidity, F18-FDG avidity, and specific pathology of the structural lesions
Indeterminate response	• Nonspecific findings on imaging studies • Faint uptake in thyroid bed on RAI scanning • Nonstimulated Tg detectable but <1 ng/mL • Stimulated Tg detectable but <10 ng/mL or	An indeterminate response should lead to: • *Continued observation* with appropriate serial imaging of the nonspecific lesions and serum Tg monitoring • Nonspecific findings that become suspicious over time can be *further evaluated* with additional imaging or biopsy • Anti-Tg antibodies stable or declining in the absence of structural or functional disease

4. **Indeterminate response**: biochemical or structural findings that cannot be classified as either benign or malignant; <1% disease-specific death

ETA/ATA—radioiodine procedure (Pacini et al. 2006a, b, 2010)

- High-risk group >100 mCi I-131 after withdrawal.
- Low-risk group 30 100 mCi I-131 after withdrawal or 100 mCi I-131 in the third day after an rhTSH 0.9 mg day 1 and 2.
- Scan before ablation may be avoided.
- TSH must be >30 mIU/L, Tg before ablation.

A low-iodine diet for approximately 1–2 weeks should be considered for patients undergoing RAI remnant ablation or treatment, even if there are no clear evidences about the benefit of strict diet. Surely, the patient should avoid medication with iodine content and contrast media; the specific region profile diet should be known and adapted. A patient coming from a region with high intake of seafood needs to know about the supplementary tests or diet restriction prior to therapy. A special attention should be considered about the use of amiodarone, where the impact on iodine uptake may influence significantly the possibility of favorable outcome; the blockade may take sometimes more than 1 year.

7.5.6 Radioactive Iodine Therapy

Radiopharmaceutical:

(I-131)NaI—sodium iodide capsules for oral administration with specific activity of 1.11, 1.85, 2.59, 3.7, and 5.55 GBq at calibration time, clearly mentioned by the producer and strictly scheduled for arriving in the department.

Principle:

This is a systemic administration of I-131 sodium iodide for selective irradiation of thyroid postsurgical remnants of differentiated thyroid carcinoma (DTC) or other nonresectable DTC or for irradiation of metastatic iodine-avid structures.

Patient Preparation:

The patient should be:

After total or near-total thyroidectomy with histopathological diagnostic of differentiated thyroid carcinoma

With a TSH value >30–40 mIU/L at 4–6 weeks after the surgery in the absence of thyroid therapy replacement

With a TSH value >40 mIU/L or a significant increment of minimum 100 times comparing the TSH value obtained under thyroid hormone treatment at 4–6 weeks of thyroid hormone withdrawal, in the case of substitutive thyroid hormonal therapy

After I.M. injection of recombinant TSH in 2 consecutive days of 0.9 mL solution, if the patient is under hormonal treatment

Fasting condition

Avoid any contact with blocking agents and iodine contrast media used for tomographic examination (at least 2–3 months!); attention to some diet restriction

In the case of female patients of childbearing potential, a routine testing for pregnancy within 72 h before the administration of I-131 must be done. When the patient history clearly indicates that pregnancy is excluded, a pregnancy test may be omitted at the discretion of the treating physician. In case of suspicious situation, a serologic analysis of beta HCG (beta human chorionic gonadotropin) may be requested.

Postoperative radioiodine will:

- Ablate the thyroid remnant, which will help in surveillance for recurrent disease.
- Eliminate suspected micrometastases.
- Eliminate known persistent disease.

If preoperative scan is performed or is needed, to avoid or reduce the stunning effect, the following have been suggested (Anderson et al. 2003; Carril 1997; Gerard and Cavalieri 2002):

- The use of I-123 or small (2 or 3 mCi) doses of I-131
- A shortened interval (of not more than 72 h) between the diagnostic I-131 dose and the therapy dose

Fixed I-131 Doses

The administration of a fixed dose of I-131 is the simplest and the most widely used method. Most clinics use this method regardless of the percentage uptake of I-131 in the remnant or metastatic lesion. Patients with tumor uptake are routinely treated with large, fixed amounts of I-131.

The dose of remnant ablation may be 30–50–70–100 mCi (1.1–1.85–2.59–3.7 GBq), according to the (Hackshaw et al. 2007):

Aggressiveness of histology

Volume of the residual tissue

The uptake, if known

The serum level of the Tg

Lymph node metastases may be treated with about 100–175 mCi (3.7–6.47 GBq) of I-131. The cancer growing through the thyroid capsule and incompletely resected is treated with 150–200 mCi (5.5–7.4 GBq). Patients with distant metastases are usually treated with 200 mCi (7.4 GBq) of I-131, which typically will not induce radiation sickness or produce serious damage to other structures but may exceed generally accepted safety limits to the blood in the elderly and in those with impaired kidney function.

Diffuse pulmonary metastases that concentrate 50% or more of the diagnostic dose of I-131 (which is very uncommon) are treated with 150 mCi or less of I-131 (5.5 GBq) to avoid lung injury, which may occur when more than 80 mCi remain in the whole body 48 h after the treatment. The administered activity of radioactive iodine (RAI) therapy should be adjusted for pediatric patients.

Quantitative Tumor I-131 Dosimetry

A second method is to use quantitative dosimetry methods to estimate the amount of radiation delivered to the lesion per unit of I-131 administered. This approach is attractive because radiation exposure from arbitrarily fixed doses of I-131 can vary substantially. It is necessary to serially measure the radiation activity in the target using a tracer dose and to estimate the tumor size to make these calculations, which is difficult to do and is impossible in the setting of diffuse or microscopic lung metastases (Tuttle et al. 2006; NCCN 2016; Schulmberger et al. 2016).

The use of I-123 or I-131 with SPECT/CT or I-124 PET-based dosimetry may facilitate whole-body and lesion dosimetry. The efficacy of RAI therapy is related to the mean radiation dose delivered to neoplastic foci and also to the radiosensitivity of tumor tissue, which is higher in younger patients, with small metastases from well-differentiated papillary or follicular carcinoma and with uptake of RAI but no or low F18-FDG uptake.

The maximum tolerated radiation absorbed dose (MTRD) is potentially exceeded in a significant number of patients undergoing empiric treatment with various amounts of I-131. Some studies found that an empirically administered I-131 activity of 200 mCi would exceed the MTRD in 8–15% of patients younger than age 70 and 22–38% of patients aged 70 years and older. These estimates imply the need for caution in administering empiric activities higher than 100–150 mCi in certain populations such as elderly patients and patients with renal insufficiency.

Blood I-131 Dosimetry

A third method is to administer a dose calculated to deliver a maximum of 200 cGy to the blood while keeping the whole-body retention less than 120 mCi (4.4 GBq) at 48 h or less than 80 mCi (2.96 GBq) in the case of diffuse pulmonary uptake.

The activity of administrated radiopharmaceutical depends on the type of surgery, the thyroglobulin values, and the volume of remnant tissue (ultrasound evaluation).

After the administration, the patient remains in fasting condition for 2 more h, and after that he/she is advised to hydrate himself.

The administration of I-131 for the treatment of DTC is performed in hospitalization conditions, and the discharge of patients is done according to national radioprotection regulation. At this moment, there are countries where the treatment may be done in ambulatory condition even with doses higher than 30 mCi (1.1 GBq) I-131.

All patients have paper and electronic information on each room about the diagnosis, the treatment options, follow-up, side effects, and personal indications about individual medication.

The rooms must have separate facilities and are continuously in surveillance by the staff, on separate cameras. At the discharging time, the patient is advised how to minimize the risk for other persons and for what period of time, depending of the dosimetry measurements at the discharging time (Willegaignon et al. 2011).

Posttreatment I-131 Imaging

When I-131 therapy is given, whole-body radioiodine imaging should be performed several days later to document I-131 uptake by the tumor. Posttreatment whole-body radioiodine imaging should be done primarily because up to 25% of such imaging show lesions that may be clinically important, which were not detected by the diagnostic imaging.

It is strongly recommended to respect the indication of surgery and of the extent of surgery, according to the risk classification and the tumor dimensions. A better presurgical diagnosis will lead to a limited number of second surgeries for the completion of thyroidectomy; it will also limit the unnecessary total thyroidectomy. The lymphadenectomy will be targeted to all the patients with clinical involvement of the lymph nodes, and the central lymph node dissection will be recommended as a routine.

Recommendations:

- Optimizing the schedule of patients for radioiodine treatments at 4–6 weeks postsurgery.
- Avoid hormonal substitution after surgery and before radioiodine, if there is the possibility to

have an optimal organization of the waiting list for therapy; use hormonal replacement if the stimulation will be done with rhTSH.

- Do not use CT with contrast media for staging; the cervical ultrasound is the best noninvasive method for correct assessment of the local extension, before the treatment.
- Avoid WBS I-131 before radioiodine treatment, unless distant metastases are suspected and important active thyroid remnant must be removed by surgery.
- Increase TSH more than 30–40 mIU/L.
- Quantitative determination of ablative doses: ultrasound volume determination, 24 h uptake of radioiodine, estimated by using less than 100 μCi I-131 or adequate dose for I-123, and serum Tg and anti-Tg levels.
- Do not use any medication that may influence the uptake of radioiodine.
- Do not use an aggressive washout of radioiodine by intensive hydration (not more than 2–2.5 L of liquids/day).
- Use WBS after therapy at 2–5 days, for a correct staging of the disease extension.
- The sialadenitis is limited by liberal hydration and by lemon juice given in the first 24–48 h after radioiodine. Our personal experience recommends 500–1000 mg of vitamin C during the first 5 days of treatment (Ceccarelli et al. 1999; Mandel and Mandel 2003; Schlumberger et al. 2004).
- The recommended activity of I-131 ranges from 1.11 to 5.55 GBq (30–150 mCi).
- Total response and disease-free is indicated by:
  - No detectable tumor mass.
  - Undetectable Tg in high TSH condition and no anti-Tg.
  - The revised guidelines for the management of thyroid disease in pregnancy include recommendations regarding the interpretation of thyroid function tests in pregnancy, iodine nutrition, thyroid autoantibodies and pregnancy complications, thyroid considerations in infertile women, hypothyroidism in pregnancy, thyrotoxicosis in pregnancy, thyroid nodules and cancer in pregnant women, fetal and neonatal considerations, thyroid disease and lactation, screening for thyroid dysfunction in pregnancy, and directions for future research.

Possible Early Adverse Events Following I-131

- Sialadenitis (lemon juice, candies, chewing gum should be used during the therapy).
- Nausea (can be minimized by prescription of antiemetics).
- Neck discomfort and swelling within a few days of I-131 may occur, especially when a large thyroid remnant is present (simple analgesics and nonsteroidal anti-inflammatory ointments for neck discomfort are recommended. A short course of corticosteroids is recommended in severe cases).
- Radiation cystitis, radiation gastritis, bleeding, and edema in metastases are all extremely rare.
- No hair loss radioiodine related.

Management of acute side effects of I-131:

- For patients with known metastatic disease, especially bone and lung metastases, consideration should be given to commencing a short course of corticosteroids to minimize peritumoral edema and an increase in local symptoms. If the patient is to receive rhTSH, then starting the corticosteroids prior to the injections is advisable.
- The total cumulative activity should be kept as low as possible.
- Monitoring of lung function for any sign of a restrictive functional deficit is recommended in patients with lung metastases.
- Acute symptoms of dyspnea and cough can be reduced with prophylactic corticosteroids.

Possible Late Adverse Events Following I-131

- Xerostomia and dysgeusia.
- Sialadenitis and lacrimal gland dysfunction may occur.
- Lifetime incidence of leukemia and second cancers is low affecting around 0.5% of patients. There are controversial studies regarding the second malignancies after I-131. Some studies showed an increased but nonsignificant risk of leukemia. The risk of leukemia increases with escalating cumulative activity and with use of additional external beam

radiotherapy (BTA 2014). Patients who have received a high cumulative I-131 activity may also be more likely to develop second solid malignancies (e.g., the bladder, colorectal, breast, and salivary glands). The author published the results on 1990 patients treated over a period of 25 years with low and medium doses of I-131, and there was no significant impact on developing second malignancies related to I-131 (Piciu et al. 2016).
- Radiation fibrosis can occur in patients who have had diffuse pulmonary metastatic disease and have received repeated doses.

Follow-up:
- The serum Tg rules out the anti-Tg: it must be undetectable after radical treatment; no measurements for 3 months after treatment.
- WBS I-131—2–3 days after 2–5 mCi I-131 and T4 withdrawal or rhTSH only at the first check up and till the first negative scan.
- Tg is measured every 6–12 months by immunometric assay in the same laboratory, for all the patients with DTC and radical treatment. Anti-Tg every time in the same determined sample (Schlumberger et al. 2004, 2016).
- Low-risk patients with radical treatment (surgery ± radioiodine), negative neck ultrasound, and TSH suppression 6 months after the treatment, and Tg stimulated after T4 withdrawal or rhTSH at 12 months with undetectable values, are uncertain for subsequent stimulated determinations (Pacini et al. 2006a; Tuttle et al. 2008; ATA 2015).
- Low-risk patients with radical treatment (surgery ± radioiodine), with negative Tg stimulated after T4 withdrawal or rhTSH, after the first WBS negative, do not need further WBS.
- If the use of human recombinant TSH is not a routine, it is recommended to be used at least for the patients with no optimum rising of TSH: circumstances in which the patient cannot elicit a sustained release of endogenous TSH include hypothalamic or pituitary dysfunction, long-term corticosteroid administration, and an unusually slow response, particularly in the elderly (Pacini et al. 2004; Tuttle et al. 2008; Chianelli et al. 2009).
- Perform morphological and functional studies with other radiotracers in case of negative WBS I-131 (see Chap. 11, PET/CT, Robbins et al. 2006).

It is very important to have a strict follow-up and early detection of the recurrence of the disease, and it is mandatory to do our best to have an accurate staging and precision of the extension.

The present studies suggest that previous administration of radioiodine therapy in female patients with well-differentiated thyroid cancer does not result in demonstrable adverse effects in subsequent pregnancies (Schlumberger et al. 1996; Ceccarelli et al. 1999; ATA/AACE 2011).

Gonadal tissue is exposed to radiation from RAI in the blood, urine, and feces. Temporary amenorrhea/oligomenorrhea lasting 4–10 months occurs in 20–27% of menstruating women after radioiodine therapy for thyroid cancer (ATA 2015). Although the numbers of patients studied are small, long-term rates of infertility, miscarriage, and fetal malformation do not appear to be elevated in women after RAI therapy (Sawka et al. 2008). One recent large retrospective cohort study showed that use of RAI was associated with delayed childbearing and decreased birthrate in later years, although it is unclear if this is due to reproductive choice or reproductive health.

In a meta-analysis, no evidence was found that I-131 treatments impaired fertility (ATA 2011), while in another meta-analysis, radioiodine therapy for thyroid cancer in young men has been associated with transient testicular dysfunction expressed as elevated serum FSH levels for up to 18 months after treatments, and some articles reported low sperm counts exceeding 1-year duration. Limited data indicate that fathering a child within 3 months of radiation exposure is not associated with an increase in congenital anomalies or fetal loss and there is no evidence of long-term reduced fertility. However, men should be advised to wait at least 3 months.

Special recommendation:

At discharge, the reports and the medical letters consist of all the identity information, diagnosis, laboratory tests, and copies of WBS, administrated activity, calibration data, and specific issues about radioprotection (ATA 2011).

Case 1: Papillary Thyroid Carcinoma

History:

A 57-year-old female, with the diagnosis of papillary thyroid carcinoma operated with total thyroidectomy and central compartment lymph nodes removal, is referred for radioiodine therapy.

T3N0M0—stage III

Clinical examination:

The examination took place at 6 weeks postsurgery, in the absence of thyroid hormonal replacement. The patient was presenting signs of myxedema.

The neck examination revealed a postthyroidectomy scar, without any palpable tumor mass or lymph nodes in the cervical area. No other signs or symptoms to be mentioned.

Examinations:

Ultrasound—no thyroid tissue remnant; no pathologic lymph nodes.

TSH—71.15 mIU/L (N.V. 0.4–4.5 mIU/L), very increased.

Tg < 0.1 μg/L (N.V. <0.1 μg/L).

Anti-Tg—12 kIU/L (N.V. <115 kIU/L), normal (Fig. 7.80).

Findings:

The patient received 90 mCi (3.33 GBq) of I-131. The WBS I-131 posttherapy showed the presence of radioiodine uptake in the thyroid area.

No distant and no locoregional pathologic uptake (Fig. 7.81).

Conclusion:

Minimal thyroid remnant with radioiodine uptake.

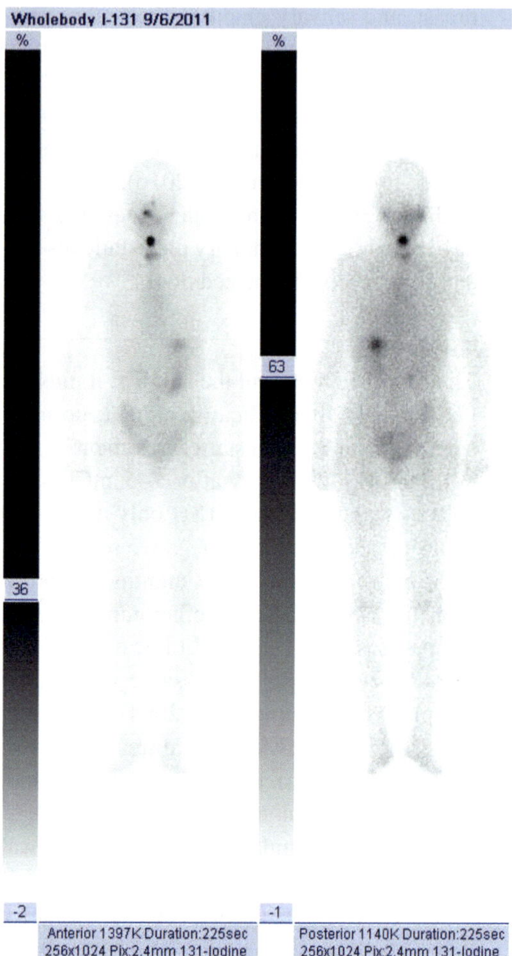

Fig. 7.81 WBS I-131 at 24 h posttherapy. Thyroid tissue remnant. No distant metastasis

Imunochimie			
Anti-tiroglobulina Electrochemiluminiscenta	12	UI/mL	≤ 115
TSH (Hormon de stimulare tiroidiana) Electrochemiluminiscenta	71.15	μUI/mL	0.27– 4.2
TG (tiroglobulina) Electrochemiluminiscenta kit 2	< 0.1	ng/mL	Valori normale: < 78ng/mL La pacienti atiroidieni: < 0.1ng/mL

Fig. 7.80 Tumor marker results (Tg and anti-Tg) 6 weeks postsurgery, without hormone replacement and with a high level of TSH

Key Points

- The decision of radioiodine therapy was made with respect to the histology and stage of the disease and of risk group.
- The patient was correctly prepared for therapy, with high TSH in the absence of hormone replacement.
- The amount of radioiodine was a fixed dose considered to the stage.
- The undetectable value of Tg, in the absence of antibodies (anti-Tg) and with stimulated TSH, might suggest the total absence of the thyroid tissue and of the disease; but the WBS I-131 posttherapy showed a positive scan.
- This discrepancy (undetectable Tg and WBS I-131 scan positive) underlines the necessity of respecting the guidelines of therapy related to the risk group.

Case 2: Follicular Thyroid Carcinoma

History:

A 60-year-old female, with the diagnosis of follicular thyroid adenoma operated 4 years before with total left lobectomy and subtotal right lobectomy. The patient is referred after the removal of solitary cerebral metastases of follicular thyroid carcinoma; she was referred for evaluation and therapy.

T × N × M1 (stage IVC)

Clinical examination:

The examination of the patient took place at 2 weeks postcraniotomy; the patient had no thyroid hormonal replacement after the thyroidectomy; no signs of hormonal disorders. The patient presented moderate motor deficiency in the lower part of the body and discrete cognitive dysfunction.

The neck examination revealed a post-thyroidectomy scar, without any palpable tumor mass or lymph nodes in the cervical area. No other signs or symptoms to be mentioned.

Examinations:

The blocks and pathology specimens were reviewed in order to reassess the correct initial diagnosis from the first operation of the thyroid. The results including the immunohistologic evaluation were negative for the diagnosis of carcinoma (Fig. 7.82).

Ultrasound—no thyroid tissue remnant; no pathologic lymph nodes.

TSH—9.88 mIU/L (N.V. 0.4–4.5 mIU/L), increased.

Tg—42,794 μg/L (N.V. <0.1 μg/L), very increased.

Anti-Tg—32 kIU/L (N.V. <115 kIU/L), normal (Fig. 7.83).

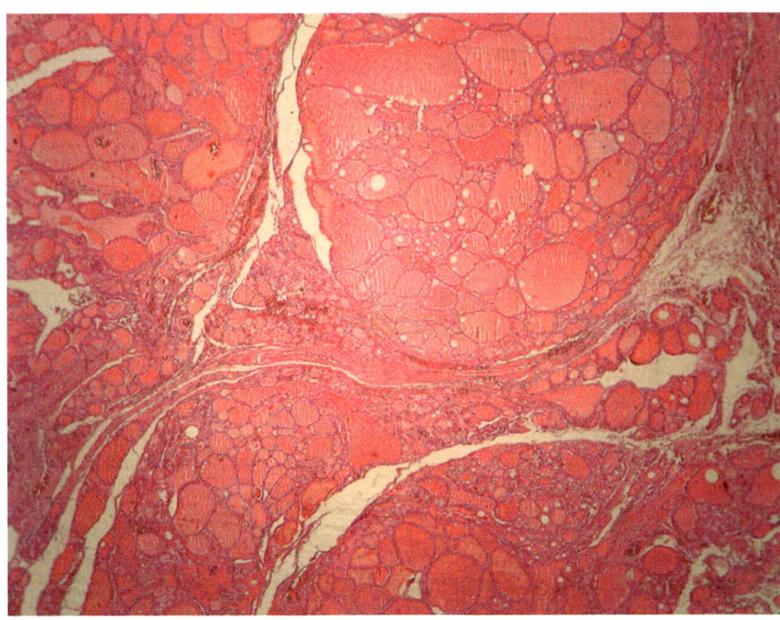

Fig. 7.82 Histology of nodular goiter

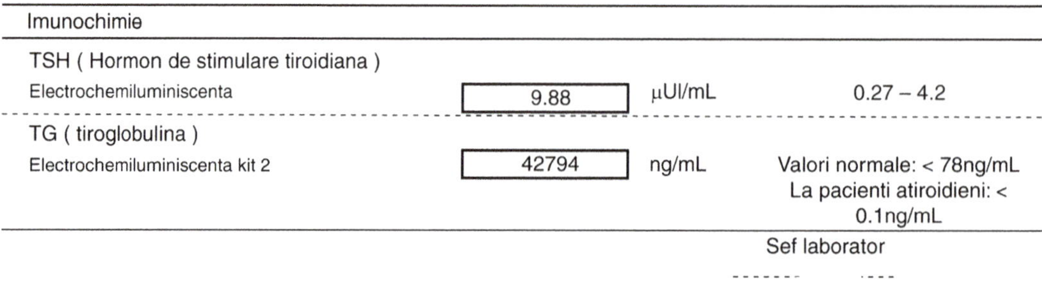

Imunochimie			
TSH (Hormon de stimulare tiroidiana)			
Electrochemiluminiscenta	9.88	µUI/mL	0.27 – 4.2
TG (tiroglobulina)			
Electrochemiluminiscenta kit 2	42794	ng/mL	Valori normale: < 78ng/mL La pacienti atiroidieni: < 0.1ng/mL
			Sef laborator

Fig. 7.83 Tumor marker results (Tg) very increased, without hormone replacement and with a high level of TSH; negative anti-Tg

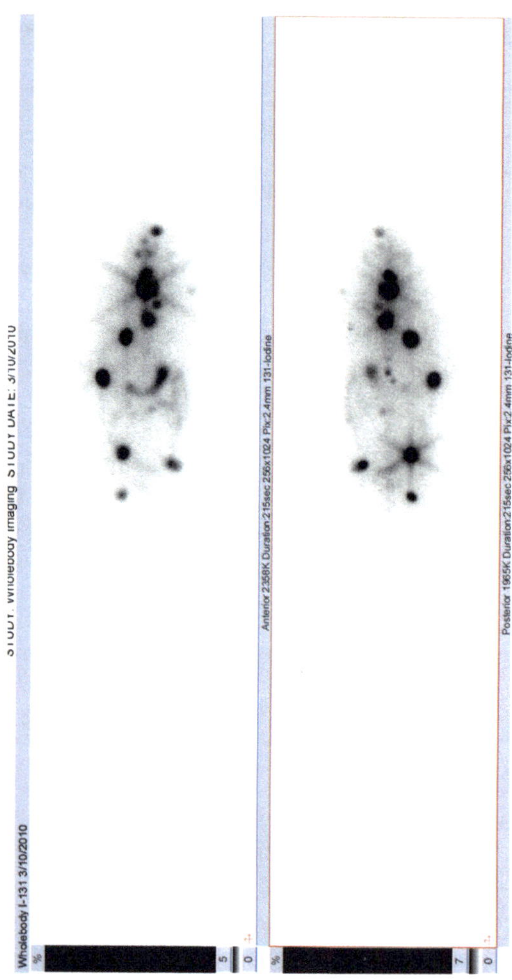

Fig. 7.84 WBS I-131 at 48 h posttherapy: thyroid recurrence with pathologic radioiodine uptake within lymph nodes and multiple distant metastases, including the skull, lungs, and bones

Findings:

The patient received 120 mCi (4.44 GBq) of I-131. The WBS I-131 posttherapy showed the presence of radioiodine uptake in the thyroid area and multiple pathologic foci of radioiodine uptake (Fig. 7.84). There are multiple distant and locoregional pathologic uptakes. The WBS I-131 after next therapy sequence, at 6 months, is presented in Fig. 7.85.

Conclusion:

Follicular thyroid carcinoma with multiple locoregional and iodine active distant metastases.

Key Points

- The case presented is essential to underline the particular feature of aggressive follicular thyroid carcinoma and the need of careful evaluation.
- The differential diagnosis between follicular carcinoma and adenoma is sometimes extremely difficult; that means that one should always judge the clinical case with respect to the cancer rule out.
- The normal hormonal status in case of total thyroidectomy, in the absence of any specific drug intake, must aware about the presence of thyroid secreting tissue (thyroid remnant, ectopic tissue, or metastases).
- In the presence of thyroid tissue, the distant metastases are dramatically less responsive to therapy; these will be much sensitive to irradiation after the destruction of thyroid remnant.
- The brain metastases should always be removed before radioiodine therapy; it is recommended to have prior external radiotherapy, in the situation of an impossible action.

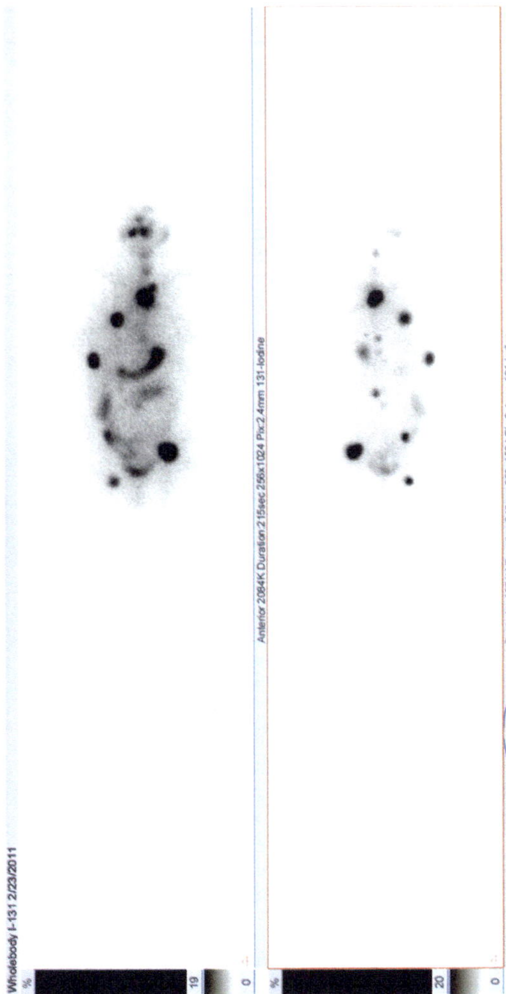

Fig. 7.85 WBS I-131 at 48 h after the second dose of I-131: favorable course at the level of the thyroid tumor recurrence and persistent distance metastases

Case 3: Follicular Thyroid Carcinoma

History:

A 51-year-old male, with the diagnosis of metastatic follicular thyroid carcinoma in the right hip, with pathologic fracture, operated 1 month before. The patient was referred after the total thyroidectomy and selective lymphadenectomy.

T4bN1bM1 (stage IVC)

Clinical examination:

The patient presented severe low back pain and right hip pain in the last 2 years, without being examined in any medical center. The pathologic fracture occurring recently determined the operation and the discovery of metastases of the follicular thyroid cancer at that level. The primary site was attributed to the thyroid. The removal of the thyroid confirmed the diagnosis. The patient presented severe motor deficiency, constant pain, and weight loss of 15 kg in the last 6 months.

The neck examination revealed a post-thyroidectomy scar, without any palpable tumor mass or lymph nodes in the cervical area.

Examinations:

CT of the pelvis—multiple osteolytic bone areas.

TSH before total thyroidectomy—0.001 mIU/L (N.V. 0.4–4.5 mIU/L), severely suppressed.

TSH—50.27 mIU/L (N.V. 0.4–4.5 mIU/L), increased.

Tg > 100,000 μg/L (N.V. <0.1 μg/L), extremely increased.

Anti-Tg—1490 kIU/L (N.V. <115 kIU/L), normal (Fig. 7.86).

Findings:

The patient received 167 mCi (6.12 GBq) of I-131. The WBS I-131 posttherapy showed the presence of pathologic radioiodine uptake in the thyroid area and multiple pathologic foci of radioiodine uptake. There are multiple distant and locoregional pathologic uptakes (Fig. 7.87). The WBS I-131 after next therapy sequence at 6 months is presented in Fig. 7.88.

Conclusion:

Follicular thyroid carcinoma with multiple locoregional and iodine active distant metastases

Key Points

- The very low TSH serum level expresses the high hormonal production by the metastatic tissues. This particular situation should be noted and not be confused with any other hyperthyroidism cases, where malignancy was not ruled out.
- The favorable response of lung metastases comparing with bone metastases underlines that in case of bone involvement, it is better, whenever is possible, to have the surgical removal, rather than I-131 irradiation.
- The severe evolution presented above is highly suggestive for the aggressive presentation of thyroid malignant disease in case of male patients.

Imunochimic			
Anti-tiroglobulina Electrochemiluminiscenta	1490	UI/mL	≤ 115
TSH (Hormon de stimulare tiroidiana) Electrochemiluminiscenta	50.27	µUI/mL	0.27 – 4.2
TG (tiroglobulina) Electrochemiluminiscenta kit 2	>100000	ng/mL	Valori normale: < 78ng/mL La pacienti atiroidieni: < 0.1ng/mL

sef laborator

Fig. 7.86 Tumor marker results (Tg and anti-Tg), without hormone replacement and with a high level of TSH

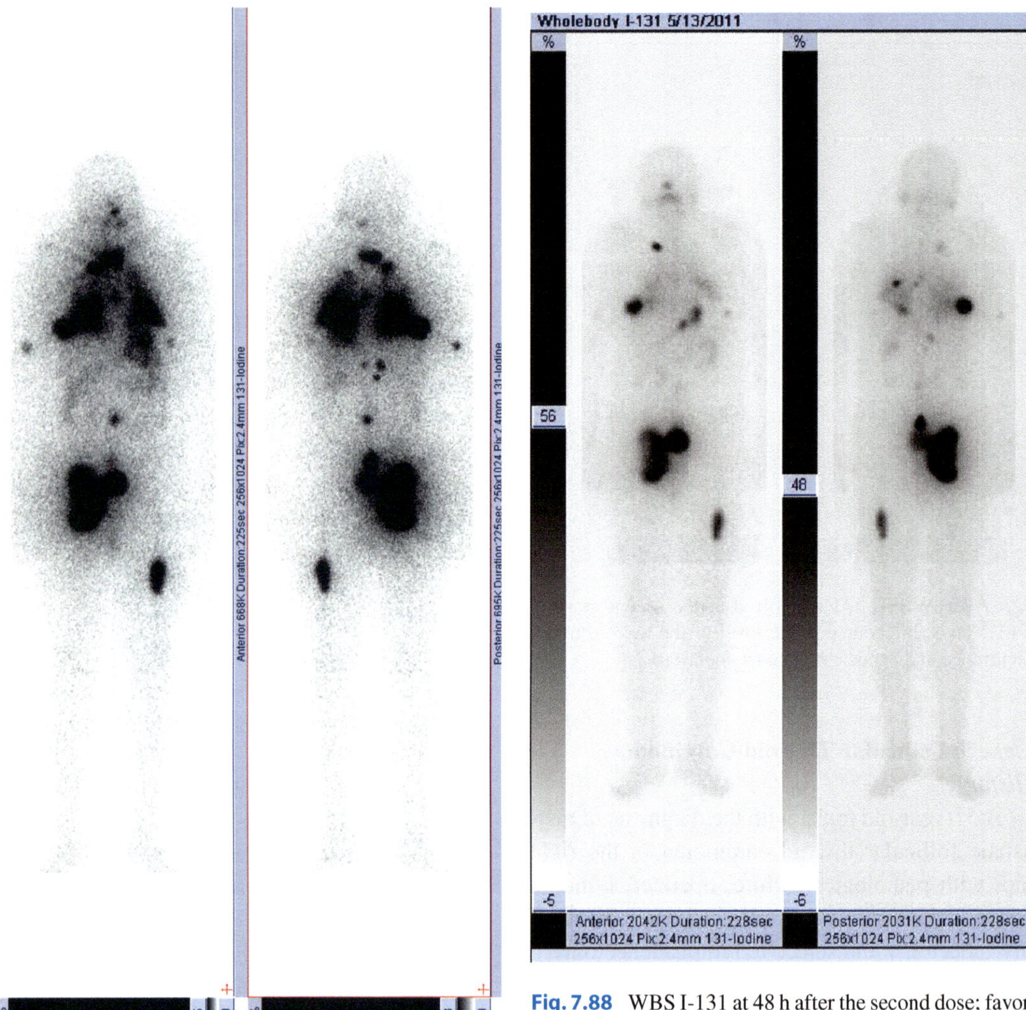

Fig. 7.87 WBS I-131 at 48 h posttherapy; mediastinum, lung, and bone distant metastases

Fig. 7.88 WBS I-131 at 48 h after the second dose; favorable course at the level of the lungs

Case 4: Lymph Node Metastases of Papillary Thyroid Carcinoma

History:

A 48-year-old female, with the diagnosis of papillary thyroid carcinoma, is operated 5 weeks before with total thyroidectomy and selective lymph node dissection. She was referred for radioiodine therapy.

T4aN1bM0—stage IVA

Clinical examination:

The patient was 6 weeks post-thyroidectomy; the patient had no thyroid hormonal replacement after the thyroidectomy; moderate signs of myxedema.

The neck examination revealed a post-thyroidectomy scar, without any palpable tumor mass or lymph nodes in the cervical area. No other signs or symptoms to be mentioned.

Examinations:

Ultrasound—no thyroid tissue remnant; a solid, hypoechogenic structure of lymph node, highly suggestive for metastases, was described in the right lateral-cervical part of the upper region (level II upper jugular nodes).

TSH—27.37 mIU/L (N.V. 0.4–4.5 mIU/L), increased.

Tg—622 μg/L (N.V. <0.1 μg/L), very increased.

Anti-Tg—78 kIU/L (N.V. <115 kIU/L), normal.

Findings:

The patient received 5 mCi (185 MBq) of I-131. The diagnosis of WBS I-131 showed very important uptake of the radioiodine in the upper mediastinum and pathologic foci of radioiodine uptake in the right upper jugular lymph nodes (Fig. 7.89).

Conclusion:

The patient presented lymph node metastases of papillary thyroid cancer and thyroid remnant in the upper mediastinum. The patient was referred to surgery for a second operation.

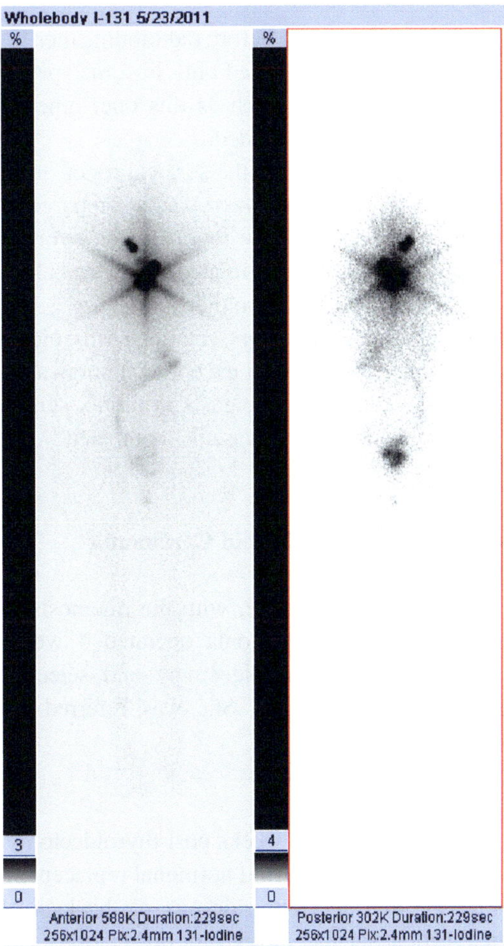

Fig. 7.89 WBS I-131 at 48 h after the diagnostic dose of I-131. Lymph node uptake in the right upper jugular lymph nodes and thyroid remnant in the upper mediastinum

Key Points

- The discrepancy between the surgical report and the high value of Tg postsurgery suggested the necessity of a diagnostic WBS I-131, which revealed the persistence of metastatic lymph nodes and the thorax extension of the thyroid tumor.

- The WBS I-131 before radioiodine therapy is recommended only in some specific situations such as this one; other way, it can be avoided.
- It is important for the surgical report to be detailed, analyzed, and compared with the pathology report; any discordance must be correlated with clinical, ultrasound, and serological findings.
- The mediastinum presentation of thyroid tumors requests an exceptional surgical protocol, with specialists in thorax surgery and/or cardiovascular competency.

Case 5: Papillary Thyroid Carcinoma

History:

A 53-year-old female, with the diagnosis of papillary thyroid carcinoma operated 4 weeks before with total thyroidectomy and selective lymph node dissection. She was referred for radioiodine therapy.

T2N0M0—stage II

Clinical examination:

The patient was 4 weeks post-thyroidectomy; the patient had no thyroid hormonal replacement after the thyroidectomy; despite of the lack of medication, she had no signs of myxedema.

The neck examination revealed a post-thyroidectomy scar, without any palpable tumor mass or lymph nodes in the cervical area. No other signs or symptoms to be mentioned.

Examinations:

The ultrasound revealed thyroid tissue remnant in both thyroid lobes.

TSH—41.7 mIU/L (N.V. 0.4–4.5 mIU/L), increased.

Tg—31 μg/L (N.V. <0.1 μg/L).

Anti-Tg < 10 kIU/L (N.V. <115 kIU/L), normal.

Findings:

The patient received 70 mCi (2.59 GBq) of I-131. WBS I-131 showed very important uptake of radioiodine in the thyroid bed and no other regional or distant pathologic uptakes (Fig. 7.90). Similar images Figs. 7.91 and 7.92.

Conclusion:

Very important thyroid remnant in the thyroid bed

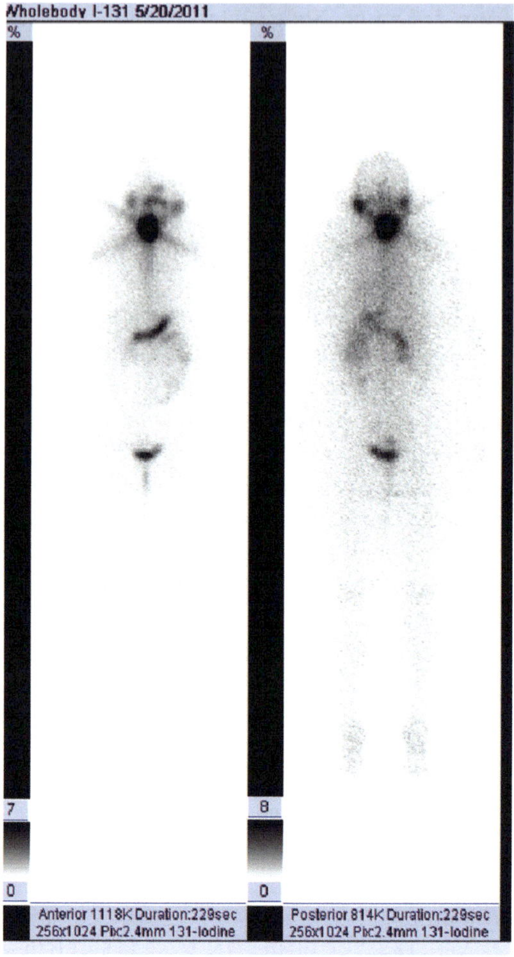

Fig. 7.90 WBS I-131 after therapeutic dose of I-131. Important thyroid remnant

Key Points

- The discrepancy between the surgical report, which frequently mentions the total thyroidectomy and the aspect of WBS posttherapy, is common in routine practice. The value of Tg and the ultrasound volume evaluation are able to suggest the necessity for reoperation.
- The important thyroid residual tissues in the neck area have a large amount of retained radioiodine; there is a characteristic "star" effect, which appears in the images, as is presented in the images above.

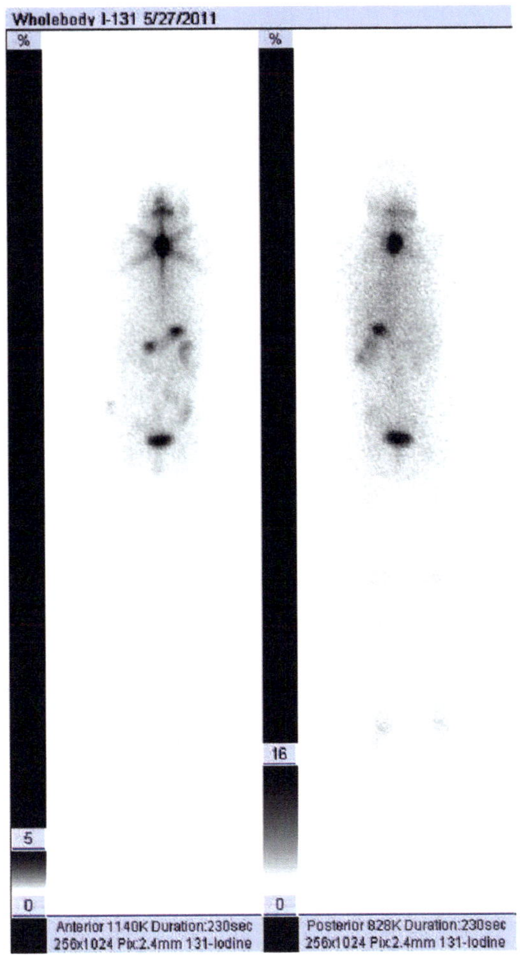

Fig. 7.91 WBS I-131 at 48 h post-administration of I-131; important thyroid remnant

Fig. 7.92 WBS I-131 at 48 h post-administration of I-131; important thyroid remnant

- Figures 7.93 and 7.94 present the usual normal WBS I-131 after total thyroidectomy, with a minimal thyroid remnant.
- Figures 7.95 and 7.96 present a less frequent situation after radical thyroid surgery; no residual thyroid tissue is observed on the scans. The images reveal an important activity in the digestive area, mainly in the stomach, which is normal at 24 h; this activity will be normally decreased if the scan is performed later at 48 h.
- The early scans obtained at 24 h show important activity in the esophagus and stomach, which may mask possible lesions in the lung, spine, etc. The activity in the esophagus needs special attention because of the possible mask of an ectopic thyroid tissue at the tongue base or because of a possible confusion with a pathologic tissue (Fig. 7.97). SPECT/CT in this situation is essential for the differential diagnosis.
- In the situation of a large or very active thyroid remnant, the activity is massively up taking; the rest of the organs physiologically passed by radioiodine and the background of the body contour do not appear on the image (Fig. 7.98).

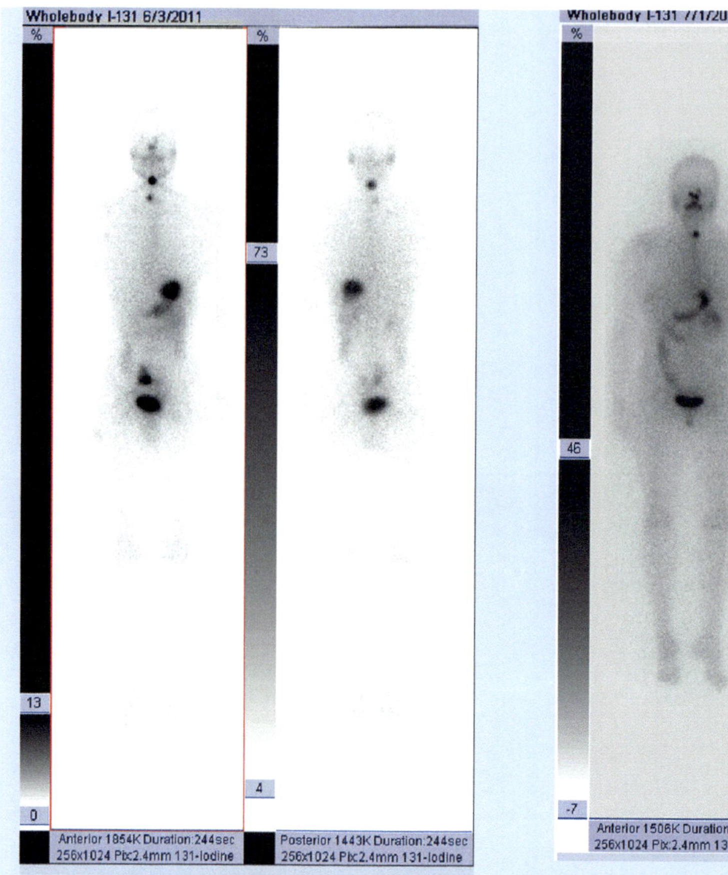

Fig. 7.93 WBS I-131 at 24 h posttherapy, with normal minimal thyroid remnant

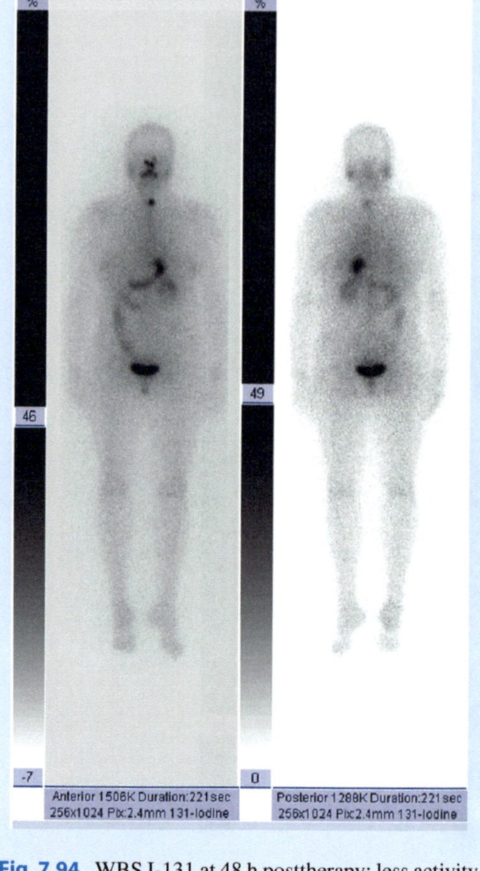

Fig. 7.94 WBS I-131 at 48 h posttherapy; less activity in the digestive area

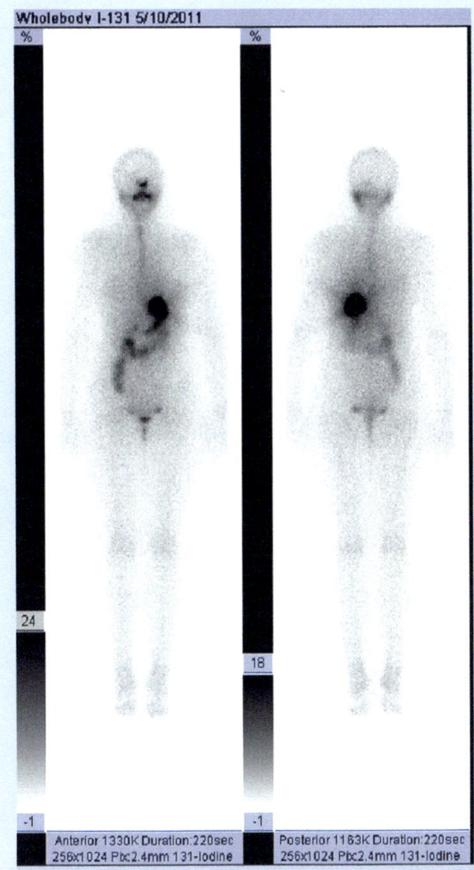

Fig. 7.95 WBS I-131 at 24 h posttherapy; no pathologic radioiodine uptake; no thyroid remnant uptake; normal visualization of the esophagus and stomach

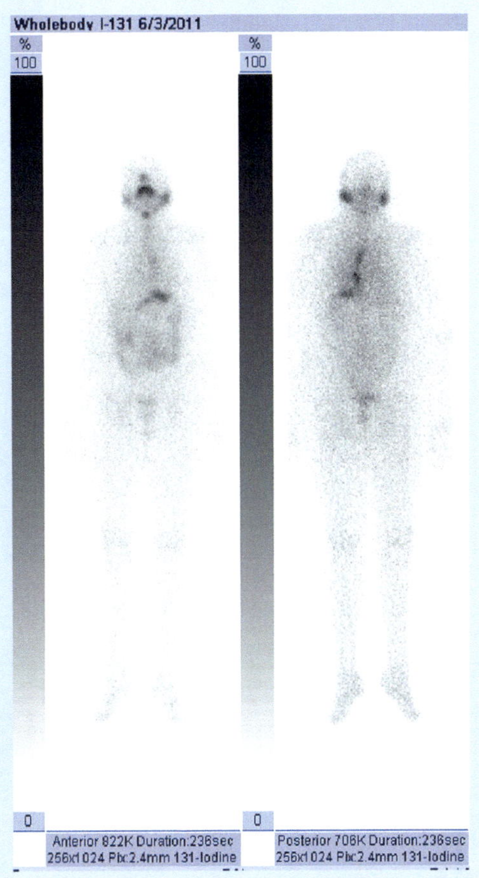

Fig. 7.96 WBS I-131 at 48 h posttherapy; no pathologic radioiodine uptake; no thyroid remnant uptake; normal visualization of the esophagus, with less activity in the stomach

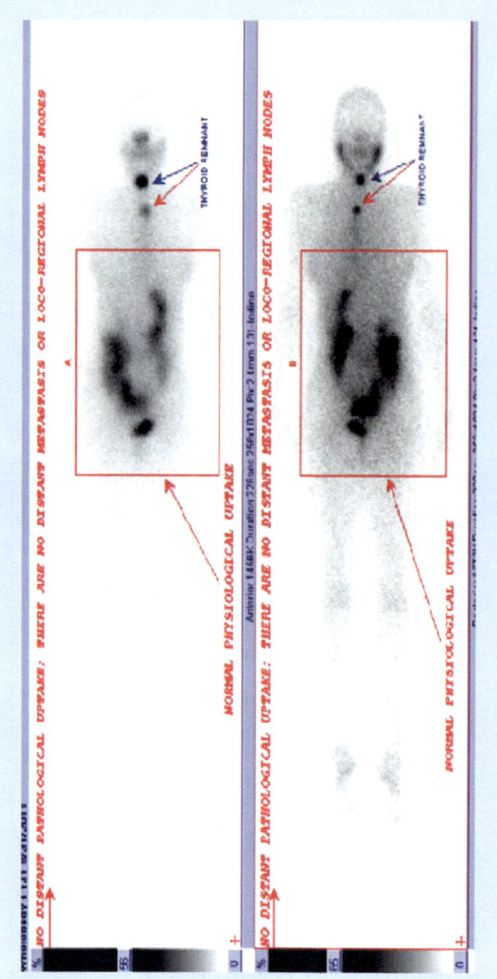

Fig. 7.97 WBS I-131—24 h. Thyroid remnant uptake and residual activity in the digestive and urinary systems

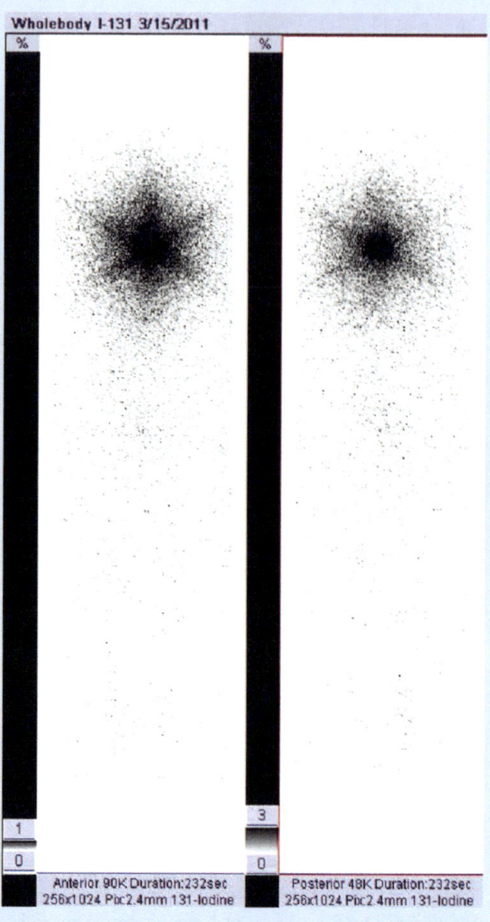

Fig. 7.98 WBS I-131 after 5 mCi (185 MBq) shows massive uptake due to an ectopic thyroid gland situated in the mediastinum. No digestive and urinary physiologic uptake

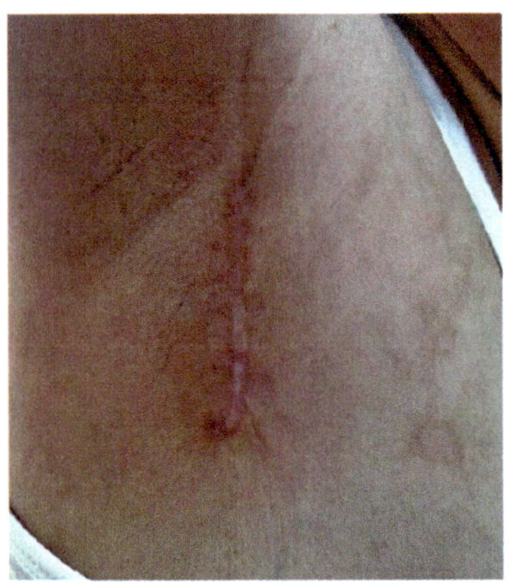

Fig. 7.99 Endoscopic axillary thyroid lobectomy

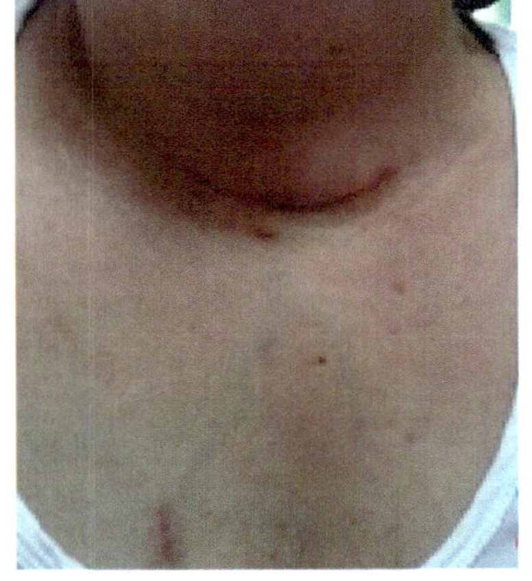

Fig. 7.100 Anterior cervical thyroidectomy

Case 6: Papillary Thyroid Carcinoma

History:

A 34-year-old female, with the diagnosis of papillary thyroid carcinoma, operated 2 months before with total right lobectomy on an endoscopic approach, via the right axilla. The pathology showed variant papillary thyroid carcinoma tall cells. Total thyroidectomy and central selective lymph node dissection were indicated.

T4aN0M0—stage I.

Clinical examination:

The patient was 3 weeks post-thyroidectomy; after thyroidectomy she had thyroid hormonal replacement, with 150 μg/day l-thyroxin; no signs of myxedema.

The right axilla presented a scar after the first endoscopic surgery of lobectomy (Fig. 7.99).

The neck examination revealed a post-thyroidectomy scar, without any palpable tumor mass or lymph nodes in the cervical area (Fig. 7.100).

No other signs or symptoms to be mentioned.

Examinations:

The ultrasound revealed no thyroid tissue remnant in thyroid area.

TSH—0.25 mIU/L (N.V. 0.4–4.5 mIU/L), under hormone replacement.

The patient had recombinant TSH (rTSH) stimulation with 0.9 mg I.M. for 2 consecutive days.

TSH—102 mIU/L (N.V. 0.4–4.5 mIU/L).

Tg—18.4 μg/L (N.V. <0.1 μg/L).

Anti-Tg < 10 kIU/L (N.V. <115 kIU/L), normal.

Findings:

Due to the histology (Fig. 7.101) and extension T4a, the patient received 70 mCi (2.59 GBq) of I-131. WBS I-131 showed minimal uptake of radioiodine in the thyroid bed and no other regional or distant pathologic uptakes (Fig. 7.102).

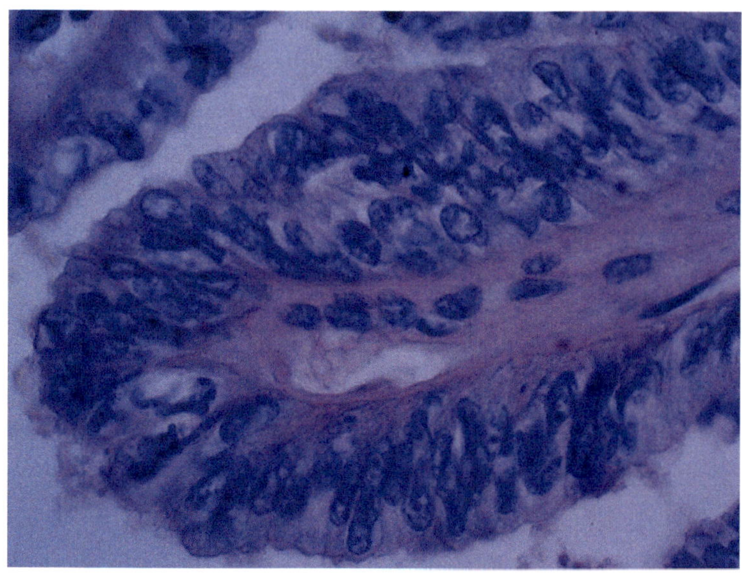

Fig. 7.101 Histology of papillary thyroid carcinoma with tall cells (HE ×400)

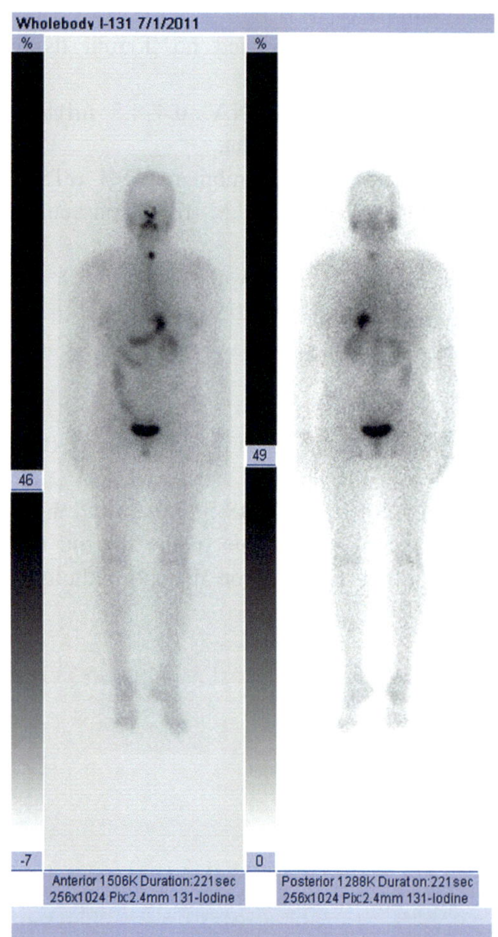

Fig. 7.102 WBS I-131 minimal thyroid remnant

Case 7: Papillary Thyroid Carcinoma

History:

A 21-year-old male, with the diagnosis of papillary thyroid carcinoma and operated with total thyroidectomy and selective right lymphadenectomy, was referred after the removal of the thyroid for evaluation and specific therapy.

T4bN1bM0 (stage I)

Clinical examination:

The patient was 5 weeks post-thyroidectomy; he had no thyroid hormonal replacement after the thyroidectomy; minimal signs of hormonal deficiency, puffy face, and fatigue.

The neck examination revealed a post-thyroidectomy scar, without any palpable tumor mass or lymph nodes in the cervical area. No other signs or symptoms to be mentioned.

Examinations:

Ultrasound—no thyroid tissue remnant; no pathologic lymph nodes

TSH—94.08 mIU/L (N.V. 0.4–4.5 mIU/L), increased.

Tg—53.44 μg/L (N.V. <0.1 μg/L), increased.

Anti-Tg > 4000 kIU/L (N.V. <115 kIU/L), very increased (Fig. 7.103).

Suspicion of distant metastases.

Findings:

The patient received 100 mCi (3.7 GBq) of I-131. The WBS I-131 posttherapy showed the presence of radioiodine uptake in the thyroid area and diffuse lung radioiodine uptake (Fig. 7.104) in March 2007. Figure 7.105 presents the WBS I-131 after next therapy sequence (July 2007). Figure 7.106 presents the tumor marker values related to the third scan performed at the end of October 2007, which was a negative scan (Fig. 7.107).

Conclusion:

Papillary thyroid carcinoma with lymph nodes and lung metastases

Key Points

- The case presented is essential to underline the potential aggressive evolution in young male patients.
- The presence of thyroglobulin's antibodies (anti-Tg) has crucial importance in the correct assessment of the disease.
- The comparative positive and negative WBS I-131 (Figs. 7.104 and 7.107) in the presence of serum high levels of anti-Tg shows how WBS I-131 may alter the therapy approaches.
- The common patterns of papillary thyroid lung metastases are the diffuse, spread, microscopic, and tuberculosis-like metastases. Sometimes the plain radiology films may be normal and highly discordant with the nuclear images. Less frequent, the lung metastases of papillary thyroid carcinoma may be macronodular as they are presented in Fig. 7.108.

Case 8: Papillary Thyroid Carcinoma

History:

A 46-year-old female, with the diagnosis of papillary thyroid carcinoma developed from a Hashimoto's thyroiditis, operated with total thyroidectomy and central compartment lymph node removal, is referred for radioiodine therapy.

T4aN0M0—stage IVA

Clinical examination:

The patient was 6 weeks postsurgery, in the absence of thyroid hormonal replacement. She was presenting signs of myxedema.

The neck examination revealed a post-thyroidectomy scar, without any palpable tumor mass or lymph nodes in the cervical area. No other signs or symptoms to be mentioned.

Examinations:

The ultrasound revealed no thyroid tissue remnant; no pathologic lymph nodes

TSH > 100 mIU/L (N.V. 0.4–4.5 mIU/L), very increased.

Tg < 0.1 µg/L (N.V. <0.1 µg/L), normal.

Anti-Tg—2774 kIU/L (N.V. <115 kIU/L), increased.

Findings:

The patient received 100 mCi (3.7 GBq) of I-131. The WBS I-131 posttherapy showed *no* radioiodine uptake in the body.

No distant and no locoregional pathologic uptake (Fig. 7.109). There will be complementary imaging tests in order to exclude the persistent disease.

Conclusion:

Negative WBS I-131

20 March 2007

Denumire	Rezultat	UM	Valori de referinta
Anti-tiroglobulina Electrochemiluminiscenta	> 4000	UI/mL	≤ 115
TSH (Hormon de stimulare tiroidiana) Electrochemiluminiscenta	94.08	µUI/mL	0.27 – 4.2
TG (tiroglobulina) Electrochemiluminiscenta kit 2	53.44	ng/mL	Valori normale: < 78ng/mL La pacienti atiroidieni: < 0.1ng/mL

Medic de laborator

Fig. 7.103 Tumor marker results (Tg and anti-Tg), without hormone replacement and with a high level of TSH

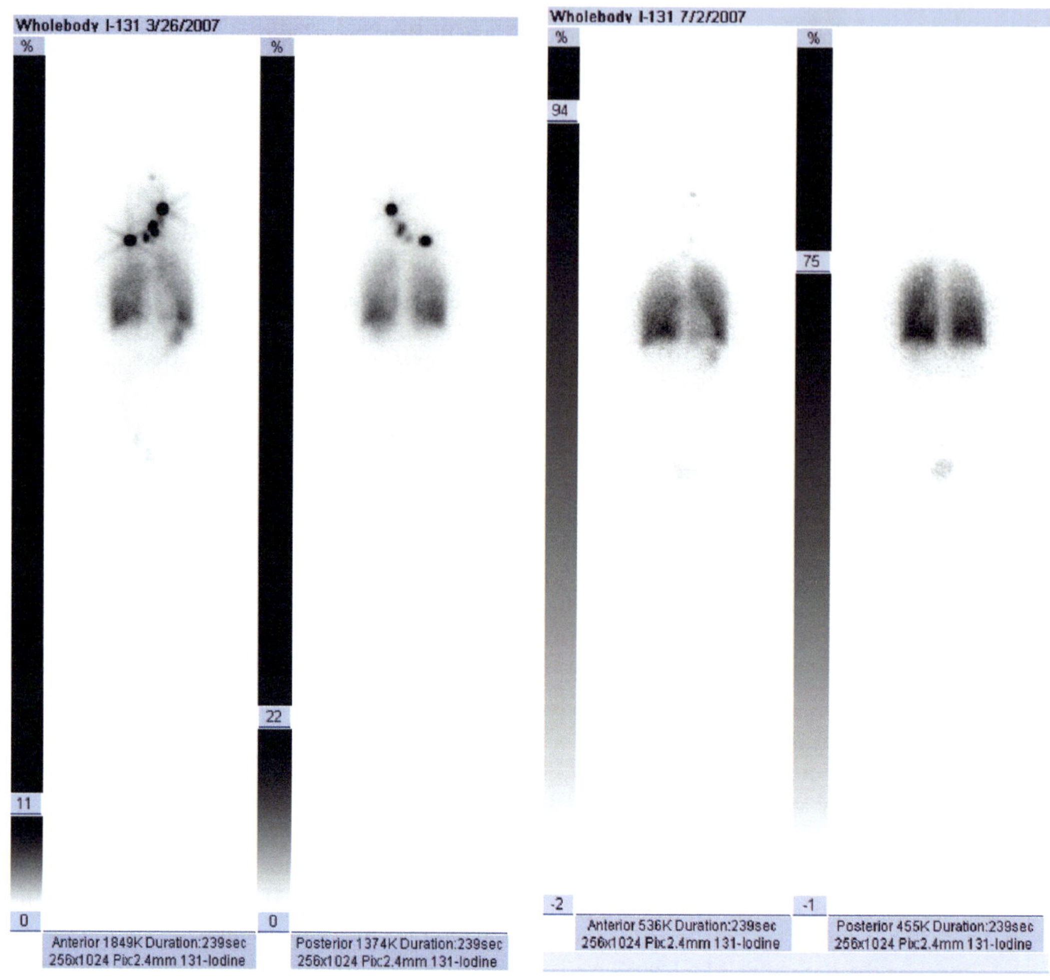

Fig. 7.104 WBS I-131—lung and lymph nodes metastases

Fig. 7.105 WBS I-131—lung metastases; favorable course at lymph node level

Denumire	Rezultat	UM	Valori de referinta
Anti-tiroglobulina Electrochemiluminiscenta	> 4000	UI/mL	≤ 115
TSH (Hormon de stimulare tiroidiana) Electrochemiluminiscenta	> 100	µUI/mL	0.27 – 4.2
TG (tiroglobulina) Electrochemiluminiscenta kit 2	2.64	ng/mL	Valori normale: < 78ng/mL La pacienti atiroidieni: < 0.1ng/mL

Medic de laborator

Fig. 7.106 Tumor marker results (Tg and anti-Tg), without hormone replacement and with a high level of TSH and anti-Tg

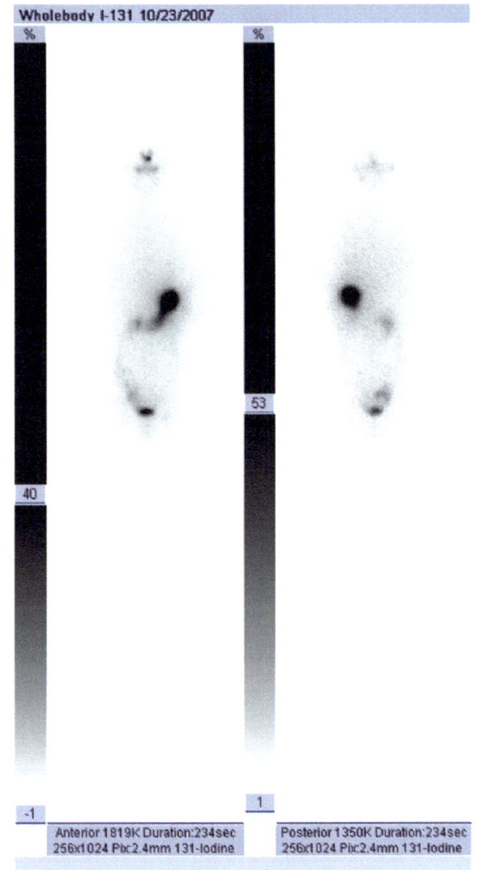

Fig. 7.107 WBS I-131—negative scan

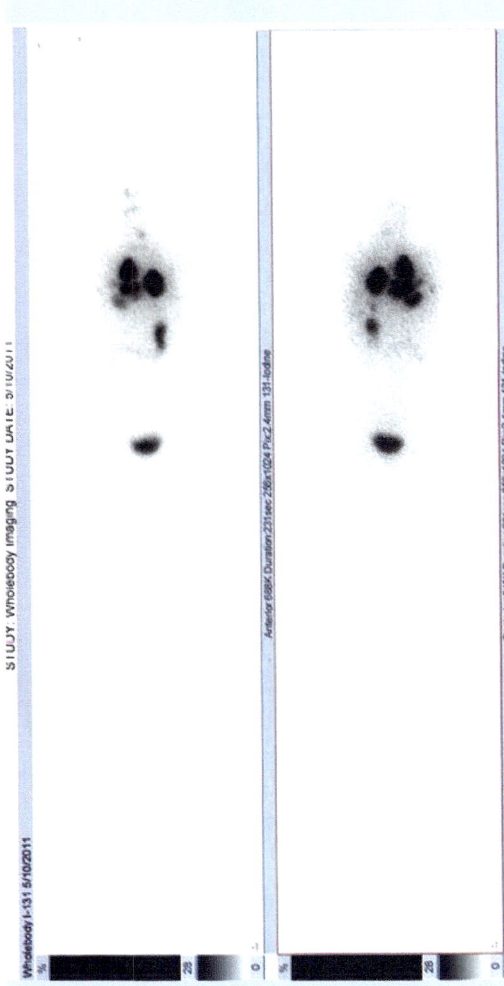

Fig. 7.108 WBS I-131 macronodular lung metastases

Key Points

- The decision of radioiodine therapy was made with respect to the histology and stage of the disease and of the risk group.
- The undetectable value of Tg in the presence of antibodies (anti-Tg) and with stimulated TSH is not sensitive for the absence of the thyroid tissue and of the disease; the WBS I-131 posttherapy showed a negative scan.
- This presence of anti-Tg requests special attention in the assessment of the disease.

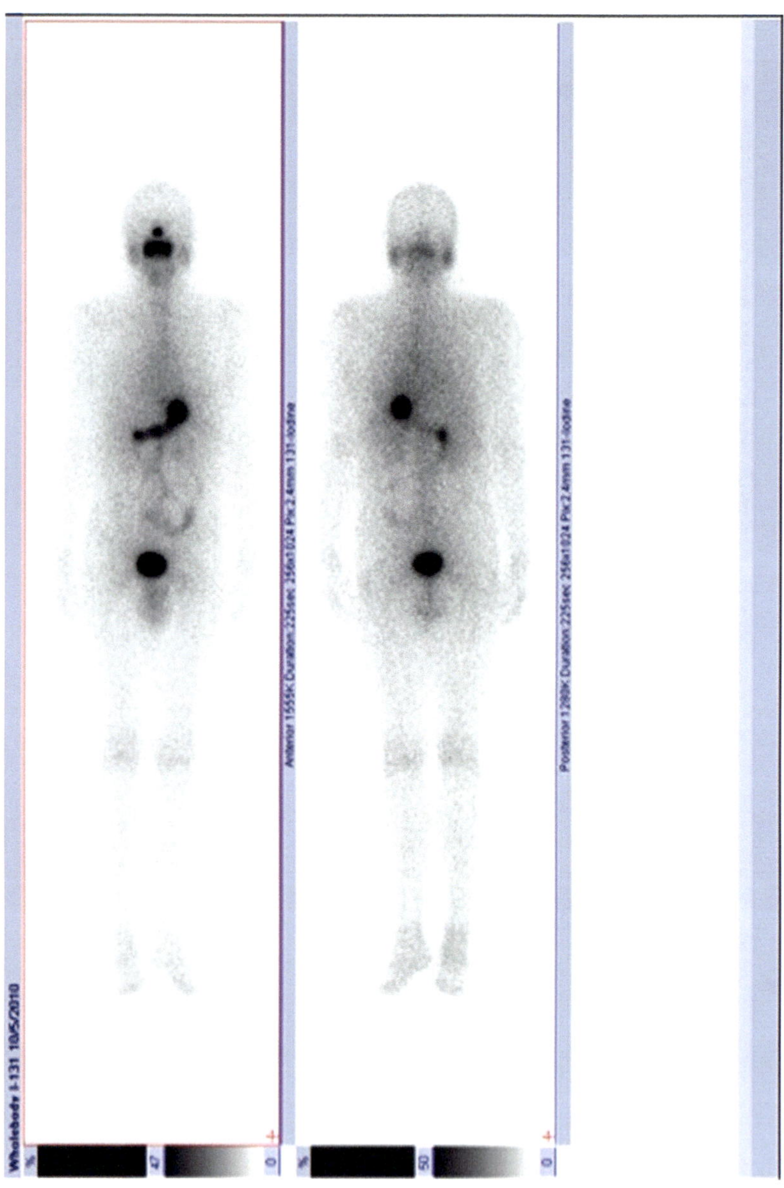

Fig. 7.109 WBS I-131 at 24 h posttherapy. No thyroid tissue remnant. No distant metastasis

Case 9: Papillary Thyroid Carcinoma

History:

A 32-year-old female, with the diagnosis of papillary thyroid carcinoma operated with affirmative total thyroidectomy and central compartment lymph node removal, is referred for radioiodine therapy.

T4aN0M0—stage I

Clinical examination:

The patient was 3 weeks postsurgery, in the absence of thyroid hormonal replacement.

The neck examination revealed a post-thyroidectomy scar, without any palpable tumor mass or lymph nodes in the cervical area. No other signs or symptoms to be mentioned.

Examinations:

The ultrasound revealed small thyroid tissue remnant in the right thyroid bed, cu microcalcification; no pathologic lymph nodes; the remnant tissue was suggesting an extension on retroclavicular area, but no further details were possible to be mentioned.

TSH > 100 mIU/L (N.V. 0.4–4.5 mIU/L), very increased.

Tg—836.2 μg/L (N.V. <0.1 μg/L), very increased considering the recent thyroidectomy.

Anti-Tg—67 kIU/L (N.V. <115 kIU/L), normal.

Findings:

Considering the value of Tg and the suspected extension in the mediastinum, the patient was submitted for a Tc-99m Pt scan, which revealed a tumor mass corresponding for a thyroid extended in the mediastinum (Fig. 7.110). No indication for WBS I-131, due to important thyroid tissue in the right retroclavicular area. The patient was submitted for reintervention in a thoracic surgery service and advised to return after for completion of the adjuvant therapies.

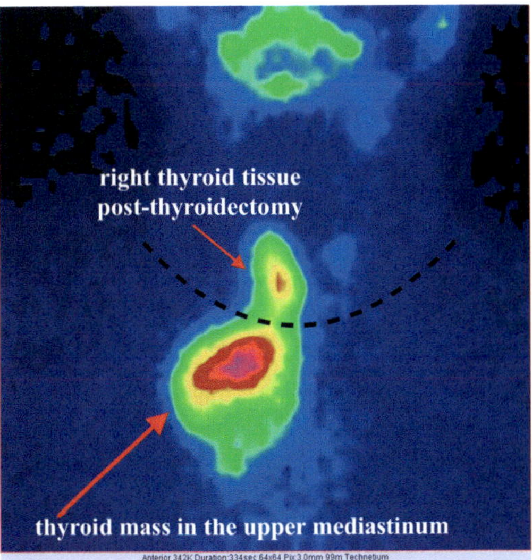

Fig. 7.110 Tc-99m Pt showing important thyroid tissue in the right retroclavicular area and upper mediastinum in a DTC case, after subtotal thyroidectomy

Key Points

- Thyroid ultrasound is the best and first option in the evaluation of DTC after surgery, before considering the I-131 therapy. It is limited for the evaluation of the disease in the mediastinum and with misinterpretation if the surgery is recent.
- A simple Tc-99m Pt scan might be a precious tool in the decision-making for a reintervention.
- In case of important thyroid mass, the WBS I-131 should be avoided, due to stunning effect B9 and to avidity of the tissue and the distant metastases frequently being not revealed.

References

Ali SZ, Cibas ES (eds) (2010) The Bethesda System for Reporting Thyroid Cytolopahology: definition, criteria and explanatory notes. Springer, New York

AACE/AME/ETA (2010) Thyroid nodule guidelines. Endocr Pract 16(suppl 1):1–43

Alexander EK, Pearce EN, Brent GA et al (2017) 2016 Guidelines of the American Thyroid Association for the Diagnosis and Management of Thyroid Disease during pregnancy and the postpartum. Thyroid. doi:10.1089/thy.2016.0457. [Epub ahead of print]

American Association of Clinical Endocrinologists. American College of Endocrinology (2002) AACE/AAES medical/surgical guidelines for clinical practice: management of thyroid carcinoma. Endocr Pract 7(3):202–220

Anderson GS, Fish S, Nakhoda K et al (2003) Comparison of I-123 and I-131 for wholebody imaging after stimulation by recombinant human thyrotropin: a preliminary report. Clin Nucl Med 28:93–96

ATA/AACE (2011) Hyperthyroidism management guidelines. Endocr Pract 17(3):1–65

Avram AM (2014) Radioiodine scintigraphy with SPECT/CT: an important diagnostic tool for thyroid cancer staging and risk stratification. J Nucl Med 53(5):754–764

Azizi G, Keller J, Lewis M et al (2013) Performance of elastography for the evaluation of thyroid nodules: a prospective study. Thyroid 23(6):734–740

Belhocine T, Rachinsky I, Akincioglu C (2008) How useful is an integrated SPECT/CT in clinical setting and research: evaluation of a low radiation dose 4 slice system. Open Med Imaging J 2:80–108

Biondi B, Filetti S, Schlumberger M (2005) Thyroid-hormone therapy and thyroid cancer: a reassessment. Nat Clin Pract Endocrinol Metab 1:32–40

Bongiovanni M, Cibas H, Faquin W (2010) The role of thyroid fine needle aspiration cytology and the Bethesda system for reporting thyroid cytopathology. Diagn Histopathol 17(3):95–105

Bojunga J, Herrmann E, Meyer G et al (2010) Real-time elastography for the differentiation of benign and malignant thyroid nodules: a meta-analysis. Thyroid 20:1145–1150

Braga M, Cavalcanti TC, Collaco LM et al (2001) Efficacy of ultrasound-guided fine-needle aspiration biopsy in the diagnosis of complex thyroid nodules. J Clin Endocrinol Metab 86:4089–4091

Braverman LE, Utiger RD (2000) The thyroid. In: Werner SC, Ingbar SH (ed). 8th edn. Lippincott, Philadelphia

Brose MS et al (2014) Sorafenib in locally advanced or metastatic, radioactive iodine-refractory, differentiated thyroid cancer: a randomized, double-blind, phase 3 trial. Lancet 384(9940):319–328

Cabanillas ME, Waguespack SG, Bronstein Y et al (2010) Treatment with tyrosine kinase inhibitors for patients with differentiated thyroid cancer: the M. D. Anderson experience. J Clin Endocrinol Metab 95(6): 2588–2595

Canchola AJ, Horn-Ross PL, Purdie DM (2006) Risk of second primary malignancies in women with papillary thyroid cancer. Am J Epidemiol 163:521–527

Carril JM, Quirce R, Serrano J et al (1997) Total-body scintigraphy with thallium-201 and iodine-131 in the follow-up of differentiated thyroid cancer. J Nucl Med 38:686–692

Ceccarelli C, Battisti P, Gasperi M et al (1999) Radiation dose to the testes after 131-I therapy for ablation of post-surgical thyroid remnants in patients with differentiated thyroid cancer. J Nucl Med 40:1716–1721

Chianelli M, Todino V, Graziano F et al (2009) Low dose (2.0 GBq; 54 mCi) radioiodine postsurgical remnant ablation in thyroid cancer: comparison between hormone withdrawal and use of rhTSH in low risk patients. Eur J Endocrinol 160:431–436

Clark OH, Duh QY (1990) Thyroid cancer. The thyroid gland. Raven Press, New York

Collins J, Rossi ED, Chandra A, Ali SZ (2015) Terminology and nomenclature schemes for reporting thyroid cytopathology: an overview. Semin Diagn Pathol 32(4):258–263

DeLellis RA, Lloyd RV, Heitz PU et al (2004) World Health Organization classification of tumours. Pathology and genetics of endocrine organs. IARC Press, Lyon, pp 49–135

DeVita VT, Hellman S, Rosenberg AS (2001) Cancer. Principles and practice of oncology, 6th edn. Lippincott, Philadelphia

Dunn JT (1994) When is a thyroid nodule a sporadic medullary carcinoma. J Clin Endocrinol Metab 78:824–825

Elisei R, Bottici V, Luchetti F et al (2004) Impact of routine measurement of serum calcitonin on the diagnosis and outcome of medullary thyroid cancer: experience in 10,864 patients with nodular thyroid disorders. J Clin Endocrinol Metab 89:163–168

Francis GL, Waguespack SG, Bauer AJ et al (2015) American Thyroid Association Guidelines Task Force. Management guidelines for children with thyroid nodules and differentiated thyroid cancer. Thyroid 25(7):716–759

Franzius C, Dietlein M, Biermann M et al (2007) Procedure guideline for radioiodine therapy and 131-iodine whole-body scintigraphy in paediatric patients with differentiated thyroid cancer. Nuklearmedizin 46:224–231

Frates MC, Benson CB, Charboneau JW et al (2005) Management of thyroid nodules detected at US: Society of Radiologists in Ultrasound consensus conference statement. Radiology 237:794–800

Gaengler S, Andrianou XD, Piciu A et al (2017) Iodine status and thyroid nodules in females: a comparison of Cyprus and Romania. Public Health 143:37–43

Gerard SK, Cavalieri RR (2002) I-123 diagnostic thyroid tumour whole-body scanning with imaging at 6, 24, and 48 hours. Clin Nucl Med 27:1–8

Giovanella L, Campenni A, Treglia G et al (2016) Molecular imaging with (99m)Tc-MIBI and molecular testing for mutations in differentiating benign from malignant follicular neoplasm: a prospective comparison. Eur J Nucl Med Mol Imaging 43:1018–1026

Goldstein RE, Netterville JL, Burkey B et al (2002) Implications of follicular neoplasms, atypia, and lesions suspicious for malignancy diagnosed by fine-needle aspiration of thyroid nodules. Ann Surg 235:656–662

Guarino E, Tarantini B, Pilli T et al (2005) Presurgical serum thyroglobulin has no prognostic value in papillary thyroid cancer. Thyroid 15:1041–1045

British Thyroid Association and Royal College of Physicians (2007) Guidelines for the management of thyroid cancer in adults, 2nd edn. Publication Unit of the Royal College of Physicians. British Thyroid Association and Royal College of Physicians, London

British Thyroid Association and Royal College of Physicians (2014) Guidelines for the management of thyroid cancer in adults (3rd ed). Publication unit of the Royal College of Physicians. British Thyroid Association and Royal College of Physicians, London. Clin Endocrinol (Oxf) 81(suppl 1):1–122

Hackshaw A, Harmer C, Mallick U et al (2007) 131I activity for remnant ablation in patients with differentiated thyroid cancer: a systematic review. J Clin Endocrinol Metab 92:28–38

Hay ID, Bergstralh EJ, Goellner JR et al (1993) Predicting outcome in papillary thyroid carcinoma: development of a reliable prognostic scoring system in a cohort of 1779 patients surgically treated at one institution during 1940 through 1989. Surgery 114:1050–1058

Hay ID, Thompson GB, Grant CS et al (2002) Papillary thyroid carcinoma managed at the Mayo clinic during six decades (1940–1999): temporal trends in initial therapy and long-term outcome in 2444 consecutively treated patients. World J Surg (8):879–885

Haugen BR, Alexander EK, Bible KC et al (2016) American Thyroid Association management guidelines for adult patients with thyroid nodules and differentiated thyroid cancer: the American Thyroid Association guidelines task force on thyroid nodules and differentiated thyroid cancer. Thyroid 26(1):1–133

Haugen BR, Sawka AM, Alexander EK et al (2017) The ATA guidelines on management of thyroid nodules and differentiated thyroid cancer task force review and recommendation on the proposed renaming of EFVPTC without invasion to NIFTP. Thyroid. doi:10.1089/thy.2016.0628. [Epub ahead of print]

Haugen BR (2017) 2015 American Thyroid Association management guidelines for adult patients with thyroid nodules and differentiated thyroid cancer: what is new and what has changed? Cancer 123(3):372–381

Hegedus L (2001) Thyroid ultrasound. Endocrinol Metab Clin North Am 30:339–360

Ho AL, Grewal RK, Leboeuf R et al (2013) Selumetinib-enhanced radioiodine uptake in advanced thyroid cancer. N Engl J Med 368:623–632

Hodgson NC, Button J, Solorzano CC (2004) Thyroid cancer: is the incidence still increasing? Ann Surg Oncol 11:1093–1097

Ito Y, Suzuki S, Ito K et al (2016) Tyrosine-kinase inhibitors to treat radioiodine-refracted, metastatic, or recurred and progressive differentiated thyroid carcinoma [Review]. Endocr J 63(7):597–602

Koizumi K, Tamaki N, Inoue T, Subcommittee on Survey of Nuclear Medicine Practice in Japan (2004) Nuclear medicine practice in Japan: a report of the 5th nationwide survey in 2002. Ann Nucl Med 18(1):73–78

Koh J, Moon HJ, Park JS et al (2016) Variability in interpretation of ultrasound elastography and gray-scale ultrasound in assessing thyroid nodules. Ultrasound Med Biol 42(1):51–59

Lee SG, Lee WK, Lee HS et al (2017) Practical performance of the 2015 American Thyroid Association Guidelines for predicting tumor recurrence in patients with papillary thyroid cancer in South Korea. Thyroid 27(2):174–181

Leger AF, Pellan M, Dagousset F et al (2005) A case of stunning of lung and bone metastases of papillary thyroid cancer after a therapeutic dose (3.7 GBq) of 131I and review of the literature: implications for sequential treatments. Br J Radiol 78:428–432

Luster M, Clarke SE, Dietlein M et al (2008) Guidelines for radioiodine therapy of differentiated thyroid cancer. Eur J Nucl Med Mol Imaging. doi:10.1007/s00259-008-0883-1

Machens A, Holzhausen HJ, Dralle H (2005) The prognostic value of primary tumour size in papillary and follicular thyroid carcinoma. Cancer 103:2269–2273

Mandel SJ, Mandel L (2003) Radioactive iodine and the salivary glands. Thyroid 13:265–271

Marqusee E, Benson CB, Frates MC et al (2000) Usefulness of ultrasonography in the management of nodular thyroid disease. Ann Intern Med 133:696–700

Mayr B, Brabant G, von zur Muhlen A (1999) Incidental detection of familial medullary thyroid carcinoma by calcitonin screening for nodular thyroid disease. Eur J Endocrinol 141:286–289

Mazzaferri EL, Jhiang SM (1994) Long term impact of initial surgical and medical therapy on papillary and follicular thyroid cancer. Am J Med 49:418–428

Mazzaferri EL, Robbins RJ, Spencer CA et al (2003) A consensus report of the role of serum thyroglobulin as a monitoring method for low-risk patients with papillary thyroid carcinoma. J Clin Endocrinol Metab 88:1433–1441

Mitchell AL, Gandhi A, Scott-Coombes D, Perros P (2016) Management of thyroid cancer: United Kingdom National Multidisciplinary Guidelines. J Laryngol Otol 130(S2):S150–S160

NCCN (2016) Clinical practice guidelines in oncology (NCCN Guidelines) Thyroid Carcinoma. Version 1.2016, 07/08/2016 © National Comprehensive Cancer Network, Inc. 2016

Nikiforov YE (2015) Thyroid cancer in 2015: molecular landscape of thyroid cancer continues to be deciphered. Nat Rev Endocrinol 12(2):67–68

Nikiforov YE, Seethala RR, Tallini G et al (2016) Nomenclature revision for encapsulated follicular variant of papillary thyroid carcinoma: a paradigm shift to reduce overtreatment of indolent tumors. JAMA Oncol 2(8):1023–1029

Pacini F, Burroni L, Ciuoli C et al (2004) Management of thyroid nodules: a clinicopathological, evidence based approach. Eur J Nucl Med Mol Imaging 31:1443–1449

Pacini F, Ladenson PW, Schlumberger M et al (2006a) Radioiodine ablation of thyroid remnants after preparation with recombinant human thyrotropin in differentiated thyroid carcinoma: results of an international, randomized controlled study. J Clin Endocrinol Metab 91:926–932

Pacini F, Schlumberger M, Dralle H et al (2006b) European consensus for the management of patients with differentiated thyroid carcinoma of the follicular epithelium. Eur J Endocrinol 154:787–803

Pacini F, Castagna MG, Brilli L et al (2010) Thyroid cancer ESMO clinical practice guideline for diagnosis, treatment and follow-up. Ann Oncol 21(5):214–219

Pacini F, Brianzoni E, Durante C et al (2016) Recommendations for post-surgical thyroid ablation in differentiated thyroid cancer: a 2015 position statement of the Italian Society of Endocrinology. J Endocrinol Invest 39(3):341–347

Piccardo A, Puntoni M, Treglia G et al (2016) Thyroid nodules with indeterminate cytology: prospective comparison between 18F-FDG-PET/CT, multiparametric neck ultrasonography, 99mTc-MIBI scintigraphy and histology. Eur J Endocrinol 174:693–703

Piciu D, Piciu A, Irimie A (2012) Thyroid cancer in children: a 20-year study at a Romanian oncology institute. Endocr J 59(6):489–496

Piciu D, Irimie A, Piciu A (2014) Investigation of thyroid carcinoma over 40 years, using the database of the Ion Chiricuta Institute of Oncology Cluj-Napoca. J BUON 19(2):524–529

Piciu D, Pestean C, Barbus E et al (2016) Second malignancies in patients with differentiated thyroid carcinoma treated with low and medium activities of radioactive I-131. Clujul Med 89(3):384–389

Pitoia F, Ward L, Wohllk N et al (2009) Recommendations of the Latin American Thyroid Society on diagnosis and management of differentiated thyroid cancer. Arq Bras Endocrinol Metabol 53(7):884–887

Rare cancers list. http://www.rarecare.eu/rarecancers/rarecancers.asp. Accessed 30 Oct 2011

Robbins J (1992) Treatment of thyroid cancer in childhood. Proceedings of a workshop National Institutes of Health, Bethesda, 1992, vol 3–61, pp 109–167

Robbins RJ, Wan Q, Grewal RK et al (2006) Real-time prognosis for metastatic thyroid carcinoma based on FDG-PET scanning. J Clin Endocrinol Metab 91:498–505

Rubino C, de Vathaire F, Dottorini ME et al (2003) Second primary malignancies in thyroid cancer patients. Br J Cancer 89:1638–1644

Russ G, Royer B, Bigorgne C et al (2013) Prospective evaluation of thyroid imaging reporting and data system on 4550 nodules with and without elastography. Eur J Endocrinol 168:649–655

Ross DS, Burch HB, Cooper DS et al (2016) American Thyroid Association guidelines for diagnosis and management of hyperthyroidism and other causes of thyrotoxicosis. Thyroid 26(10):1343–1421

Sassolas G, Hafdi-Nejjari Z, Remontet L et al (2009) Thyroid cancer: is the incidence rise abating? Eur J Endocrinol 160(1):71–79

Sawka AM, Lakra DC, Lea J et al (2008) A systematic review examining the effects of therapeutic radioactive iodine on ovarian function and future pregnancy in female thyroid cancer survivors. Clin Endocrinol (Oxf) 69:479–490

Schlumberger M, Pacini F (1999) Thyroid tumours. Nucleon, Paris

Schulmberger M, Pacini F, Tuttle RM (2016) Thyroid tumours, 4th edn. IME, Paris

Schlumberger M, De Vathaire F, Ceccarelli C et al (1996) Exposure to radioactive iodine-131 for scintigraphy or therapy does not preclude pregnancy in thyroid cancer patients. J Nucl Med 37:606–612

Schlumberger M, Pacini F, Wiersinga WM et al (2004) Follow-up and management of differentiated thyroid carcinoma: European perspective in clinical practice. Eur J Endocrinol 151:539–548

Shah JP, Loree TR et al (1992) Prognostic factors in differentiated carcinoma of the thyroid gland. Am J Surg 164:658–661

Sipple JR (1961) The association of pheocromocitoma with cancer of thyroid gland. Am J Med 31:163–166

Staging & Grading Thyroid Carcinoma (2010) AJCC cancer staging handbook, 7th edn. Springer, New York

Stokkel MPM, Handkiewicz Junak D, Lassmann M et al (2010) EANM procedure guidelines for therapy of benign thyroid disease. Eur J Nucl Med Mol Imaging 37:2218–2228. doi:10.1007/s00259-010-1536-8

Takami H, Ito Y, Okamoto T et al (2014) Revisiting the guidelines issued by the Japanese Society of Thyroid Surgeons and Japan Association of Endocrine Surgeons: a gradual move towards consensus between Japanese and western practice in the management of thyroid carcinoma. World J Surg 38(8):2002–2010

The American Thyroid Association Guidelines Taskforce (2006) Management guidelines for patients with thyroid nodules and differentiated thyroid cancer. Thyroid 2(16):3–34

The American Thyroid Association Guidelines Taskforce on Thyroid Nodules and Differentiated Thyroid Cancer (2009) Revised American thyroid association management guidelines for patients with thyroid nodules and differentiated thyroid cancer. Thyroid 19:1195–1214

The American Thyroid Association Guidelines Task Force (2009) Medullary thyroid cancer: management guidelines of the American Thyroid Association. Thyroid 19(6):565–612

The American Thyroid Association Taskforce on Radioiodine Safety (2011) Radiation safety in the treatment of patients with thyroid diseases by radioiodine 131I: practice recommendations of the American Thyroid Association. Thyroid 21(4):1–12

Tuttle RM, Haugen B, Perrier ND (2017) Updated American Joint Committee on Cancer/Tumor-Node-Metastasis Staging System for Differentiated and Anaplastic Thyroid Cancer (Eighth Edition): what changed and why? Thyroid 27(6):751–756. doi: 10.1089/thy.2017.0102. Epub 19 May 2017. PubMed PMID: 28463585; PubMed Central PMCID: PMC5467103

Tuttle RM, Leboeuf R, Robbins RJ, Qualey R, Pentlow K, Larson SM, Chan CY (2006) Empiric radioactive iodine dosing regimens frequently exceed maximum tolerated activity levels in elderly patients with thyroid cancer. J Nucl Med 47(10):1587–1591

Tuttle RM, Brokhin M, Omry G et al (2008) Recombinant human TSH-assisted radioactive iodine remnant ablation achieves short-term clinical recurrence rates similar to those of traditional thyroid hormone withdrawal. J Nucl Med 49:764–770

Velzen van AJM, Chemaly CR (2005) A survey on radioisotope production capabilities, therapeutic radioisotope usage in Europe, expected trends in terms of research activities. European Commission report, pp 1–328

Verburg FA, Stokkel MP, Düren C et al (2010) No survival difference after successful (131) I ablation between patients with initially low-risk and high-risk differentiated thyroid cancer. Eur J Nucl Med Mol Imaging 37:276–283

Willegaignon J, Saptenza M, Ono C et al (2011) Outpatient radioiodine therapy for thyroid cancer. Clin Nucl Med 36(6):440–446

Yi KH (2016) The revised 2016 Korean Thyroid Association guidelines for thyroid nodules and cancers: differences from the 2015 American Thyroid Association guidelines. Endocrinol Metab (Seoul) 31(3):373–378

Zimmermann D, Hay ID, Gough IR (1988) Papillary thyroid carcinoma in children and adults: long-term follow-up of 1039 patients conservatively treated at one institution during three decades. Surgery 104:1157–1166

The Parathyroid Glands

8

Nature does nothing uselessly.

Aristotle (Antique philosopher 384–322 B.C.E)

8.1 Anatomy of the Parathyroid Glands

The parathyroid glands are located on the posterior surface of the thyroid gland.

These four glands produce the parathyroid hormone (PTH), which helps to maintain calcium homeostasis by acting on the renal tubule as well as calcium stores in the skeletal system and by acting indirectly on the gastrointestinal tract through the activation of vitamin D (Beierwaltes 1991).

The parathyroid glands have a distinct, encapsulated, smooth surface that differs from the thyroid gland, which has a more lobular surface.

The superior parathyroid glands are most commonly located in the posterior-lateral aspect of the superior pole of the thyroid gland at the cricothyroid cartilage junction. They are most commonly found 1 cm above the intersection of the inferior thyroid artery and the recurrent laryngeal nerve.

The inferior parathyroid glands are more variable in location and are most commonly found near the lower pole of the thyroid.

8.1.1 Embryology

The parathyroid glands develop from the endoderm of the third and fourth pharyngeal pouches. The inferior parathyroid glands are derived from the dorsal part of the third pharyngeal pouch, and the thymus arises from the ventral part of the third pharyngeal pouch. As the inferior parathyroid glands and the thymus migrate together toward the mediastinum, they eventually separate. In most cases, the inferior parathyroid glands become localized near the inferior poles of the thyroid, and the thymus continues to migrate toward the mediastinum.

The superior parathyroid glands are derived from the fourth pharyngeal pouch. The superior parathyroid glands migrate a shorter distance than the inferior glands, which results in a relatively more constant location in the neck.

8.1.2 Parathyroid Vascularity

The inferior parathyroid glands that descend into the anterior mediastinum are usually vascularized by the inferior thyroid artery. If a parathyroid is positioned low in the mediastinum, a thymus branch of the internal thoracic artery or even a direct branch of the aortic arch may supply it.

The superior parathyroid gland is usually supplied by the inferior thyroid artery or by an anastomotic branch between the inferior thyroid and the superior thyroid artery.

The location of the inferior parathyroid glands exhibits a greater degree of variability than the superior parathyroid glands. If the inferior glands

D. Piciu, *Nuclear Endocrinology*, DOI 10.1007/978-3-319-56582-8_8

fail to separate or separation from the thymus is delayed during their descent, the inferior glands may have ectopic locations within the superior mediastinum.

In rare cases, there is possible to have an intrathyroid localization. After adhering to the thyroid capsule, the parathyroid gland may actually enter the thyroid gland and embed there rather than remaining outside the gland. This situation results in an intrathyroidal parathyroid gland.

8.2 Physiology and Pathophysiology of the Parathyroid Glands

The main role of the parathyroid glands is to produce the parathyroid hormone (PTH). The secretion of PTH is stimulated by low serum calcium concentration and inhibited by high serum calcium. The role of phosphate is not yet clear: high concentration stimulates secretion of PTH; this effect may also be an indirect consequence of the high phosphate levels, causing a reduction of serum calcium concentration (Arnold et al. 2002; Beierwaltes 1991).

The two forms of vitamin D (D2-ergocalciferol and D3-cholecalciferol) are both activated to the calcitriol form. The calcitriol has an important role in the long-term regulation of plasma calcium levels and therefore regulates the PTH production.

PTH acts on the kidney and the bone as targeted organs.

The effects of PTH on the kidney:

- Increases the reabsorption of calcium from the urine
- Increases the excretion of phosphates
- Increases the expression of the enzyme 1α-hydroxylase, which activates vitamin D

The effects of PTH on the bone:

- High levels increase bone resorption by stimulating the activity of osteoclasts.
- Low levels increase bone formation by stimulating the activity of osteoblasts.

8.2.1 Pathophysiology

More than 80% of the patients are asymptomatic or have nonspecific symptoms (AACE/AAES Task Force 2005), while less than 15% of the patients are presenting renal stones.

Primary hyperparathyroidism results from a solitary adenoma in over 80% of the cases. Diffuse hyperplasia occurs less frequently and very rarely, parathyroid carcinoma accounting for about 4%.

The treatment is surgical with a high success rate of 90–95%, even if preoperative localization procedures fail sometimes in identifying the lesion. Recurrent and persistent hyperparathyroidism is usually related to aberrant or ectopically located glands or recurrent hyperplasia. Re-exploration is technically difficult with a higher morbidity and poorer success rate than initial surgery. Diffuse hyperplasia accounts for approximately 15% of the cases of primary hyperparathyroidism, and a substantial proportion of these may occur in association with the multiple endocrine neoplasias (MEN syndromes).

Secondary hyperparathyroidism is associated with chronic renal failure being also related to diffuse hyperplasia; it may require surgical therapy due to progressive bone disease. Secondary hyperparathyroidism is consequent to a chronic hypocalcemic condition that can be caused also by gastrointestinal malabsorption, dietary rickets, and ingestion of drugs, like phenytoin, phenobarbital, and laxative, which generate a decreased intestinal absorption of calcium. The continuous stimulus to produce and to secrete PTH results in parathyroid gland hyperplasia. Secondary hyperparathyroidism is a frequent and serious complication in hemodialysis patients. Because all the parathyroid tissue is stimulated, the presence of unsuspected supernumerary glands has major impact in terms of surgical failure.

Tertiary hyperparathyroidism occurs during dialysis. Tertiary hyperparathyroidism is a condition where parathyroid hyperplasia, secondary to chronic hypocalcemia, becomes autonomous with development of hypercalcemia. This condition generally does not regress after the correction of the underlying cause that generated chronic hypocalcemia. Usually, in tertiary hyperparathyroidism, we find asymmetrical parathyroid gland hyperplasia. Tertiary hyperparathyroidism is also used to designate hyperparathyroidism that persists or develops after renal transplantation.

The Parathyroid Center from Tampa General Hospital, Florida, USA, led by one of the most experienced parathyroid surgeons, Professor Jim Norman, has created a brief description of the main features of pathologic parathyroid gland known as: "The ten parathyroid rules of Norman" (Norman 1998b).

8.2.2 The Ten Parathyroid Rules of Norman

1. There are no drugs that will treat parathyroid disease.
2. Most (>95%) parathyroid patients have symptoms.
3. Symptoms of parathyroid disease do not correlate with the level of calcium in the blood.
4. All patients with parathyroid disease have fluctuating calcium levels and PTH levels.
5. All patients with hyperparathyroidism will develop osteoporosis.
6. The drugs for osteoporosis do not treat parathyroid disease.
7. Parathyroid disease will get worse with time in all patients.
8. There is only one treatment for primary hyperparathyroidism: surgery.
9. Most parathyroid patients can be cured with a minimal operation.
10. The success rate and complication rate for parathyroid surgery are very dependent upon the surgeon's experience.

8.3 Diagnosis of the Parathyroid Glands

8.3.1 Clinical Examination

The parathyroid glands are less accessible to clinical inspection than is the thyroid gland. Despite this, the very specific determination of the parathyroid hormone (PTH) gives the physicians the possibility to find the suggestive elements for parathyroid disorders, in patient's history.

8.3.1.1 History

The parathyroid glands require a careful anamnestic interview with the aim to discover signs and symptoms that might be related to hypo- or hypercalcemia (Silverberg et al. 1999). Parathyroid pathology may have genetic determinism; primary hyperparathyroidism is possible to occur in association with other endocrine diseases, in the so-called multiple endocrine neoplasias (MENs). The history is one of the first steps in the patient evaluation.

Due to severe increasing of nodular goiter and extensive thyroid surgery, the pathology of accidental parathyroidectomy is frequent nowadays. The hypocalcemia mainly due to deficient intake or surgery complications does not represent a topic in the present chapter. The area of interest will be the identification of parathyroid glands responsive for primary hyperparathyroidism.

History will bring information related to:

- Age (elder patients need special attention, firstly because of more frequent bone pathologies)
- Gender (female are more frequently affected by osteoporosis, and the differential diagnosis to parathyroid involvement is crucial for the evolution of the disease)
- Signs/symptoms of hyper-/hypothyroidism; the thyroid pathology may be associated
- Rapid evolution of osteoporosis severity
- Digestive disorders due to hypercalcemia (ulcers)
- Kidney lithiasis and gallbladder lithiasis occurring in familial aggregation

History may report association of parathyroid pathology into other syndromes:

- Found to have association with medullary thyroid cancer (MTC) in MEN II syndrome (parathyroid adenoma, MTC, and pheochromocytoma)

- Pituitary adenoma, parathyroid adenoma, and pancreatic islet cell tumors (MEN I—Wermer syndrome)

History elements suggestive for malignancy:

- Rapid progressive enlargement of cervical area
- Hoarseness
- Dysphagia
- Dyspnea
- Lymph nodes
- Familial history of other thyroid cancers

8.3.1.2 Clinical Examination

The situation of parathyroid glands in the posterior face of the thyroid gland makes the inspection almost impossible. The lymph node palpation of the neck should be carefully done undergoing the known pathways of lymphatic drainage: lateral-cervical, supraclavicular, and submental. This is important for the situation of associated thyroid tumors; parathyroid cancer is very unusual, so the signs determined by this pathology are very rare.

The inspection will focus mainly on the signs and symptoms produced by hypercalcemia or by other neuroendocrine mediators secreted by the associated tumors.

General signs:

- Bone pain with different degrees of impairment of motion and bone abnormalities
- Diarrhea if it is in association with carcinoid tumors
- Anxiety, depression, lethargy, and other mental disorders
- Weight loss
- Muscle weakness
- Extreme fatigue
- Other symptoms dictated by associated neuroendocrine tumors

All these signs and symptoms come to design a clinical, very severe presentation that may very seriously affect the patient's status and which frequently is discovered late.

8.3.2 Laboratory Serum Testing

8.3.2.1 Calcium, Phosphorus, and Vitamin D

With primary hyperparathyroidism, people will generally have high calcium and high PTH levels, while phosphorus levels are often low. Secondary hyperparathyroidism is usually due to kidney failure, and phosphorus may not be excreted efficiently, disrupting its balance with calcium. Kidney disease may also make those affected unable to produce the active form of vitamin D, and this means that they are unable to properly absorb calcium from the diet. As phosphorus levels build up and calcium levels fall, PTH is secreted. Secondary hyperparathyroidism can also be caused by any other condition that causes low calcium, such as malabsorption of calcium due to intestinal disease and vitamin D deficiency.

8.3.2.2 Parathyroid Hormone

PTH is ordered to help diagnose the reason for a low or high calcium level and to help distinguish between parathyroid-related and non-parathyroid-related causes. A doctor will evaluate both calcium and PTH results together to determine whether the levels are appropriate and are in balance as they should be.

Calcium-PTH relationship (AACE/AAES 2005)

- If calcium levels are low and PTH levels are high, the parathyroid glands respond, as they should, and produce appropriate amounts of PTH. A low calcium level must be investigated by further measurement of vitamin D, phosphorus, and magnesium levels.
- If calcium levels are low and PTH levels are normal or low, then PTH is not responding, and the person tested probably has hypoparathyroidism. It may be due to a variety of conditions and may be persistent, progressive, or transient. Those affected will generally have low PTH levels, low calcium levels, and high phosphorus levels.
- If calcium levels are high and PTH levels are high, then the parathyroid glands are producing inappropriate amounts of PTH. This is the current presentation of hyperparathyroidism.

- If calcium levels are high and PTH levels are low, then the parathyroid glands are responding properly, but the doctor is likely to perform further investigations to check for non-parathyroid-related reasons for the elevated calcium.

PTH levels will vary during the day, peaking at about 2 a.m. Specimens are usually drawn about 8 a.m. Drugs that may increase PTH levels include phosphates, anticonvulsants, steroids, isoniazid, lithium, etc. PTH can be measured in the blood in several different forms, intact PTH, N-terminal PTH, mid-molecule PTH, and C-terminal PTH, and different tests are used in different clinical situations. The average PTH level is of 10–60 ng/L.

Insulin, glucagon, calcitonin, prolactin, gastrin, chromogranin A, serotonin, metanephrine, etc., all these hormones may be determined in the serum level having a contribution in the clinical status of parathyroid association in other endocrinopathies.

8.3.3 Imaging Tests

8.3.3.1 Plain Films

In the parathyroid pathology are indicated hands films and other bone radiographies for the diagnosis of bone abnormalities

8.3.3.2 Dual-Energy X-Ray Absorptiometry

DEXA may be useful in assessing chronic bone mineral loss. Significant bone loss—absolute (*T* score) and age-related (*Z* score)—may be an indicator for parathyroid surgery, in primary hyperparathyroidism, even in the absence of other clinical symptoms or marked hypercalcemia.

8.3.3.3 CT and MRI

The association with different other endocrine tumors makes the imagistic tests for parathyroid to be complex:

- Parathyroid glands: neither CT nor MRI are imaging tests of first line, due to the low sensitivity comparing with nuclear tests.
- Thyroid gland: ultrasound and FNAB in case of suspicious MTC.
- Pituitary tumors: Magnetic resonance imaging (MRI), with attention to the sella turcica region, is the test of choice when biochemical evidence of pituitary disease is found. Some tumors may not be functioning; however, asymptomatic patients should also be screened regularly (every 3–5 years).
- Gastrinomas: Somatostatin receptor scintigraphy is the imaging procedure of choice for gastrinomas. Its sensitivity range is 70–90%. Somatostatin receptor scintigraphy can be enhanced by selective arterial secretagogue test with secretin or calcium infusion (in 10% of the cases of gastrinomas secretin, it is not diagnostically useful). Operative intervention should be preceded by a computed tomography (CT) or MRI scan. Endoscopic ultrasonography detects tumors in the pancreatic head but rarely in the duodenal wall. It is more sensitive than the CT or the transabdominal ultrasound.
- Insulinomas: CT scan and MRI are recommended first. Somatostatin receptor scintigraphy findings may be positive in up to 50% of patients with insulinomas. It is best used in conjunction with single-photon emission CT (SPECT). Endoscopic ultrasonograph has a reported detection sensitivity of up to 94%.

8.3.3.4 Nuclear Medicine Tests

Thallium-201 chloride was the first agent used to successfully image the parathyroid glands in the 1980s. Tc-99m MIBI (Chudzinski et al. 2005; Mitchell 1996; Lavely et al. 2007) was first described for parathyroid localization involving the subtraction technique using I-123 to outline the thyroid. I-123 has the advantage of being a compound that is both trapped and organified by the thyroid. However, it is expensive and normally requires a delay of some hours between administration and imaging, with a lengthening of the entire procedure. The uptake of Tc-99m MIBI per gram of parathyroid tissue was lower than for thallium, but the ratio between the parathyroid and thyroid tissue was higher. Tc-99m tetrofosmin has also been investigated for imaging parathyroid tissue since it is a similar class of radiopharmaceutical as Tc-99m MIBI. Positron emission tomography (PET) tracers have met variable success. 18-Fluoro-2-deoxy-D-glucose (FDG) has been found useful by some authors for the identification of parathyroid adenomas, although others have not had this success. C-11 methionine seems promising although there is still limited experience. In the latest years, PET/CT with F18-choline showed interesting results in identifying parathyroid adenoma. Nevertheless, it is useful when there are problems in the identification of a parathyroid site with conventional scintigraphy.

Thallium, MIBI, and tetrofosmin are all cardiac imaging agents. In the neck, they are taken up by the salivary tissue as well as by the thyroid and parathyroid glands. In the chest, the heart is clearly visualized, but the mediastinum should be clear of focal uptake with only a low-grade blood pool depending on the imaging time. For the PET tracers, FDG has low-grade uptake in the mediastinum as a result of blood pool and can have low-grade focal uptake in lymph nodes of benign cause.

8.3.3.5 Parathyroid Scintigraphy Dual-Tracer Technique (Subtraction Scanning) Tc-99m Pt/I-123 and Tc-99m MIBI/Tc-99m Tetrofosmin/Tl-201 Chloride

Radiopharmaceuticals:

- I—Technetium-99m pertechnetate (Tc-99m Pt) or I-123 for thyroid phase
- II—Technetium-99m MIBI or Tc-99m tetrofosmin or thallium-201 chloride

Principle:

The examination is based on the differential washout of Tc-99m MIBI or Tc-99m tetrofosmin or thallium-201 chloride from the thyroid tissue compared with abnormal parathyroid tissue. The rate of washout from the abnormal parathyroid tissue, such as parathyroid adenoma, is much slower than that of the normal thyroid tissue (Hindie et al. 2009).

The distributions of the two tracers can be visually compared. The thyroid scan can be digitally subtracted from the parathyroid scan; removing the thyroid activity enhances the visualization of the parathyroid tissue. Lower sensitivity of Tl-201 together with higher radiation dose compared to Tc-99m MIBI made its use for parathyroid scanning less frequent.

Tc-99m tetrofosmin is an alternative to Tc-99m MIBI for parathyroid subtraction scanning. Absence of differential washout in the thyroid and parathyroid has not allowed its use as a single agent for double-phase study. However, because only early imaging is required with subtraction imaging, Tc-99m tetrofosmin can be an appropriate tracer.

Indications:

- Diagnosis of parathyroid adenomas.
- To detect recurrent or persistent disease both in primary hyperparathyroidism (PHPT) and secondary hyperparathyroidism.
- To improve results of initial surgery in PHPT.
- To select patients with PHPT for unilateral surgery or focused surgery, instead of the conventional bilateral neck exploration.
- The use of Tc-99m MIBI scanning before initial surgery of secondary hyperparathyroidism is controversial.

Technique:

- Patient preparation:
  - No need for fasting.
  - No need for thyroid hormone withdrawal in case of Tc-99m, but in case of I-123, attention to all blocking agents.
  - Influence of other drugs: calcium intake, drugs for osteoporosis must be interrupted at least 1 week before examination.
  - Attention to breastfeeding patients, children, and potential fetal exposure.
- The administered activity is of 370–555 MBq (10–15 mCi)/patient of Tc-99m MIBI.
- The average activity of I-123 is of 15 MBq (400 μCi).
- The activity of the used Tc-99m pertechnetate depends on the protocol: about 60–100 MBq is used if the protocol starts by thyroid imaging, and 150 MBq is given if thyroid imaging is done at the end of the Tc-99m MIBI procedure.
- 185 MBq (5 mCi) of Tc-99m tetrofosmin or Tl-201 chloride.
- Dose calibration.
- Injected I.V.

Procedure for simultaneous dual-tracer Tc-99m MIBI and I-123 scanning (planar)

- I-123 is given.
- Two hours later, the patient is placed under the gamma camera, and the Tc-99m MIBI is injected.
- Images are acquired simultaneously using appropriate windows without energy overlap.
- Imaging can start 3–5 min after Tc-99m MIBI injection with a broad field of view of the neck and mediastinum extending from the submandibular salivary glands to the upper part of the myocardium to ensure detection of ectopic glands.
- Digital data are acquired in a 256 × 256 matrix using a LEHR collimator.
- The acquisition procedure may also use a pinhole collimator.
- An image analysis computer program is used to subtract a progressively increasing percentage of the I-123 image from the Tc-99m MIBI.
- Delayed images (2–4 h postinjection) are not useful and do not increase the sensitivity of the subtraction protocol.
- Additional image acquisition may be useful.
- When ectopic uptake is observed (in mediastinum or submandibular), an additional SPECT acquisition is useful.
- SPECT/CT images should be used whenever is possible, due to higher sensitivity.

Procedure for double-tracer Tc-99m-pertechnetate and Tc-99m MIBI with successive acquisition

A subtraction scan based on sequential image acquisition of these two tracers can be carried out in many different ways:

1.
   - The patient is injected I.V. with 185 MBq Tc-99m Pt.
   - After 20 min, the thyroid image is acquired.
   - At the end, keeping the patient in the same position, 300 MBq of Tc-99m MIBI is administrated I.V., and a 20 min dynamic acquisition is performed.
   - This protocol has good sensitivity and specificity, but it has a drawback: high count rates from the thyroid gland do not allow, after the subtraction, the identification of a small parathyroid hyperfunctioning gland located behind the thyroid.
2.
   - Tc-99m Pt 40–60 MBq I.V.
   - Twenty minutes after the injection, a 10 min image is obtained.
   - Then, without moving the patient, 370–600 MBq of Tc-99m MIBI is injected.
   - Five minutes after the injection, a pinhole image of the neck is recorded for 15 min (or a 20/35 min dynamic acquisition).
3.
   - The technique suggested by Rubello et al. (2003). This procedure consists in the oral administration of 400 mg potassium perchlorate immediately before starting the acquisition of the thyroid scan, with the aim of inducing rapid Tc-99m Pt washout from the thyroid and reducing its interference on the Tc-99m MIBI.
   - 150–200 MBq of Tc-99m Pt and 550–600 MBq of Tc-99m MIBI are injected.
   - A matrix size of 128 × 128 is adequate.
   - A large field of view image with parallel hole collimator is always necessary to detect aberrant parathyroids and should include the submandibular salivary glands and the upper part of the myocardium.
   - Realignment of images is sometimes needed to correct the patient motion between the two sets of images.

Clinical applications:
- Diagnosis of hyperparathyroidism

Necessary additional examinations:
- Clinical examination; remember to discuss and to examine the patient *BEFORE* the injection, in order to limit the hazardous radiation exposure.
- Thyroid and parathyroid ultrasound.
- Serologic tests: serum level of PTH, serum and urinary level of calcium and phosphates, and alkaline phosphate.

Comments:
- The place of scintigraphy in the assessment of hyperparathyroidism is being largely

controversial, related to the finding of the best radiotracer and to the important limitation of other imagistic and structural diagnostic methods.

- To reach a high sensitivity in detecting multiglandular disease with subtraction techniques, the degree of subtraction should be monitored carefully. Over-subtraction can easily delete additional foci and provide a wrong image suggestive of a single adenoma.
- The use of SPECT/CT improved specificity, but unfortunately could not improve sensitivity. The role of dual-tracer SPECT/CT should be investigated in recurrent hyperparathyroidism as it allows correlation with morphological information, but clearly, low sensitivity in the thyroid bed area compared to pinhole subtraction imaging precludes its routine use before the first operation.

Reports:

- The reports respect the general format of the department with all the identification data of the patient, the institution, and the physician; the technical data related to the radiopharmaceutical, the dose used, the type of gamma camera, the acquisition data, and the estimation of absorbed dose due to this examination.
- The report will include the positive diagnosis of parathyroid adenoma and the lateralization and if it is possible the most accurate localization.

Normal image of parathyroid scan in dual-phase-tracer technique: adding the subtraction procedure, if there is no pathology in the parathyroid area, the glands will not appear in the image (Fig. 8.1).

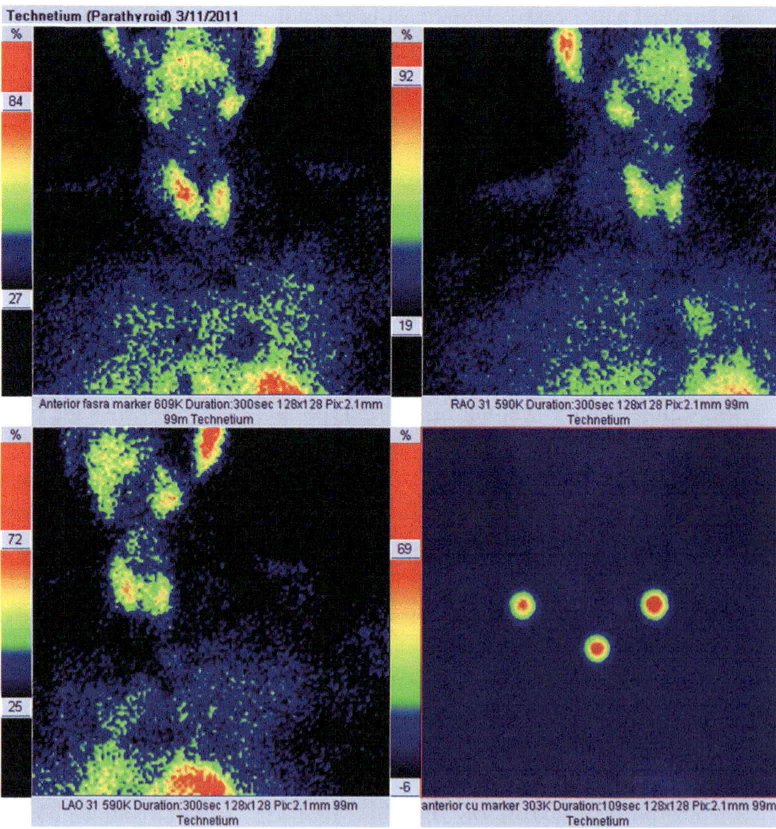

Fig. 8.1 Normal dual-tracer parathyroid scan with subtraction. The image with markers (*right bottom*) shows the thyroid "clean" area, with no tracer uptake

Case 1: Inferior Right Parathyroid Adenoma

History:

A 44-year-old female, with previous history of reno-ureteral lithiasis and gastric ulcer, is referred.

Clinical examination:

Symptoms: extreme fatigue, muscle pain and weakness, insomnia, and weight loss of 4 kg in 2 months

The neck examination does not reveal any pathological findings. No clinical evidence of lymph nodes.

Examinations:

The ultrasound revealed a solid, hypoechogenic nodule in the inferior pole of the right thyroid lobe. The nodule had regular contour and reduced vascularity. No pathologic lymph nodes.

Serum level of PTH—223 ng/L (N.V. 15–65 ng/L), high

TSH—1.38 mIU/L (N.V. 0.2–4.2 mIU/L)—normal

Calcium serum level—10.8 mg/dL (N.V. 8.6–10.2 mg/dL)

Findings:

The scintigraphy with Tc-99m Pt/Tc-99m MIBI showed:

- I phase of Tc-99m Pt—an intense uptake of the radiotracer in the entire inferior pole of the right thyroid lobe ("hot" nodule), corresponding to the ultrasound finding. The rest of the gland presents homogenous uptake, but clear reduced compared with the right lobe (Fig. 8.2).
- II phase of Tc-99m MIBI—subtraction of image—the right inferior pole of the thyroid bed presents an intense uptake, while the thyroid gland has cleaned its area (Fig. 8.3).

Conclusion:

The diagnosis was right inferior parathyroid adenoma, confirmed at surgery (Figs. 8.4 and 8.5).

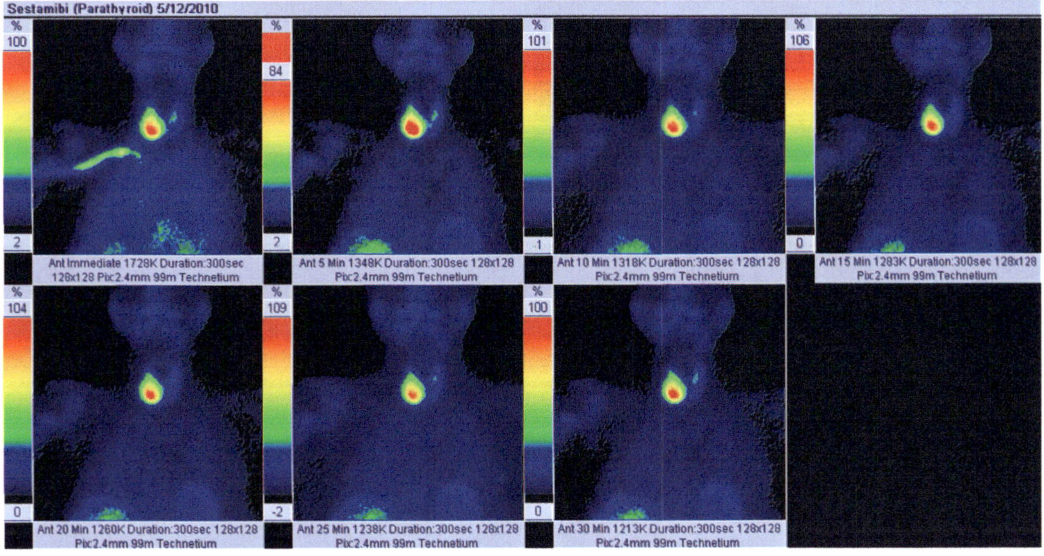

Fig. 8.2 Phase I of parathyroid scan

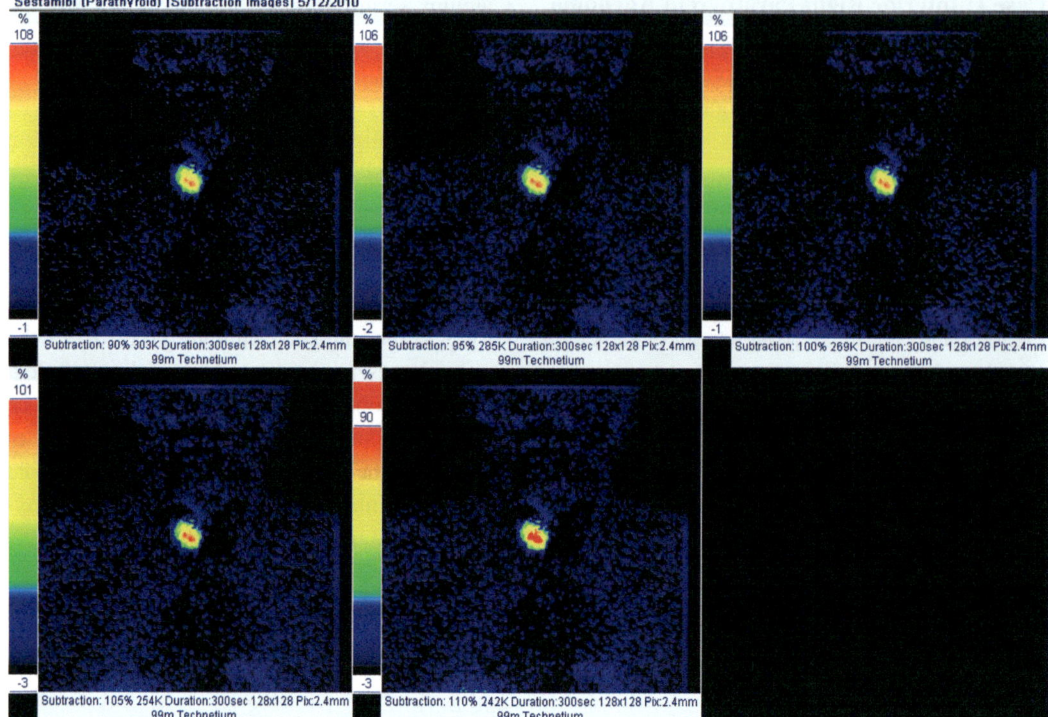

Fig. 8.3 The phase II of a parathyroid scan; subtraction of the thyroid; inferior right parathyroid adenoma

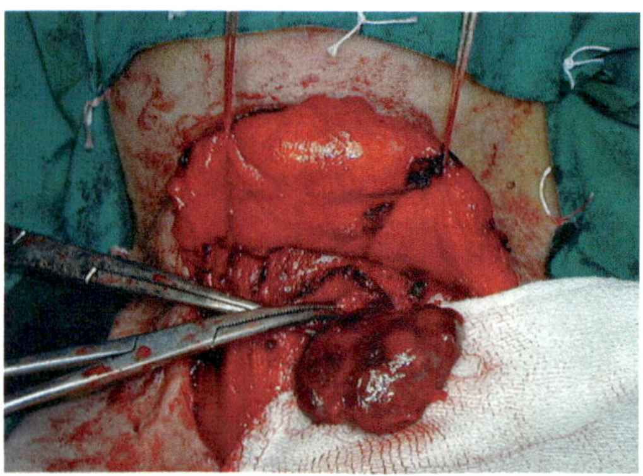

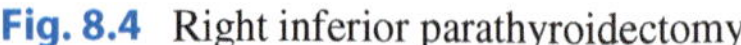

Fig. 8.4 Right inferior parathyroidectomy

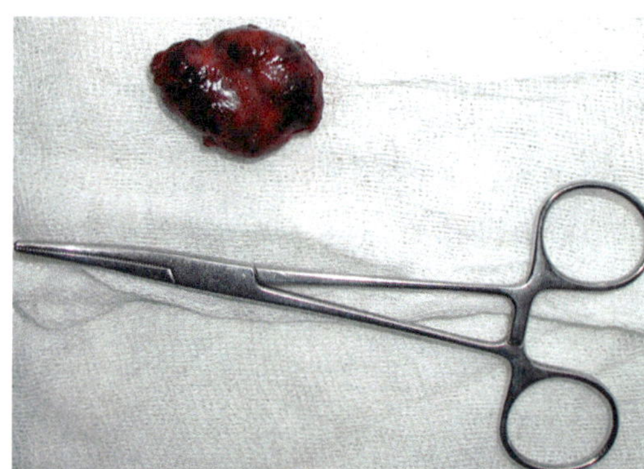

Fig. 8.5 The parathyroid adenoma

Key Points

- The signs or symptoms of hypercalcemia impose the check of PTH serum level; even if serum level of calcium is not high or significantly high, one should not forget about the possibility of normocalcemic hyperparathyroidism.
- The thyroid and parathyroid ultrasound sometimes fails to discover parathyroid adenomas mainly in the situation of nodular goiter association or in case of ectopy.
- The most sensitive method in the diagnosis of primary hyperparathyroidism is the nuclear test of parathyroid glands; the best tracers and procedure are subject of debates and are strictly related to the experience of the physician and availability.
- Adding SPECT/CT to planar images will improve significantly the sensitivity of the method and the accuracy.

Case 2: Ectopic, Mediastinum Left Parathyroid Adenoma

History:

A 28-year-old male, with previous history of right parathyroid adenoma operated 2 years ago with parathyroidectomy

Clinical examination:

Symptoms: fatigue, severe impairment of movement, gallbladder stones, and osteoporosis

The neck examination does not reveal any pathological findings, except the scar of the previous surgical neck incision. No clinical evidence of lymph nodes.

Examinations:

The neck ultrasound revealed no pathological findings and no pathologic lymph nodes.

Serum level of PTH—174 ng/L (N.V. 15–65 ng/L), increased

Serum level of calcium—11.3 mg/L (N.V. 8.6–10.2 mg/dL)

25-HO-D-vitamin—62 ng/mL (N.V. deficiency, <10 ng/mL; insufficient level, 10–30 ng/mL; optimum level, 30–100 ng/mL; toxicity, >100 ng/mL), normal

Findings:

The scintigraphy with Tc-99m Pt/Tc-99m MIBI showed:

- I phase of Tc-99m Pt—normal uptake of the radiotracer in the entire thyroid gland, corresponding to the thyroid phase of the test.
- II phase of Tc-99m MIBI—subtraction of image—in the left mediastinum, an ectopic intense uptake is present, while the thyroid gland is completely washed out (Fig. 8.6).

Conclusion:

Left ectopic mediastinum parathyroid adenoma

Key Points

- The parathyroid adenoma may be ectopic, the nuclear test being by far the most suitable method to diagnose it.
- The examination with large-field gamma camera and the acquisition of images extended to the thorax area are mandatory.
- The persistent postsurgery hyperparathyroidism is an expression of an improper evaluation and suboptimal surgery.
- The parathyroid glands may be ectopic; according to their embryogenetic development, these sites are limited to the central mediastinum with the lower limit to heart basis.

8.3.3.6 Parathyroid Scintigraphy Single-Tracer (Dual-Phase) Technique Tc-99m MIBI

Radiopharmaceuticals:

- Technetium-99m MIBI

Principle:

The examination is based on the differential washout of Tc-99m MIBI from the thyroid tissue compared with the abnormal parathyroid tissue. The rate of washout from abnormal parathyroid tissue, such as parathyroid adenoma, is much slower than that of the normal

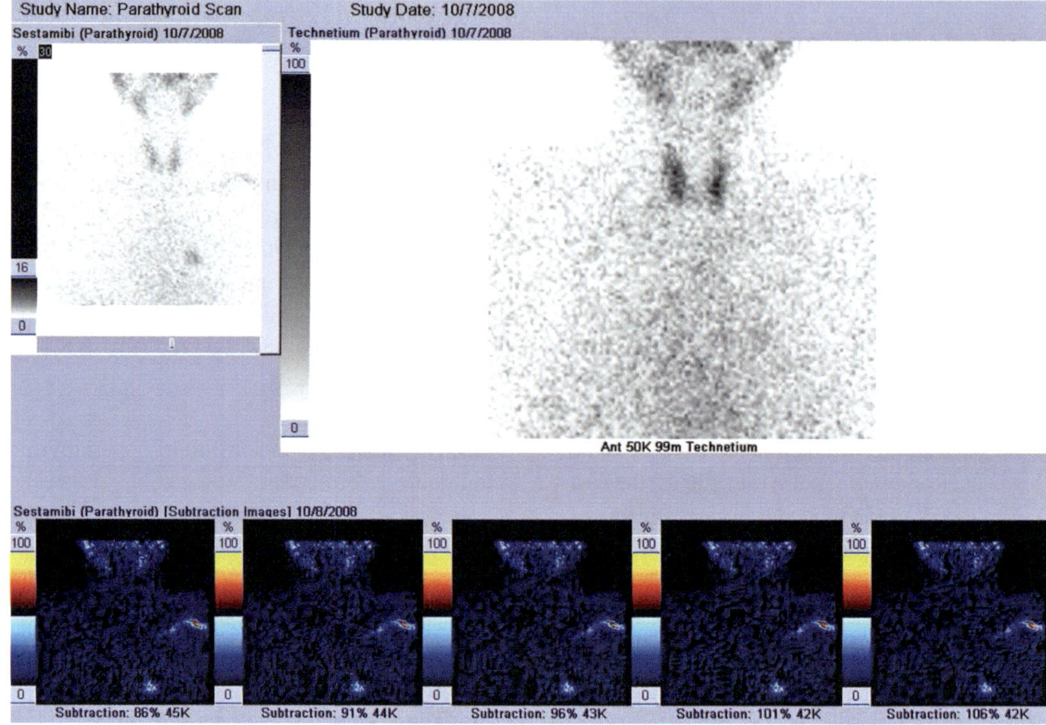

Fig. 8.6 Left ectopic mediastinum parathyroid macroadenoma

thyroid tissue. The retention is presumably related to the oxyphil cells of parathyroid lesions, which are rich in mitochondria.

The dual-phase technique of one single tracer consists in obtaining early images at 15 min and delayed images at 1.5–2 h even 3 h depending on the thyroid washout.

Technique:

- Patient preparation:
  - No need for fasting
  - No need for thyroid hormone withdrawal
  - Influence of other drugs: calcium intake, drugs for osteoporosis
  - No influence of recent procedures with iodine contrast substances
  - Attention to breastfeeding patients, children, and potential fetal exposure (see the chapter of radioprotection)
- Dose—370–555–925 MBq (10–15–25 mCi)/patient of Tc-99m MIBI obtained from generator of Tc-99m and labeled in the department, respecting the quality control rules and labeled with MIBI.
- Dose calibration.
- Injected I.V.
- The initial early image is obtained 10–15 min after the injection; this step is called the thyroid phase of the study because Tc-99m MIBI is rapidly concentrated in the thyroid gland at this time. The delayed image is obtained 1.5–3 h after the injection; this step is called the parathyroid phase.
- Patient position: supine, slightly neck extension.
- Gamma camera:
  - Daily calibration and valid quality control tests.
  - Low-energy high-resolution (LEHR) collimator.
  - Incidence: Anterior-posterior (AP) over the patient's neck, as close to the neck as possible, avoiding the influence of resolution by an inadequate distance. The field must cover the area of the superior mediastinum permitting the registration of any ectopic parathyroid gland.

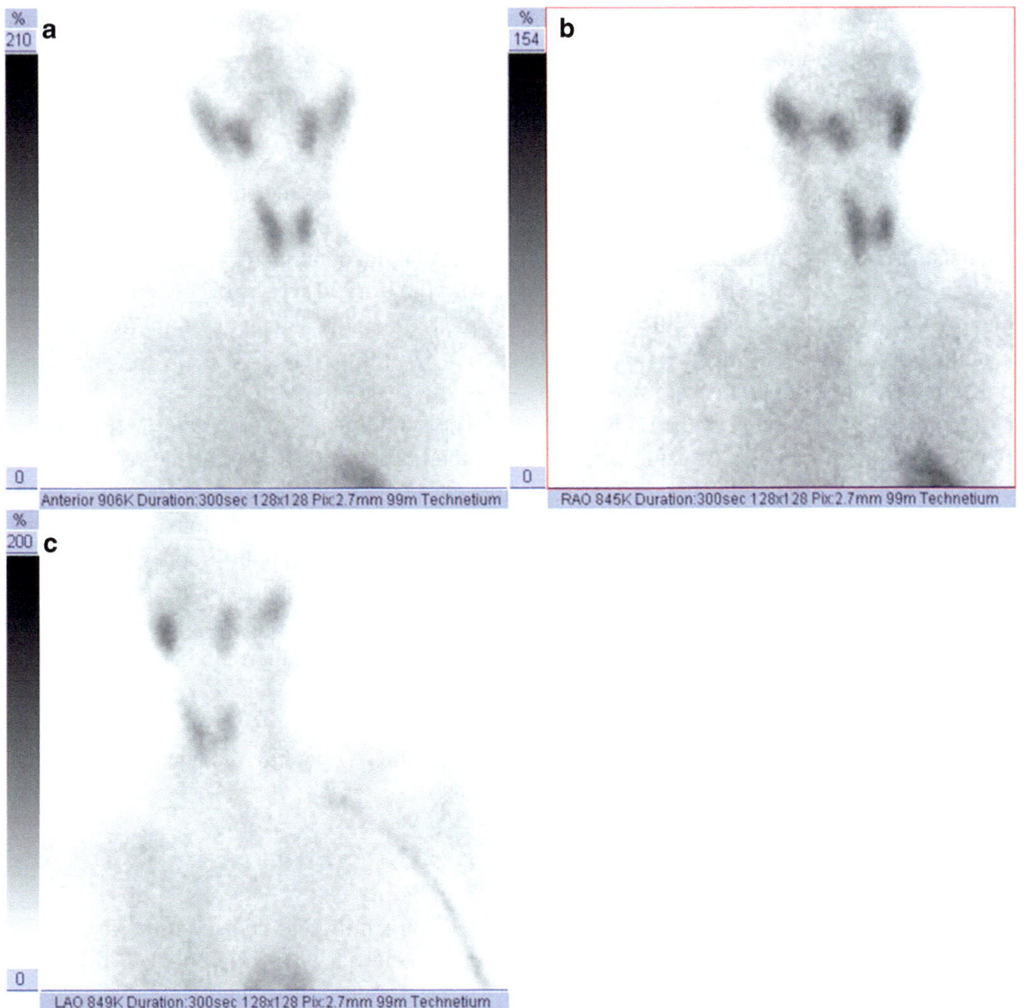

Fig. 8.7 Normal parathyroid Tc-99m MIBI single tracer ((**a**), AP incidence; (**b**, **c**) lateral oblique incidences). No pathologic uptake beside the thyroid area

- Acquisition:
  - Dynamic planar acquisition from the first minute to 10 min; this sequence is followed by static acquisition at 15, 60, 120, and if necessary at 180 min.
  - Selected energy 140 keV.
  - Window 15–20%.
  - 128 × 128 matrix.
  - Minimum 250,000 counts/image.
  - Mark the suprasternal notch, with a point source of Tc-99m Pt or Cobalt-57; this mark will be registered on the images.
  - Oblique-lateral images must be obtained.
  - Any palpable nodule should be marked on the images, during the acquisition, giving the physician the facility to position the nodule.
- Processing: there are special PC programs; there are special templates available for processing the image.
- Normal image is shown in Fig. 8.7 (a, anterior; b, right lateral oblique; c, left lateral oblique).

Clinical applications:

- Diagnosis of hyperparathyroidism

Necessary additional examinations:

- Clinical examination; remember to discuss and to examine the patient *before* the injection, in order to limit the hazardous radiation exposure.

- Thyroid and parathyroid ultrasound.
- Serologic tests: serum level of PTH, serum and urinary level of calcium and phosphates, and alkaline phosphate.

Comments:
- This procedure is the simplest and fastest in the localization of parathyroid lesions.
- The single-tracer scintigraphy in the assessment of hyperparathyroidism is the only one examination accepted by some of the most prestigious centers for parathyroid, such as the Norman Parathyroid Center in the USA.
- Please note the advantages of using SPECT/CT while this test is performed.

Reports:
- The reports respect the general format of the department with all the identification data of the patient, the institution, and the physician; the technical data related to the radiopharmaceutical, the dose used, the type of gamma camera, the acquisition, the data, and the estimation of the absorbed dose due to this examination.
- The report will include the positive diagnosis of parathyroid lesion and the lateralization and will mention the localization as accurate as possible.

Case 1: Inferior Right Parathyroid Adenoma

History:

A 33-year-old female, with previous history of papillary thyroid carcinoma with total thyroidectomy and radioiodine therapy, 4 years ago

Clinical examination:

Symptoms: extreme fatigue, muscle weakness, severe impairment of movement, insomnia, constipation, and depression

The neck examination does not reveal any pathological findings. No clinical evidence of lymph nodes.

Examinations:

The neck ultrasound revealed a solid, hypoechogenic nodule in the inferior pole of the right thyroid bed area of 1.8/3.1 cm. The results suggested the possible recurrence of the thyroid disease in the area; no pathologic lymph nodes.

Serum PTH level—1641 ng/L (N.V. 15–65 ng/L), very increased

Serum calcium level—12.2 mg/L (N.V. 8.6–10.2 mg/dL)

25-HO-D-vitamin—48 ng/mL (N.V. deficiency, <10 ng/mL; insufficient level, 10–30 ng/mL; optimum level, 30–100 ng/mL; toxicity, >100 ng/mL), normal

TSH—0.07 mIU/L (N.V. 0.2–4.2 mIU/L), suppression on the 150 μg/day L-thyroxine

Findings:

The scintigraphy with Tc-99m MIBI showed the total absence of uptake of the radiotracer in the entire thyroid gland, corresponding to the total thyroidectomy previously performed. Tc-99m MIBI was rapidly trapped in the early images in the right inferior pole of thyroid bed; the intense uptake also persisted in the delayed sequences, while the thyroid gland is completely absent (Fig. 8.8).

Conclusion:

Right inferior parathyroid adenoma (Figs. 8.9 and 8.10)

Key Points
- The parathyroid adenoma may be also associated with differentiated thyroid carcinomas, not only with medullary forms.
- The absence of the thyroid gland makes easier the visualization of the parathyroid glands pathologically modified.
- In the situation of a patient with history of thyroidectomy and suspected hyperparathyroidism, we should carefully analyze the images, in order to avoid a misinterpretation. The thyroid remnant tissue visualized on early and frequently on delayed images in the anterior cervical region may alter the correct diagnosis; there is a high probability of confusion, and therefore a SPECT/CT might be essential in the differential diagnosis (Fig. 8.11).

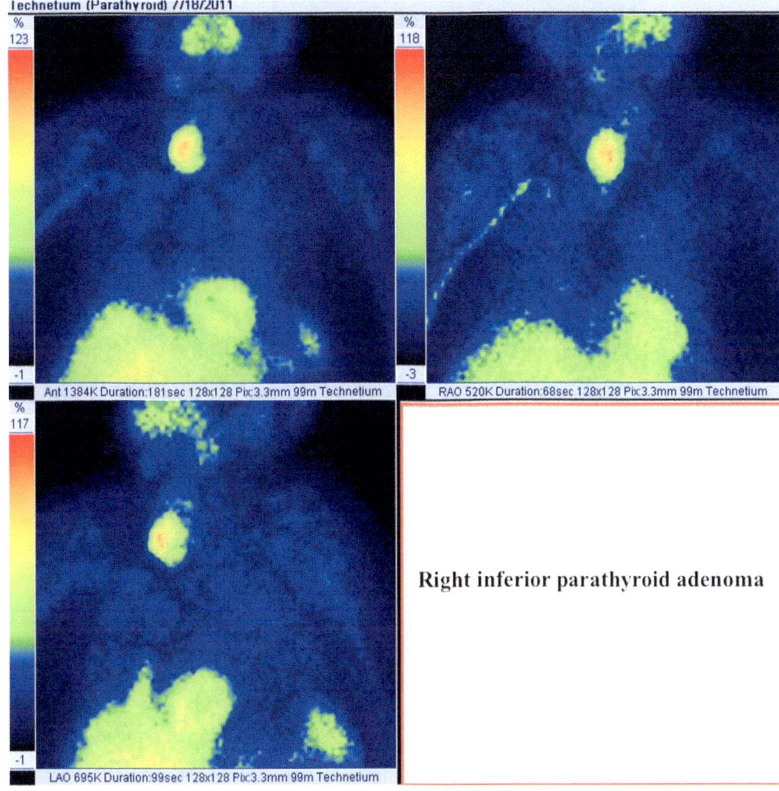

Fig. 8.8 Right inferior parathyroid macroadenoma

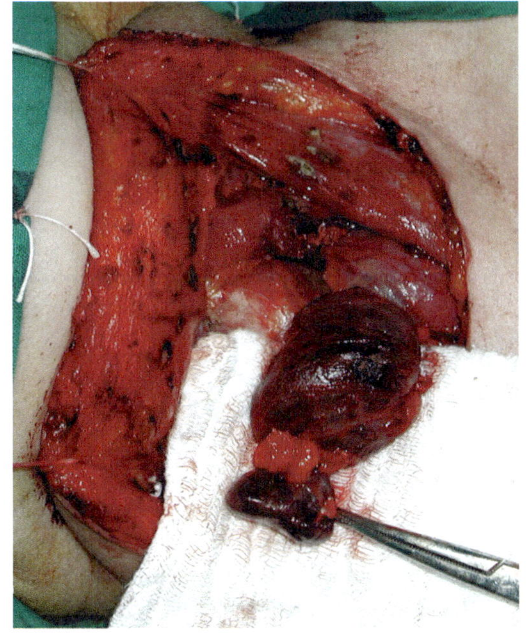

Fig. 8.9 Parathyroid macroadenoma; surgical specimen

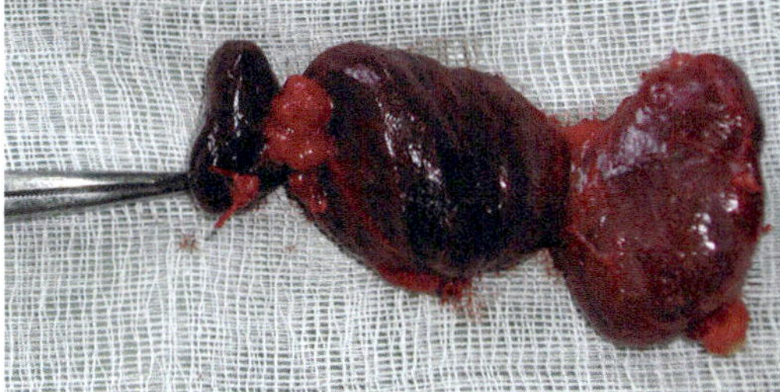

Fig. 8.10 Parathyroid adenoma

Case 2: Inferior Right Parathyroid Adenoma *History*:

A 54-year-old female, with recent history of severe osteoporosis

Clinical examination:

Symptoms: muscle weakness and very severe diffuse bone pain

The neck examination does not reveal any pathological findings. No clinical evidence of lymph nodes.

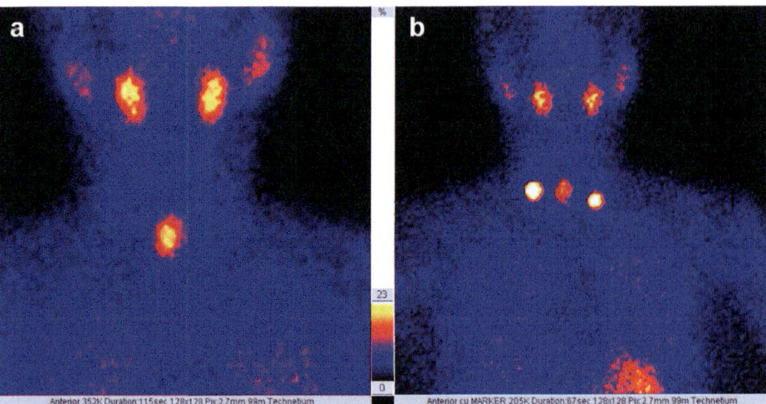

Fig. 8.11 Thyroid remnant tissue after thyroidectomy for DTC, highly probable to be misinterpreted as parathyroid adenoma, in the case of suspected primary hyperparathyroidism. The early images (**a**) show Tc-99m MIBI uptake in the cervical anterior area. The delayed images (**b**) with markers on both clavicles showed the persistence of the uptake

Examinations:

The neck ultrasound revealed a diffuse enlargement of the thyroid gland, having a structure with multiple nodules in the entire area, but with no ultrasound features suggesting a malignancy. In the inferior right lobe, it was suggested that the presence of a nodule of 0.9 cm probably related to the parathyroid, with no pathologic lymph nodes.

Serum level of PTH—101 ng/L (N.V. 15–65 ng/L), increased
TSH—1.6 mIU/L (N.V. 0.2–4.2 mIU/L), normal
Serum calcium level—9.3 mg/L (N.V. 8.6–10.2 mg/L)

Findings:

The scintigraphy with Tc-99m MIBI showed in the early phase the enlargement of the thyroid gland and a discrete increase of the uptake in the inferior right thyroid lobe. The delayed images showed the clearance of the thyroid radiotracer and the persistency of the tracer in the mentioned right area (Fig. 8.12). The skin markers permitted to accurately determine the distances between the anatomic regions and the localization of the parathyroid lesion; this will help the strategy of surgeons in case of minimally invasive parathyroidectomy.

Conclusion:

Right inferior parathyroid adenoma

Key Points

- The serum calcium level in case of primary hyperparathyroidism may be also normal; do not miss the fact that the calcium and PTH level may be fluctuant during the evolution.
- The symptom severity is not always related to the PTH serum level.

Similar cases (Figs. 8.13 and 8.14).

Case 3: Inferior Right Parathyroid Adenoma

History:

A 29-year-old female suffering from chronic renal failure with recent left inferior parathyroidectomy

Clinical Examination:

Symptoms: muscle weakness, very severe diffuse bone pain, impossibility of self-movement, and symptoms due to chronic renal failure

The neck examination revealed a scar after previous parathyroidectomy.

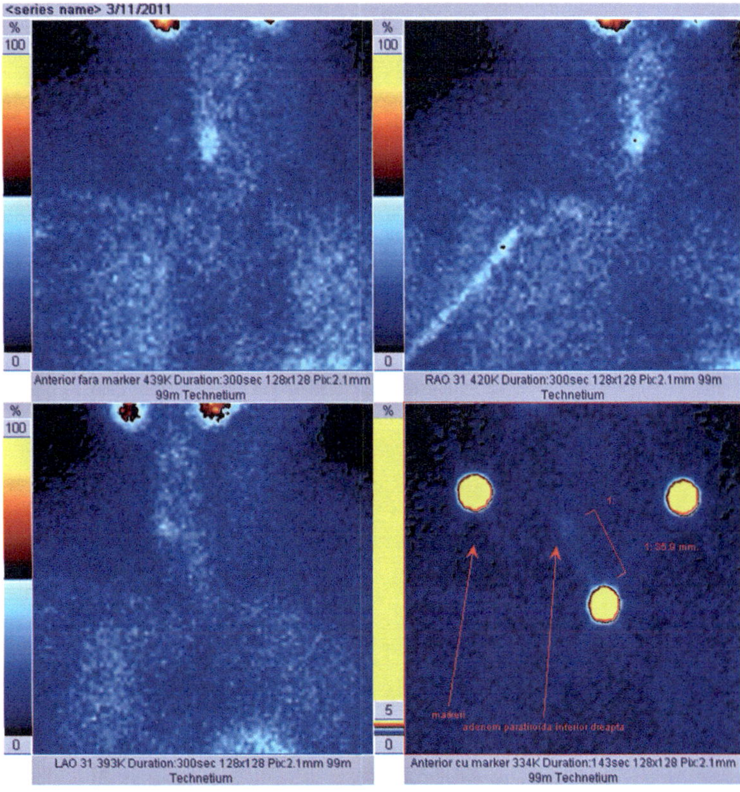

Fig. 8.12 Right inferior parathyroid adenoma

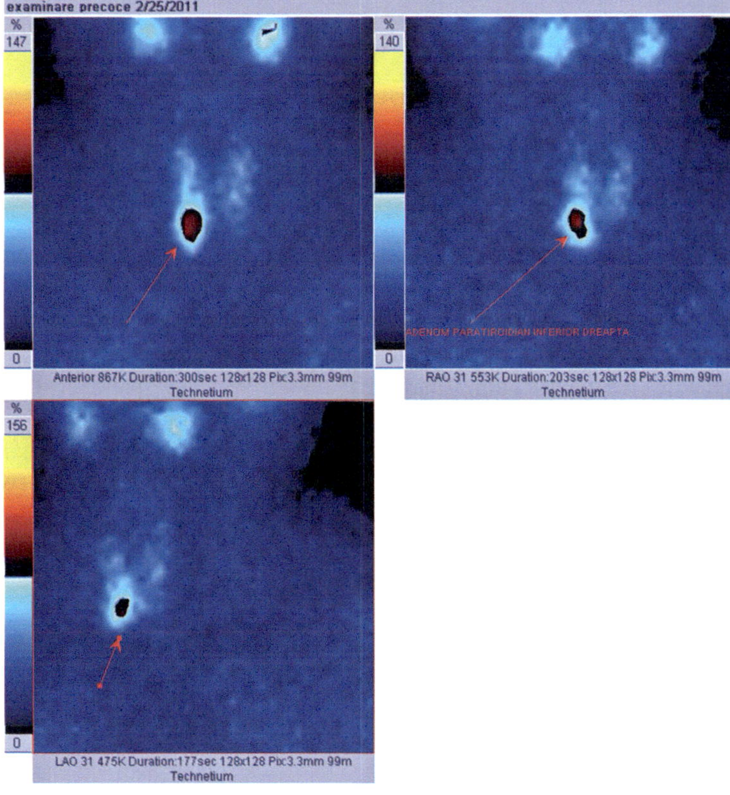

Fig. 8.13 Right inferior parathyroid adenoma

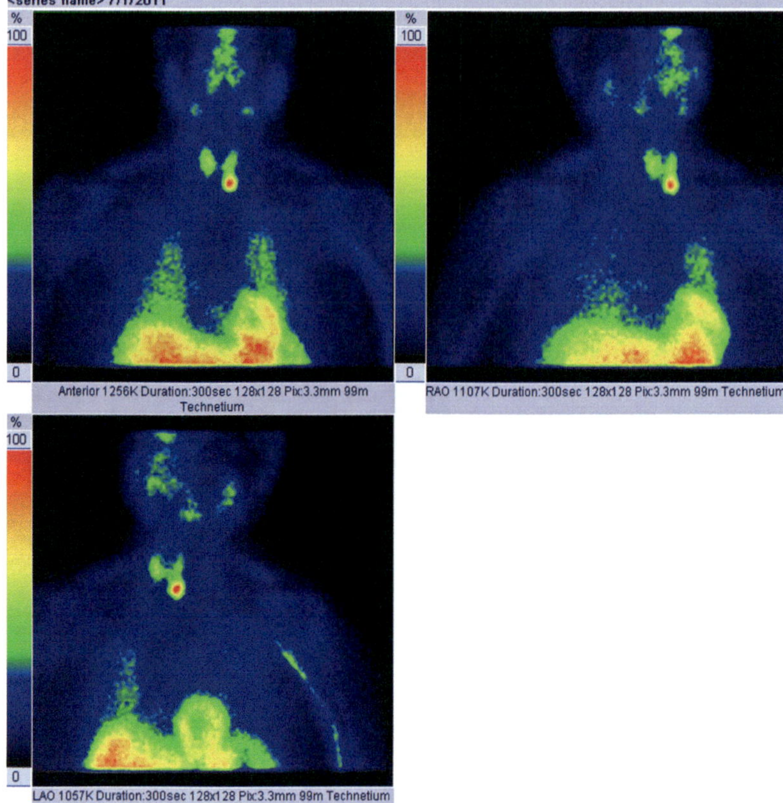

Fig. 8.14 Left inferior parathyroid adenoma

Examinations:

Serum level of PTH—231 ng/L (N.V. 15–65 ng/L), increased

Serum calcium level—13.5 mg/L (N.V. 8.6–10.2 mg/L)

Findings:

The scintigraphy with Tc-99m MIBI showed in the early phase the increase of the uptake in the inferior right thyroid lobe and also the ectopic uptake in the mediastinum (Fig. 8.15).

Conclusion:

Ectopic mediastinum parathyroid adenoma

Key Points

- The high PTH serum and calcium level in the case of a previously operated primary hyperparathyroidism is firstly due to the lack of identifying the adenoma (frequent multiple and ectopic), rather than to the recurrence.
- In this particular case, the delayed images would be extremely useful to assess the presence of the possible right inferior parathyroid adenoma; the early images show only the increased uptake, both attributed to thyroid or parathyroid.

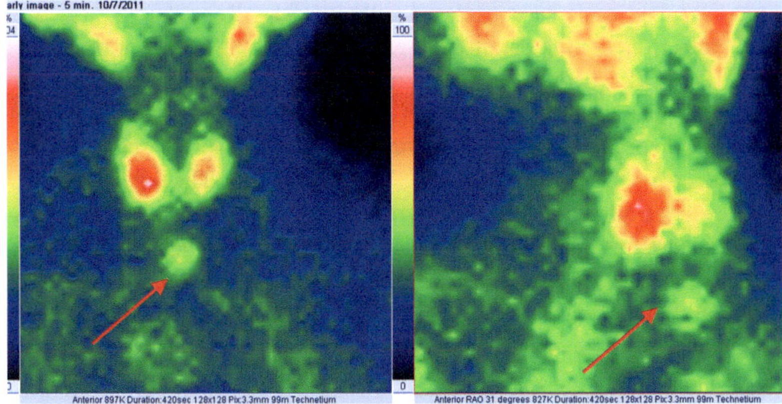

Fig. 8.15 Ectopic mediastinum parathyroid adenoma

8.3.3.7 Parathyroid Scintigraphy SPECT and SPECT/CT

Radiopharmaceuticals:

- Technetium-99m MIBI in double tracer or single tracer

Principle:

The examination is based on the intention to have a better anatomy localization of parathyroid disease, improving the sensitivity and sensibility of the nuclear tests in hyperparathyroidism diagnosis.

Technique:

- The preparation of the patient is realized according to the tracers used.
- The SPECT, SPECT/CT, and pinhole SPECT have been used and have the ability to locate more precisely the sites of the hyperfunctioning parathyroid than simple planar imaging and allow the detection of smaller lesions.
- The SPECT study should be acquired immediately following early planar acquisitions (to avoid false-negative results due to parathyroid adenomas with rapid washout) with the patient in the same position, using a matrix of 128 × 128 for 120 projections every 3° (360° rotation) and with an imaging time of 15–25 s per projection and suitable zoom factor.
- SPECT/CT provides fused images of functional and anatomical modalities, which considerably improve the interpretation of findings of individual procedures.
- Pinhole SPECT study should be acquired immediately following early planar acquisitions with the patient in the same position with 32 projections over 180° with a circular orbit. The acquisition time per step may be set to 40 s. The main characteristics of the pinhole collimator are a 3 mm aperture and an inner focal length of 205 mm.
- Processing:
  - No special processing for planar images is needed.
  - For SPECT processing, transaxial tomograms are reconstructed by filtered back-projection using a low-pass filter without attenuation correction. Attenuation correction can be useful when using SPECT/CT.
  - The two sets of planar images (early and delayed) are visually inspected. Focal areas of increased uptake, which show either a relative progressive increase over time or a fixed uptake, which persisted on delayed

imaging, must be considered pathological hyperfunctioning parathyroid glands.
 - The SPECT or SPECT/CT images give information about the correct position of the hyperfunctioning gland, especially if deep in the neck or ectopic. The use of volume rendering of parathyroid SPECT images might be helpful for visualization.

Clinical applications:
- Diagnosis of hyperparathyroidism

Necessary additional examinations:
- Clinical examination; remember to discuss and to examine the patient *before* the injection, in order to limit the hazardous radiation exposure.
- Thyroid and parathyroid ultrasound.
- Serologic tests: serum level of PTH, serum and urinary level of calcium and phosphates, and alkaline phosphate.

Reports:
- The reports respect the general format of the department with all the identification data of the patient, the institution, and the physician.
- The report should include the timing of acquisition of the images. Planar images must be labeled to show the type of projection and the region imaged. SPECT should include the reconstruction of images in the three axes (coronal, sagittal, and transaxial) (Figs. 8.16 and 8.17).
- The report will include the positive diagnosis of parathyroid adenoma and the lateralization and if possible the most accurate localization (Figs. 8.18 and 8.19).

In view of new findings since the Fourth International Workshop on the Management of Asymptomatic PHPT, guidelines for management have been revised (Bilezikian et al. 2014).

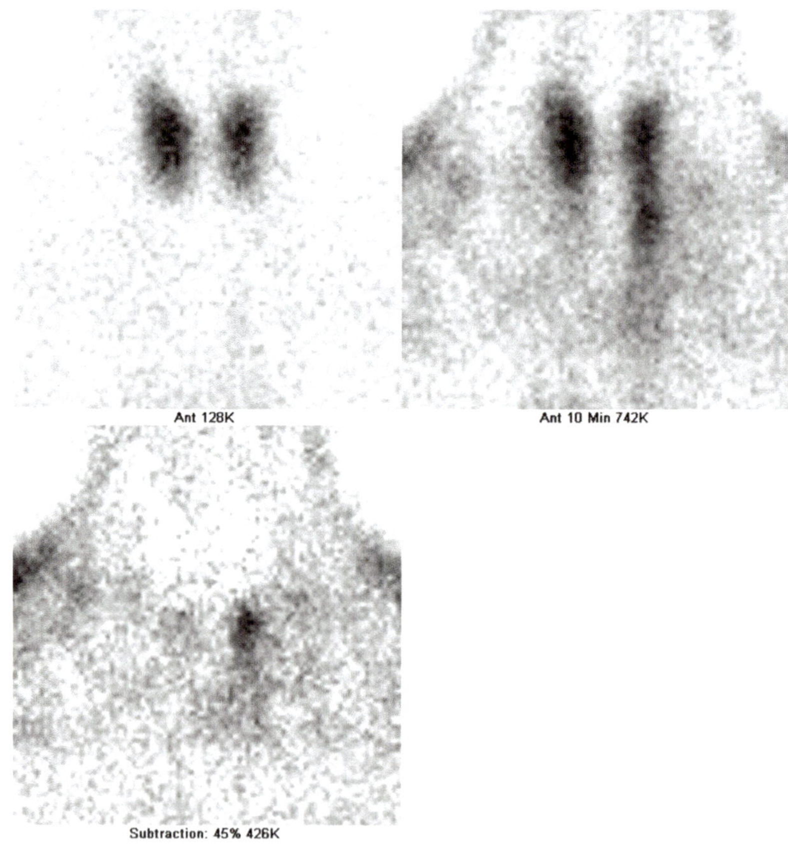

Fig. 8.16 Tc-99m MIBI planar scan; inferior left parathyroid adenoma

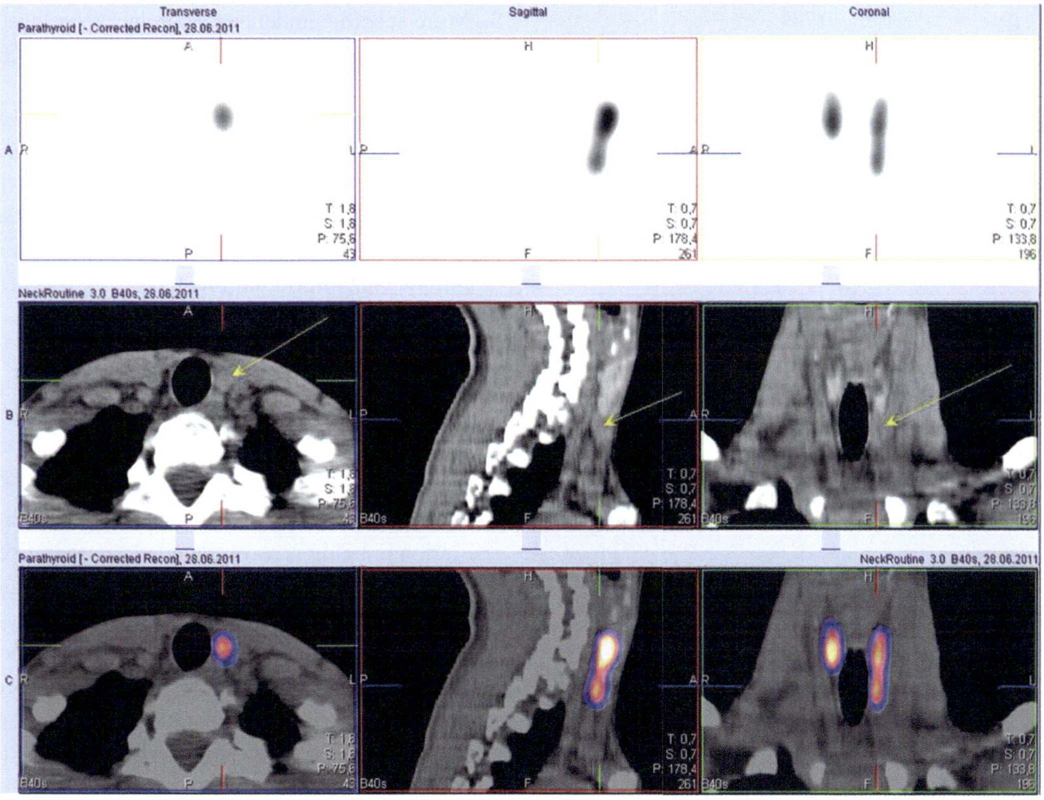

Fig. 8.17 SPECT/CT Tc-99m MIBI (with the courtesy of Dr. Andries G.—County Hospital Cluj-Napoca)

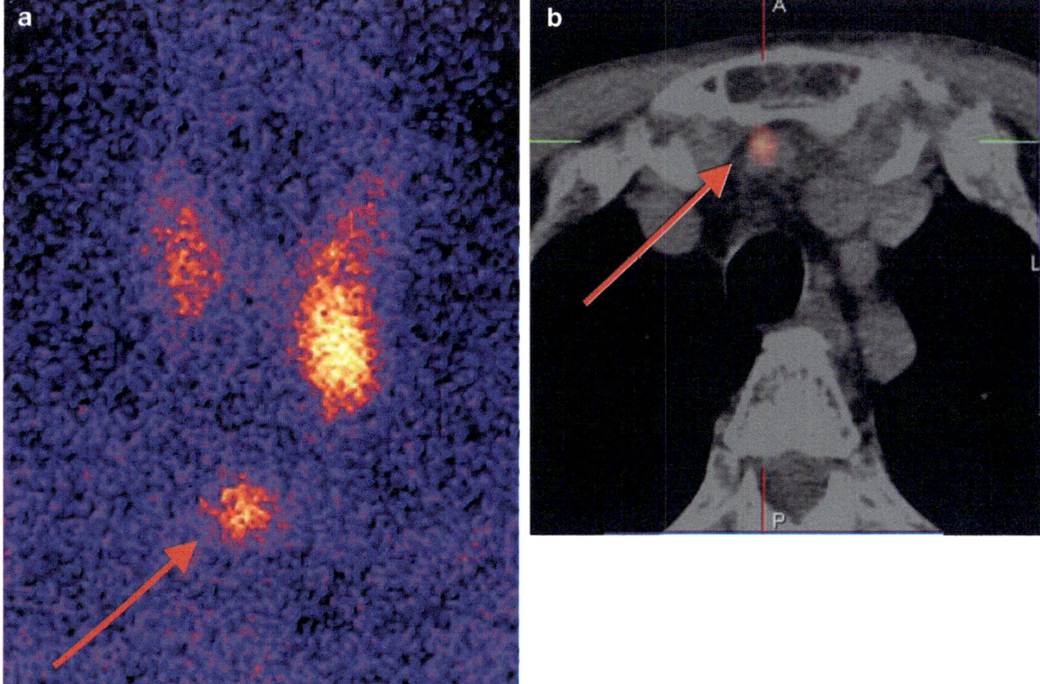

Fig. 8.18 Parathyroid scintigraphy Tc-99m MIBI ((**a**) planar image showing an ectopic parathyroid adenoma and (**b**) SPECT/CT transversal section, on the specific region of the ectopic adenoma)

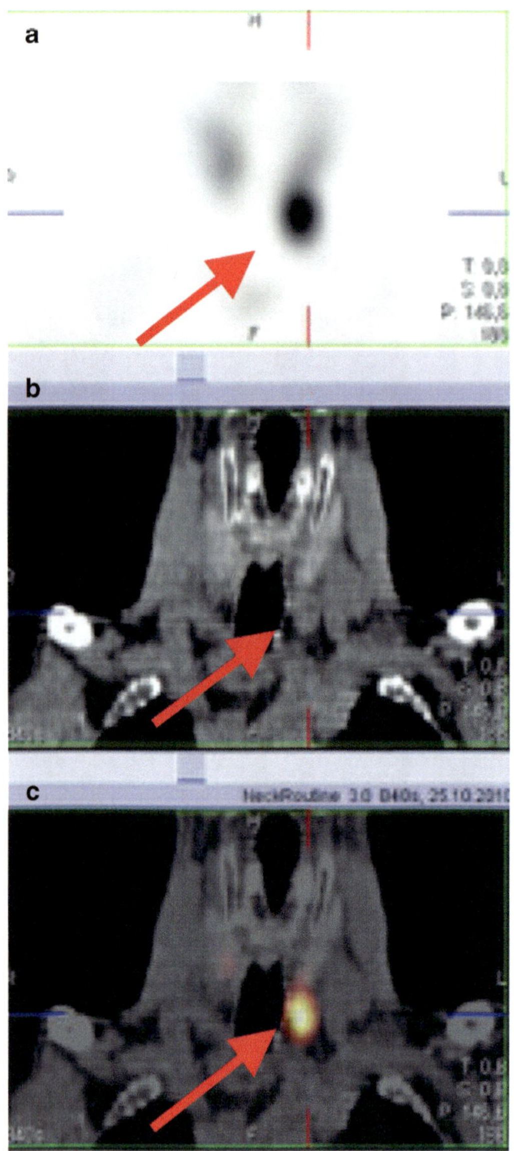

Fig. 8.19 SPECT/CT Tc-99m MIBI ((**a**) coronal section SPECT, (**b**) CT coronal and (**c**) coronal fused image SPECT/CT) shows a parathyroid adenoma of the left inferior parathyroid gland

The revised guidelines include:

1. Recommendations for more extensive evaluation of the skeletal and renal systems
2. Skeletal and/or renal involvement as determined by further evaluation to become part of the guidelines for surgery
3. More specific guidelines for monitoring those who do not meet guidelines for parathyroid surgery

These guidelines should help endocrinologists and surgeons caring for patients with PHPT (Bilezikian et al. 2014; Khan et al. 2017; Wilhelm et al. 2016).

Initial evaluation should include:

- 25-Hydroxyvitamin D measurement
- 24-hour urine calcium measurement
- Dual-energy X-ray absorptiometry (DEXA)
- Supplementation for vitamin D deficiency

Cervical ultrasonography or other high-resolution imaging is recommended for operative planning. Patients with nonlocalizing imaging remain surgical candidates. Preoperative parathyroid biopsy should be avoided. Surgeons who perform a high volume of operations have better outcomes. The possibility of multigland disease should be routinely considered. Both focused, image-guided surgery (minimally invasive parathyroidectomy) and bilateral exploration are appropriate operations that achieve high cure rates. For minimally invasive parathyroidectomy, intraoperative parathyroid hormone monitoring via a reliable protocol is recommended. Minimally invasive parathyroidectomy is not routinely recommended for known or suspected multigland disease. Ex vivo aspiration of resected parathyroid tissue may be used to confirm parathyroid tissue intraoperatively.

Clinically relevant thyroid disease should be assessed preoperatively and managed during parathyroidectomy. Devascularized normal parathyroid tissue should be autotransplanted. Patients should be observed postoperatively for hematoma, evaluated for hypocalcemia and symptoms of hypocalcemia, and followed up to assess for cure defined as normocalcemic at more than 6 months. Calcium supplementation may be indicated postoperatively. Familial PHPT, reoperative parathyroidectomy, and parathyroid carcinoma are challenging entities that require special consideration and expertise.

Diagnosis

1. Confirmed if serum calcium is elevated (total calcium corrected for albumin or elevated ionized calcium) in the presence of an elevated or inappropriately normal PTH in the absence of conditions mimicking PHPT (e.g., thiazide diuretics or lithium).
2. Familial hypocalciuric hypercalcemia (FHH)—three variants now identified.
3. Consider evaluation of familial PHPT.

Imaging:

1. Imaging is not used for the diagnosis of PHPT, which is based on biochemical profile.
2. Identification of abnormal parathyroid tissue is enhanced with single-photon emission computed tomography (SPECT) study in combination with a computed tomography (CT) study and is particularly valuable in repeat surgical cases.
3. Ultrasound and Tc99m-sestamibi scintigraphy continue to be useful localization tools; however, they can miss small adenomas and hyperplasia.
4. Additional imaging or localization tools for those failing surgery or suspected of having an ectopic parathyroid gland include CT scans, MRI, and C11-methionine or F18-choline PET/CT parathyroid scan (see Chap. 11).

Presentation:

1. In developed countries—approximately 85% of patients present with asymptomatic disease and 20% present with renal complications (kidney stones, nephrocalcinosis), skeletal complications (fracture, osteitis fibrosa cystica, bone pain), or symptomatic hypercalcemia.
2. In developing countries, the majority of patients present with symptomatic disease.

Indications for Parathyroid Surgery

Parathyroidectomy is indicated:

1. For all symptomatic patients
2. Should be considered for most asymptomatic patients
3. Is more cost-effective than observation or pharmacologic therapy Asymptomatic PHPT—surgery is a valuable option particularly in those meeting criteria for surgical intervention.

Criteria for surgical intervention:

1. Age <50 years.
2. Serum calcium >1 mg/dL or >0.25 mmol/L of the upper limit of the reference interval for total calcium and >0.12 mmol/L for Ca^{2+}.
3. BMD T-score ≤−2.5 at the lumbar spine, femoral neck, the total hip, or the 1/3 radius for postmenopausal women or males >50 years. A prevalent low-energy fracture (i.e., in the spine) is also considered an indication for surgery, which requires a routine X-ray of the thoracic and lumbar spine (or vertebral fracture assessment by DXA).
4. A glomerular filtration rate (GFR) of <60 mL/min. Further evaluation of asymptomatic patients with renal imaging (X-ray, CT, or ultrasound) in order to detect silent kidney stones or nephrocalcinosis is advised. A complete urinary stone risk profile should be performed in those individuals whose urinary calcium excretion is >400 mg/day. If stone(s), nephrocalcinosis, or high stone risk is determined, surgery should be recommended.

Medical Management

1. Vitamin D deficiency/insufficiency should be corrected and is effective in lowering serum PTH without further elevating serum calcium. Correct serum 25OHD to >50 nmol/L.
2. Amino-bisphosphonates are effective in preventing decreases in BMD and lowering bone remodeling.
3. Cinacalcet is effective in lowering serum calcium and should be considered for symptomatic PHPT when surgery is not an option. Amino-bisphosphonates may be used in combination with cinacalcet in selected patients.
4. Data with medical therapy currently is short term and insufficient to justify medical therapy as an alternative to surgery. There is no fracture data with any of the existing medical therapies.

8.4 Radio-Guided Surgery of the Parathyroid Glands

8.4.1 Overview

The first successful parathyroidectomy was performed in 1925 by Mandl F. and consists in the bilateral neck exploration; until nowadays surgery remained the standard treatment of primary hyperparathyroidism. The success with this approach, as measured by the return to normal calcium levels, depends primarily on the experience and the judgment of the surgeon in recognizing the difference between enlarged or normal-sized glands.

The difficulty of parathyroid surgery consists not only in reduced size and delicate location of glands among important nerves and vessels but also in distinguishing an adenoma from hyperplasia, a distinction that can be difficult not only intraoperatively but sometimes also histopathologically (Carty et al. 1997). This surgery requests the most experienced surgeons being able to make the difference of the normal glands from abnormal ones, by evaluating the size, shape, and color of the parathyroid glands during surgery (Gauger et al. 2001; Henry et al. 2001). In the absence of a reliable pre- or intraoperative imaging study to identify or localize abnormal parathyroid glands, conventional four-gland exploration is mandatory.

Ectopic parathyroid tumors and unrecognized multiglandular parathyroid disease are major causes of surgical failure. Reoperation is always a riskier and technically difficult procedure due to fibrosis and deformed normal anatomy.

The accepted surgical methods for parathyroid surgery are:

- Bilateral neck exploration
- Unilateral neck exploration
- Limited dissection under local anesthesia
- Endoscopic (video-assisted) parathyroidectomy
- Minimally invasive surgery

The scientific community made efforts to develop new diagnosis and treatment procedures to replace the classic extensive neck exploration, with the intention to reduce the surgical risk and to have minimal morbidity, no mortality, low recurrence rates, and a reasonable cost.

The approach to parathyroid surgery changed dramatically after the use of Tc-99m MIBI for preoperative imaging of primary hyperparathyroidism (PHPT). Radio-guided minimally invasive surgery for hyperparathyroidism using a gamma probe facilitates the surgical exploration; several papers were published about its usefulness after the initial reports of J. Norman (1998a, b). Alternative arguments have also been reported in the following years, until nowadays the best approach being direct related to the experience of the entire team involved in treatment.

8.4.2 Minimally Invasive Parathyroidectomy

With the introduction of Tc-99m MIBI scintigraphy having the purpose to identify and locate the parathyroid adenoma preoperatively, it began the era of focused exploration and minimally invasive parathyroidectomy, the radio-guided surgery, and novel endoscopic techniques (Monchik et al. 2002). In case of primary hyperparathyroidism, the goal of surgery is to return the patient's calcium level to normal.

The success of the surgical treatment depends on the localization and identification of the abnormal glands. These procedures may be done as outpatient surgery, even with local anesthesia.

Introduction of intraoperative quick PTH assays opened also new ways of approaches in the management of primary hyperparathyroidism. This assay measures intact PTH levels in the patient's plasma using an immunochemiluminometric technique and can be performed during the operation. Therefore, a significant drop in quick PTH level is observed 5–10 min after removal of the abnormal gland. The fall of quick PTH level of about 50% of the preoperative level is considered indicative of successful removal. Under these conditions, the quick PTH assay has a sensitivity and a specificity of 98% and 94%, respectively, and an overall accuracy of 97% in predicting success of surgery (Irvin and Carneiro 2000).

8.4.3 Gamma Probe-Guided Operation Technique

1. Minimally Invasive Approach

   After the induction of the chosen anesthesia (local/general), a gamma probe survey is done over the skin to locate the hotspot and make a mark over the skin (skin marking can also be done in the nuclear medicine department under the gamma camera by using a cobalt pen during scintigraphy). Then, a small incision (less than 2 cm) is done through this point and, after, the dissection of strap muscles; the underlying space is explored using the gamma probe (Costello and Norman 1999; Norman 1998a). The gamma probe's auditory and digital signals guide the surgeon to find the hyperactive gland. An in vivo parathyroid to thyroid ratio greater than 1.5 and parathyroid to background ratio greater than 2.5–4.5 strongly suggest the presence of parathyroid adenoma. After the excision of the radioactive suspected tissue, ex vivo counts are obtained, and the 20% rule is applied, with the limitations previously cited.
2. Bilateral Cervical Exploration

   Radio-guided surgery is also useful when performing a standard bilateral approach (Burkey et al. 2002). If bilateral cervical exploration is going to be performed, before skin incision, counts over four quadrants in the neck, as well as over the mediastinum, are obtained with the gamma probe. A standard collar incision and a bilateral cervical exploration are performed. Suspected tissues with high in vivo gamma probe counts compared with background counts are excised, and ex vivo counts are recorded. The exploration of the neck is terminated after a post-resection gamma probe survey of all four quadrants.

8.4.4 The Radio-Guided Minimally Invasive Parathyroidectomy

The radio-guided technique introduced and patented by one of the most experienced parathyroid surgeons, Jim Norman, consists in the exploration of all four parathyroid glands that have previously retained the Tc-99m MIBI injected preoperative (Norman 1998a, 2011).

Radio-guided parathyroidectomy is indicated in:

- PHPT due to parathyroid adenomas.
- Reoperation for persistent or recurrent hyperparathyroidism.
- Ectopic adenomas.
- In patients with multinodular goiter, dual-phase Tc-99m MIBI scintigraphy combined with ultrasound examination or double-tracer subtraction protocols is recommended before planning the surgery to demonstrate MIBI-avid thyroid nodules.
- The gamma probe-guided surgery may also be used in patients undergoing bilateral neck exploration with a negative preoperative scintigraphy because it decreases operation time and gives more guarantees about the pathological parathyroid tissue removal.

The following steps are performed in this operation:

1. Injection of Tc-99m MIBI 15–20 mCi (555–740 MBq) intravenously.
2. Image of the parathyroid glands on gamma camera after 10–15 min in the AP incidence and oblique lateral left and right. Normal parathyroid glands become dormant when the calcium is high; thus normal parathyroid glands do not uptake significantly the radioactive tracer.
3. The surgeon knows which general area of the neck to operate doing a 3/4 in. incision in the lower neck, which is typically made for the minimal parathyroid operation. The surgery may start immediately after the scan and delayed for a period of about 3–4 h, the radiotracer still being active at optimal level.

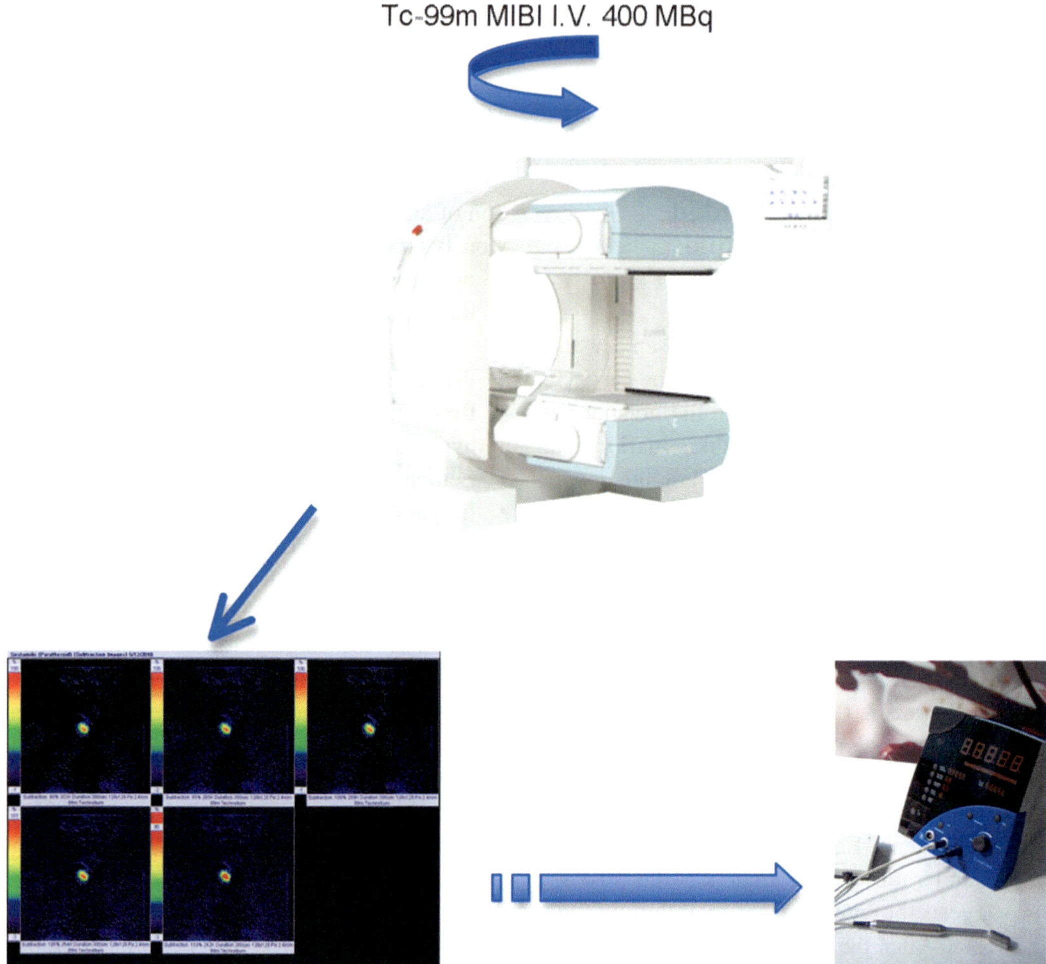

Fig. 8.20 The sequences of parathyroid adenoma diagnosis and radio-guided parathyroid surgery

4. A miniature handheld radiation-detecting probe (gamma probe) is used to find the radioactive parathyroid. This probe will emit an audio signal when it is placed near the parathyroid gland because it detects radioactivity. The next step is for the surgeon to dissect the overactive parathyroid tumor away from the rest of the neck structures and remove it (Fig. 8.20).
5. Measure the radioactivity in the parathyroid tumor to make sure that the patient is cured of his disease. Once the enlarged parathyroid gland is out, the probe is placed on it to make sure that the radioactive tumor has been removed. Performed correctly, this method is much more accurate than measuring PTH levels during the operation (over 99% accuracy!). Using all of this information, the experience of the surgeon will determine whether more operating is needed or not.
6. Typically, at least one or more parathyroid glands are inspected visually, and their radioactivity is measured, while the other two are checked with the probe (without dissecting them).

Tc-99m MIBI I.V. 400 MBq

To optimize the parathyroid-thyroid count ratio, different protocols have been introduced.

1. Norman and Chheda's (1997) protocol consists of dual-phase Tc-99m MIBI scintigraphy

on the day of the surgery, and gamma probe-guided surgery begins at the end of the scintigraphy, about 2.5–3 h after the injection of the radioactivity. According to this protocol, the standard activity of dual-phase scintigraphy that must be used is about 740 MBq (see the dedicated section).

2. Casara et al. (2000) performed gamma probe-guided surgery using a separate-day protocol: Tc-99m MIBI diagnostic imaging is performed before the surgery, preferably with double-tracer protocol. On the day of the surgery, a smaller activity of Tc-99m MIBI is injected in the operating room just before the operation, about 37 MBq. This protocol reduces the surgery team's exposure and allows the localization of the parathyroid tissue with rapid washout timing (less than 2.5–3 h).
3. Bozkurt et al. (2007) performed a patient-specific optimal time to surgery method. In their protocol, double-phase MIBI scintigraphy was performed on a separate day before surgery including a dynamic Tc-99m MIBI acquisition to obtain a time-activity curve showing differential parathyroid to thyroid ratio to determine the optimum time to surgery.
4. Several other groups use a modified separate-day protocol in which a higher Tc-99m MIBI activity (370 MBq) is injected to reach a higher target to the background ratio. This procedure is useful to identify ectopic parathyroid adenomas.

Comments:

- Different protocols have their own advantages and disadvantages like scheduling of the operating room for the surgery and cooperation between nuclear medicine and surgery departments (Desiato et al. 2016).
- A different-day protocol is probably preferable in iodine-deficient geographic areas with a high prevalence of nodular goiter in order to better select the patient for gamma probe-guided surgery.
- Injected radioactivity differs according to the protocol chosen. If a same-day protocol including double-phase imaging followed by surgery is planned, 740 MBq is usually administrated. In a separate-day protocol, in order to decrease the dose to the patient and surgical staff in the operating room, a lower dose of Tc-99m MIBI (37 MBq) can be used with satisfactory results.
- Ex vivo radioactivity counting "20% rule" (Murphy and Norman 1999). Measurement of the radioactivity in the excised tissue allows the physician to distinguish parathyroid adenoma from normal parathyroid tissue and other neck structures in order to make the appropriate operative decisions. This method which is also called the "20% rule" implicates that any excised tissue containing more than 20% of background radioactivity at the operative basin is a parathyroid adenoma and additional frozen section is not required. According to Murphy and Norman (1999), the hyperplastic glands will not accumulate more than 18% of background radioactivity whatever their size.

8.4.5 Radiation Safety Considerations

In order to decrease the radiation dose of the operating room personnel, the lowest dose of Tc-99m MIBI that is necessary to effectively remove the pathological parathyroid tissue should be given (ALARA principles). The radiation dose rates from the excised specimens are quite low and would not result in significant radiation exposure to pathology personnel.

Surgeons and operating room personnel are accepted as non-radiation workers and have an annual dose limit of 1 mSv.

For the single-day protocol (injection of 740 MBq Tc-99m MIBI 2.5–3 h before surgery), the surgeons reach the annual limit doing 20 patients/year. Instead, with the 2-day protocol (injection of lower dose of 37 MBq on the day of operation), the radiation exposure of the surgeon is very low: 400 patients/year are needed to reach the limit.

References

AACE/AAES Task Force on Primary Hyperparathyroidism (2005) The American Association of Clinical Endocrinologists and the American Association of Endocrine Surgeons Position Statement on the diagnosis and management of primary hyperparathyroidism. Endocr Pract 11(1):49–54

Arnold A, Shattuck TM, Mallya SM et al (2002) Molecular pathogenesis of primary hyperparathyroidism. J Bone Miner Res 17(Suppl 2):N30–N36

Beierwaltes WH (1991) Endocrine imaging: parathyroid, adrenal cortex and medulla, and other endocrine tumours. Part II. J Nucl Med 32:1627–1639

Bilezikian JP, Brandi ML, Eastell R et al (2014) Guidelines for the management of asymptomatic primary hyperparathyroidism: summary statement from the Fourth International Workshop. J Clin Endocrinol Metab 99(10):3561–3569

Bozkurt M, Ugur O, Pinar K (2007) Gamma probe guided parathyroidectomy: factors affecting lesions detectability. J Nucl Med 48(Suppl 2):269P

Burkey SH, van Heerden JA, Farley DR et al (2002) Will directed parathyroidectomy utilizing the gamma probe or intraoperative parathyroid hormone assay replace bilateral cervical exploration as the preferred operation for primary hyperparathyroidism? World J Surg 26:914–920

Carty SE, Worsey J, Virji MA et al (1997) Concise parathyroidectomy: the impact of preoperative SPECT 99mTc sestamibi scanning and intraoperative quick parathormone assay [with discussion]. Surgery 122:1107–1116

Casara D, Rubello D, Piotto A et al (2000) Tc99m-MIBI radio-guided minimally invasive parathyroid surgery planned on the basis of a preoperative combined 99mTc-pertechnetate/99mTc-MIBI and ultrasound imaging protocol. Eur J Nucl Med 27:1300–1304

Chudzinski W et al (2005) P-Glycoprotein expression influences the result of Tc-99m – MIBI scintigraphy in tertiary hyperparathyroidism. Int J Mol Med 16:215–219

Costello D, Norman J (1999) Minimally invasive radioguided parathyroidectomy. Surg Oncol Clin N Am 8:555–564

Desiato V, Melis M, Amato B et al (2016) Minimally invasive radioguided parathyroid surgery: a literature review. Int J Surg 28(Suppl 1):S84–S93

Gauger PG, Agarwal G, England BG et al (2001) Intraoperative parathyroid hormone monitoring fails to detect double parathyroid adenomas: a 2-institution experience. Surgery 130:1005–1010

Henry JF, Raffaelli M, Iacobone M et al (2001) Video-assisted parathyroidectomy via the lateral approach vs conventional surgery in the treatment of sporadic primary hyperparathyroidism: results of a case-control study. Surg Endosc 15:1116–1119

Hindie E, Ugur O, Fuster D et al (2009) EANM parathyroid guidelines. Eur J Nucl Med Mol Imaging 36:1201–1216

Irvin GL III, Carneiro DM (2000) Management changes in primary hyperparathyroidism. JAMA 284:934–936

Khan AA, Hanley DA, Rizzoli R et al (2017) Primary hyperparathyroidism: review and recommendations on evaluation, diagnosis, and management. A Canadian and international consensus. Osteoporos Int 28:1. doi:10.1007/s00198-016-3716-2

Lavely WC et al (2007) Comparison of SPECT/CT, SPECT, and planar imaging with single- and dual-phase Tc-99m-Sestamibi parathyroid scintigraphy. J Nucl Med 48:1084–1089

Mitchell BK (1996) Mechanism of technetium 99m sestamibi parathyroid imaging and the possible role of P-glycoprotein. Surgery 120:1039–1045

Monchik JM, Barellini L, Langer P et al (2002) Minimally invasive parathyroid surgery in 103 patients with local/regional anesthesia, without exclusion criteria. Surgery 131:502–508

Murphy C, Norman JG (1999) The 20% rule: a simple, instantaneous radioactivity measurement defines cure and allows elimination of frozen sections and hormone assays during parathyroidectomy. Surgery 126:1023–1029

Norman JG (1998a) Minimally invasive radio-guided parathyroidectomy: an endocrine surgeon's perspective. J Nucl Med 39:15N–24N

Norman JG (1998b) http://parathyroid.com/10_parathyroid_rules.htm. Accessed Aug 2011

Norman JG (2011) http://parathyroid.com/sestamibi.htm. Accessed 18 Aug 2011

Norman JG, Chheda H (1997) Minimally invasive parathyroidectomy facilitated by intraoperative nuclear mapping. Surgery 122:998–1004. doi:10.1016/S0039-6060(97),90201-4

Rubello D, Casara D, Pelizzo MR (2003) Optimization of preoperative procedures. Nucl Med Commun 24:133–140. doi:10.1097/00006231-200302000-00005

Silverberg SJ, Shane E, Jacobs TP et al (1999) A 10-year prospective study of primary hyperparathyroidism with or without parathyroid surgery. N Engl J Med 341:1249–1255

Wilhelm SM, Wang TS, Ruan DT et al (2016) The American Association of Endocrine Surgeons guidelines for definitive management of primary hyperparathyroidism. JAMA Surg 151(10):959–968

9 The Adrenal Glands

"If anything is sacred, the human body is sacred"

Walt Whitman, (poet 1819–1892)

9.1 Overview

The two suprarenal glands, which are also called adrenal glands, are retroperitoneal organs that lie on the upper poles of the kidneys. They are surrounded by renal fascia but are separated from the kidneys by the perirenal fat. The combined weight of suprarenal glands in human adults ranges from 7 to 10 g. The right suprarenal gland is pyramid shaped and caps the upper pole of the right kidney. It lies behind the right lobe of the liver and extends medially behind the inferior vena cava. It rests posteriorly on the diaphragm. The left adrenal is crescent shaped and lies medial to the kidney above the left renal vein. It lies behind the pancreas, the lesser sac, and the stomach and rests posteriorly on the diaphragm.

A conjunctive capsule wraps the adrenal gland, composed of two distinct parts:

- Cortex—the peripheral area
- Medulla—the core area

The cortex represents 80–90% and is composed of cords of epithelial cells that are directly related to the blood vessels (capillary sinusoids). These epithelial cells are grouped so that different adrenal cortex shows a characteristic layering in three areas arranged as follows:

- Zone glomerulosa—a thin layer of cells that lies just underneath the capsule, constitutes about 15% of the adrenal cortex. These cells are the only ones in the adrenal gland capable of secreting significant amounts of aldosterone because they contain the enzyme aldosterone synthase, which is necessary for the synthesis of aldosterone. The secretion of these cells is mainly controlled by the extracellular fluid concentrations of angiotensin II and potassium, both of which stimulate aldosterone secretion.
- Zone fasciculata—the middle and widest layer, constitutes about 75% of the adrenal cortex and secretes the glucocorticoids cortisol and corticosterone, as well as small amounts of adrenal androgens and estrogens. The secretion of these cells is controlled in large part by the hypothalamic-pituitary axis via the adrenocorticotropic hormone (ACTH).
- Zone reticularis—the deep layer of the cortex, secretes the adrenal androgens dehydroepiandrosterone (DHEA) and androstenedione, as well as small amounts of estrogens and some glucocorticoids. ACTH also regulates secretion of these cells, although other factors such as cortical androgen-stimulating hormone, released from the pituitary, may also be involved.

D. Piciu, *Nuclear Endocrinology*, DOI 10.1007/978-3-319-56582-8_9

Some of the actions produced by these hormones include:

- Cortisol hormone—also known as hydrocortisone, controls the body's use of fats, proteins, and carbohydrates.
- Corticosterone—this hormone, together with cortisol hormones, suppresses inflammatory reactions in the body and also affects the immune system.
- Aldosterone hormone—this hormone inhibits the level of sodium excreted into the urine, maintaining blood volume and blood pressure.
- Androgenic steroids (androgen hormones)—these hormones cause retention of Na (protein anabolic effect) and stimulate osteogenesis and somatic development.

The suprarenal medulla (*MSR*) is the core of the gland and represents 20% of it, and the cortex surrounds it.

MSR is composed of chromaffin cells, arranged in groups or in columns in which there are large capillary sinusoids and veins of different sizes. Among the chromaffin cells, scattered sympathetic ganglion cells are found, alone or in groups. These cells are neurons which have lost their axons and gained secretory properties and therefore can be considered as a medullosuprarenal sympathetic ganglion.

Medullosuprarenal hormones are called catecholamines, and they are represented by adrenalin (80%) and noradrenalin (20%):

- *Adrenalin* (also called epinephrine)—This hormone increases the heart rate and force of heart contractions, facilitates blood flow to the muscles and brain, causes relaxation of smooth muscles, and helps with conversion of glycogen to glucose in the liver and other activities.
- *Noradrenalin* (also called norepinephrine)—This hormone has little effect on the smooth muscle, metabolic processes, and cardiac output but has strong vasoconstrictive effects, thus increasing blood pressure.

9.2 Pathophysiology

9.2.1 Pathologies of the Adrenal Cortex

9.2.1.1 Hypoadrenalism (Adrenal Insufficiency): Addison's Disease

This disease results from an inability of the adrenal cortices to produce sufficient adrenocortical hormones, and this in turn is most frequently caused by primary atrophy or injury of the adrenal cortices. In about 80% of the cases, the atrophy is caused by autoimmunity against the cortices. The adrenal gland hypofunction is also frequently caused by tuberculosis destruction of the adrenal glands or by cancer invasion of the adrenal cortices.

The symptoms of Addison's disease develop insidiously. The most common symptoms are fatigue, lightheadedness upon standing or while upright, muscle weakness, fever, weight loss, difficulty in standing up, anxiety, nausea, vomiting, diarrhea, headache, sweating, changes in mood and personality, and joint and muscle pains. Some have marked cravings for salt or salty foods due to the urinary losses of sodium. Affected individuals may note increased tanning since adrenal insufficiency is manifested in the skin primarily by hyperpigmentation, specifically due to the decrease in cortisol and subsequent increase in ACTH levels.

9.2.1.2 Hyperadrenalism: Cushing's Syndrome

Hypersecretion by the adrenal cortex causes a complex cascade of hormone effects called the *Cushing's syndrome*. Many of the abnormalities of Cushing's syndrome are ascribable to abnormal amounts of cortisol, but excess secretion of androgens may also cause important effects. Hypercortisolism can occur from multiple causes, including:

- Adenomas of the anterior pituitary that secrete large amounts of ACTH, which then causes adrenal hyperplasia and excess cortisol secretion
- Abnormal function of the hypothalamus that causes high levels of corticotropin-releasing hormone (CRH), which stimulates excess ACTH release
- "Ectopic secretion" of ACTH by a tumor elsewhere in the body, such as an abdominal carcinoma
- Adenomas of the adrenal cortex

When the Cushing's syndrome is secondary to excess secretion of ACTH by the anterior pituitary, this is referred to as *Cushing's disease*.

A special characteristic of Cushing's syndrome is the mobilization of fat from the lower part of the body, with concomitant extra deposition of fat in the thoracic and upper abdominal regions, giving rise to a buffalo torso. The excess secretion of steroids also leads to an edematous appearance of the face, and the androgenic potency of some of the hormones sometimes causes acne and hirsutism (excess growth of facial hair). The appearance of the face is frequently described as a "moon face." About 80% of patients have hypertension, presumably because of the mineralocorticoid effects of cortisol.

9.2.2 Pathologies of the Adrenal Medulla: The Pheochromocytoma

Pheochromocytoma is a neuroendocrine tumor of the medulla of the suprarenal glands originating in the chromaffin cells and secrets excessive amounts of catecholamines, usually noradrenalin, and adrenalin to a lesser extent. In general, they are benign tumors, but there are situations when they might be malignant.

The signs and symptoms of a pheochromocytoma are those of sympathetic nervous system hyperactivity, including:

- Skin rash
- Flank pain
- Elevated heart rate; elevated blood pressure, including paroxysmal (sporadic, episodic) high blood pressure, which sometimes can be more difficult to detect
- Orthostatic hypotension
- Anxiety often resembling that of a panic attack
- Excessive sweating
- Headaches
- Elevated blood glucose level (due primarily to catecholamine stimulation of lipolysis (breakdown of stored fat) leading to high levels of free fatty acids and the subsequent inhibition of glucose uptake by muscle cells; further, stimulation of beta-adrenergic receptors leads to glycogenolysis and gluconeogenesis and thus elevation of blood glucose levels)

The diagnosis can be established by measuring catecholamines and metanephrines in plasma (blood) or through a 24-h urine collection, and surgical resection of the tumor is the treatment of first choice, either by open laparotomy or else laparoscopy.

The evaluation of adrenal disorders has been simplified by the development of sensitive and specific biochemical tests and by the availability of high-resolution CT and MR imaging. On the other hand, the exquisite spatial resolution of these imaging modalities has produced the diagnostic conundrum of the adrenal incidentaloma. The scintigraphic assessment of disorders of the adrenal cortex, such as Cushing's syndrome, primary aldosteronism, and adrenal hyperandrogenism, is only infrequently required, whereas the disease in patients with pheochromocytoma has resulted in an expanding clinical role for adrenal medullary imaging.

9.3 Adrenal Cortical Scintigraphy

I-131-6β-Iodomethyl-19-norcholesterol (also known as iodocholesterol or NP-59) is the current radiopharmaceutical of choice for adrenal cortical imaging. The main disadvantage of iodocholesterol scintigraphy is the high radiation dose, due to beta component of I-131. The uptake of these agents into adrenocortical cells is related to the precursor status of cholesterol for adrenal steroid synthesis and to the transportation of cholesterol and radiocholesterol by low-density lipoprotein (LDL). An increase in the serum cholesterol reduces the uptake by downregulating LDL receptors. Any increase in circulating ACTH results in increased radiocholesterol uptake. Although radiocholesterol is stored in adrenal cortical cells, it is not esterified and therefore not incorporated into adrenal hormones. Several medications, including glucocorticoids, diuretics, spironolactone, ketoconazole, and cholesterol-lowering agents, may interfere with radiocholesterol uptake. Following injection, the uptake of the radiocholesterols is progressive over several days, and there is prolonged retention within the adrenal cortex, permitting imaging over a period of days to weeks. Although adrenal uptake for all of these agents is ≤0.2% per gland, total body exposure is relatively high:

- *Radiopharmaceutical*: I-131—iodocholesterol
- *Activity administered*: 37 MBq (1 mCi)
- *Effective dose equivalent*: 105 mSv (10 rem)
- *Patient preparation*: thyroid blocked
- *Gamma camera*:
- Collimator—high energy, general purpose, parallel hole
- Images of the abdomen acquired: posterior, lateral, anterior, and oblique
- Images acquired at about 4 and 7 days postinjection
- 20-min exposure per image

Emphasis is given to the posterior view of the abdomen, and lateral views may be required to differentiate gallbladder uptake from activity in the right adrenal gland. Due to problems with soft tissue attenuation and relatively high variability of percentage uptake between normal glands, the quantitation of differential uptake is troublesome. Only when uptakes differ by more than 50% should they be considered abnormal.

Although radiotracer uptake reaches its maximum by 48 h, imaging is usually delayed to day 4 or 5 to allow clearance of background activity. The right adrenal gland frequently appears more intense than the left one due to its more posterior location and the superimposition of hepatic activity. Visualization of the liver, colon, and gallbladder is physiological.

9.3.1 Cushing's Syndrome

The diagnostic accuracy of iodocholesterol scintigraphy for detecting adrenal hyperplasia, adenoma, or carcinoma as the cause of glucocorticoid excess is approximately 95%. However, it is rarely necessary in the evaluation of Cushing's syndrome. Biochemical testing combined with CT and/or MRI is usually successful in localizing the site of ACTH secretion without scintigraphy, except in occasional cases of ectopic ACTH syndrome.

Virtually all adrenocortical carcinomas are detected by F-18 FDG PET and can be accurately staged by PET as well. In patients with recurrent Cushing's syndrome following prior bilateral adrenalectomy, adrenal scintigraphy may be the most sensitive means of localizing functional adrenal remnants.

9.3.2 Primary Aldosteronism

The differentiation of adenoma from bilateral hyperplasia is difficult with biochemical testing without performing bilateral adrenal vein sampling. Aldosteronomas are typically less than 2 cm in diameter and cannot be differentiated from nonfunctioning adenomas by CT or MRI; hyperplasia is often inferred by the absence of a detectable mass.

Aldosterone is not regulated by pituitary ACTH secretion. An adenoma cannot be diagnosed on a baseline scan because both adrenal glands are visualized in all patients with primary aldosteronism, and the degree of asymmetry may be identical in patients with bilateral hyperplasia or adenoma. To increase the specificity, it is necessary to have a dexamethasone suppression scan. Dexamethasone suppression, 4 mg for 7 days before and continued for 5–7 days postinjection, results in scans in which the normal cortex is visualized no earlier than the fifth day after the iodocholesterol injection:

- Unilateral adrenal visualization before the fifth day postinjection or marked asymmetrical activity thereafter is consistent with adenoma.
- Bilateral adrenal visualization before the fifth day suggests bilateral adrenal cortical hyperplasia.
- Bilateral uptake after the fifth day may occur in normal subjects.

Accuracy of the dexamethasone suppression scan exceeds 90%.

9.3.3 Hyperandrogenism

Dexamethasone suppression radiocholesterol scintigraphy has been successfully used to identify an adrenal source of androgen hypersecretion. Because cholesterol is the precursor for synthesis of gonadal steroids, iodocholesterol imaging has successfully localized sources of excess androgen secretion.

9.4 Adrenal Medullary Scintigraphy

Pheochromocytomas are catecholamine-secreting neoplasms arising from chromaffin cells.

There is a well-known rule of “ten.” Approximately:

- 10% are malignant.
- 10% are bilateral.
- 10% occur in children.
- 10–20% are extra-adrenal in origin (paragangliomas), usually in the abdomen or pelvis but occasionally in the neck or mediastinum.

Because anatomical imaging studies are nonspecific and may not be sensitive for the presence of extra-adrenal foci, bilaterality, or metastatic disease, adrenal medullary scintigraphy may play a major role in the diagnosis of patients with pheochromocytoma, paraganglioma, or neuroblastoma. This is especially important in view of the severalfold higher perioperative complication rate associated with reoperation.

Radiopharmaceuticals:
- Metaiodobenzylguanidine (MIBG-iobenguan) is a guanethidine analogue similar to norepinephrine that is taken up by adrenergic tissue via expressed plasma membrane norepinephrine transporters and intracellular vesicular monoamine transporters.
- The uptake may be inhibited by a variety of pharmaceuticals including sympathomimetics, antidepressants, and some antihypertensives, especially labetalol. These must be withheld for an appropriate length of time before MIBG administration.
- The radiopharmaceutical may be labeled as I-123 MIBG or I-131 MIBG.

Activity administered:
- 400 MBq (approximately 10 mCi) I-123 MIBG
- 20 MBq (approximately 0.5 mCi) I-131 MIBG

Effective dose equivalent:
- 6 mSv (600 mrem) I-123 MIBG
- 3 mSv (300 mrem) I-131 MIBG

Patient preparation:
- I-123 MIBG: Lugol’s solution or (6 drops/day) a saturated solution of potassium iodide (100 mg twice a day) begun the day prior to the administration of the radiopharmaceutical and continued for 4 days afterward.
- I-131 MIBG: Lugol’s solution or (6 drops/day) a saturated solution of potassium iodide (100 mg twice a day) begun the day prior to

the administration of the radiopharmaceutical and continued for 7 days afterward. The pediatric doses are 25–50% lower than those of adults, related to age and weight.

Gamma camera:

- I-123 MIBG: collimator—low energy, high resolution, parallel hole
- Images acquired: whole-body images, anterior and posterior, 10 min per step, at 24 h (and 48 h as needed)
- I-131 MIBG: collimator—high energy, general purpose, parallel hole (I-131 MIBG)
- Images acquired: SPECT of the abdomen; whole-body images, anterior and posterior, 20 min per step, at 24 and 48 h (and 72 h as needed)

Although both I-131 and I-123 have been used to label MIBG, I-123 is preferred because of its favorable dosimetry and imaging characteristics. Plasma clearance of MIBG is rapid, with 50–70% of the dose excreted unchanged into the urine within 24 h. Due to the release of free radioiodine from the radiopharmaceutical, the co-administration of stable iodine to block thyroid uptake is necessary.

Physiological activity is typically seen within the liver, spleen, bladder, and salivary glands. Faint activity is seen in the normal adrenal medulla in 16% of cases using I-131 MIBG and in over 25% of the cases using I-123 MIBG.

Relatively faint activity is also seen in the myocardium and lungs, especially in early images. Free radioiodine will localize to the gastric mucosa and later in the colon. The uterus may be visualized during menstruation. Importantly, no skeletal activity is normally present. Anatomical variations in the renal collecting system may lead to false-positive imaging results.

9.4.1 Clinical Applications

The diagnosis of pheochromocytoma is made by the laboratory demonstration of elevated catecholamines in the plasma and/or urine. However, in patients with suspected pheochromocytoma who have negative imaging findings with CT and MRI, MIBG scintigraphy can be very useful, especially in view of its high negative predictive value. However, malignant pheochromocytoma may dedifferentiate and thus no longer accumulate MIBG. In these instances, F-18 FDG PET imaging or In-111 octreotide scintigraphy may better demonstrate the extent of metastatic disease.

Most neuroendocrine tumors express somatostatin receptors, and somatostatin receptor scintigraphy (SRS) using In-111 octreotide or Tc-99m Tektrotyd has been reported to be highly sensitive (>90%) for the detection of head and neck paragangliomas. However, SRS has been reported to have sensitivity as low as 25% for the detection of primary adrenal pheochromocytoma. SRS is at least as sensitive as MIBG imaging for the detection of metastatic pheochromocytoma (87% versus 57% of lesions). Therefore, SRS is not recommended as a first-line modality for detection of suspected primary pheochromocytoma.

I-123 MIBG imaging may be especially useful in children who more frequently have hereditary syndromes (multiple endocrine neoplasia, von Hippel-Lindau, neurofibromatosis, familial pheochromocytoma, and Carney's triad) and are at higher risk for multi-focality, extra-adrenal disease, and malignant disease. Bilateral uptake due to medullary hyperplasia may be demonstrated by MIBG scintigraphy, but sensitivity is insufficient to exclude contralateral disease. It must be remembered that MIBG imaging, SRS, and F-18 FDG PET may detect other neuroendocrine tumors such as medullary thyroid carcinoma, carcinoid, and islet cell tumors as well as neuroblastoma and small cell lung carcinoma.

Case 1: Left Pheochromocytoma

History:

A 33-year-old male, with previous history of medullary thyroid carcinoma, with total thyroidectomy suffered 4 years ago.

Clinical examination:

Symptoms: fatigue, tremor, rush, palpitation, crisis of high blood pressure.

The neck examination does not reveal any pathological findings; presence of a scar after thyroidectomy. No clinical evidence of lymph nodes.

Examinations:

The abdominal ultrasound revealed solid, hypoechogenic nodule in the left adrenal gland.

Metanephrine in plasma—1200 ng/L (N.V. <90 ng/L), very increased.

Calcitonin—<2 ng/L (N.V. <13 ng/L)—excludes the recurrence of medullary thyroid cancer.

Findings:

The scintigraphy with I-131 MIBG showed an uptake of the radiotracer in the left adrenal gland (Fig. 9.1).

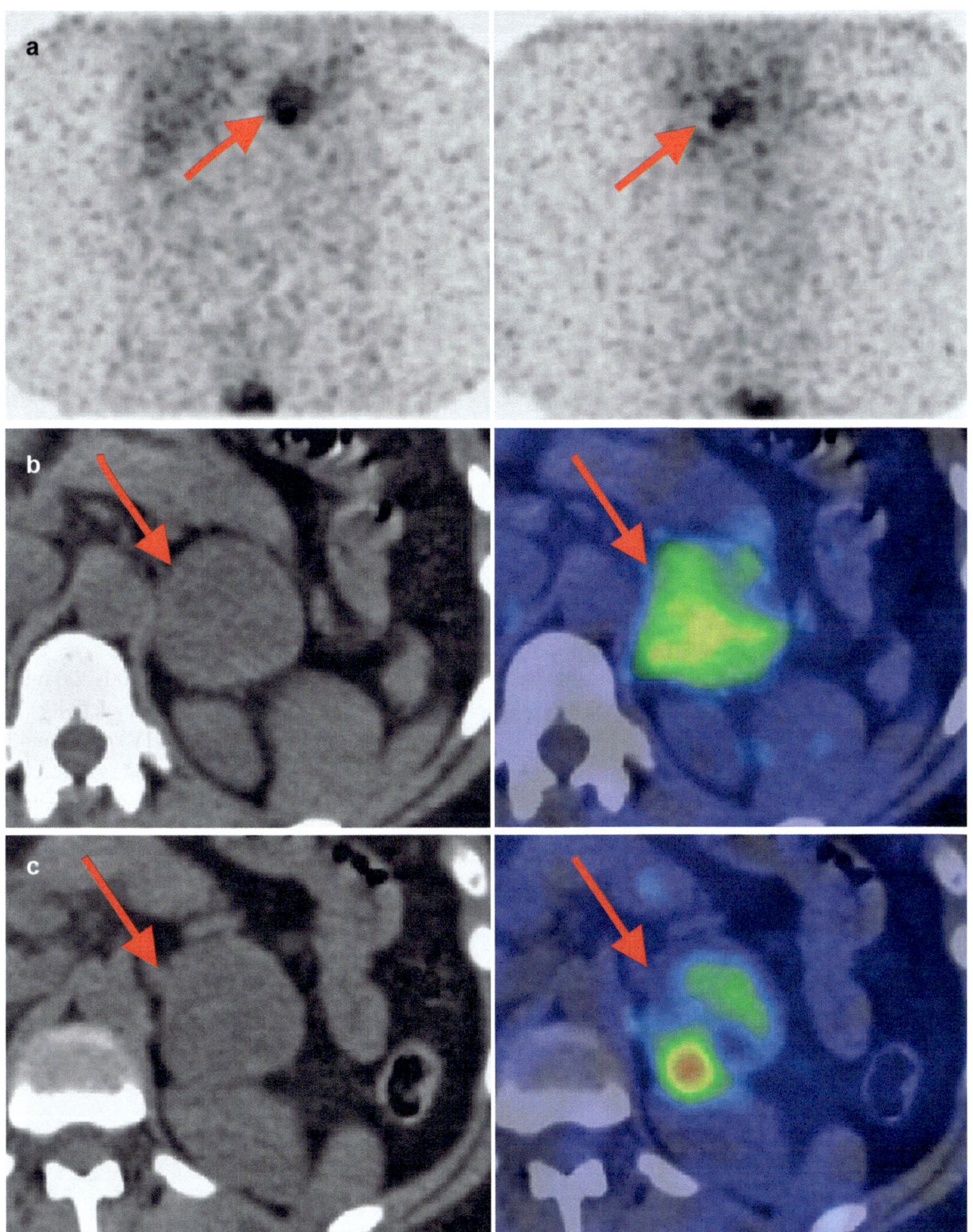

Fig. 9.1 Left pheochromocytoma. SPECT/CT I-131 MIBG (**a**, transversal CT; **b**, transversal SPECT/CT; **c**, transversal SPECT/CT) (University of Debrecen-Scanomed, with the courtesy of L. Szabados, M.D.)

Conclusion:
Left pheochromocytoma.

Key Points
The pheochromocytoma may be associated with medullary thyroid cancers in the MEN IIA and MEN IIB syndromes, so special attention must be accorded to this pathology.

Even if CT or MRI is able to frequently discover the disease, the role of the nuclear scan is firstly in recurrence and in the presence of ectopia.

9.5 Nuclear Therapy of Malignant Pheochromocytoma

Radiopharmaceutical:

- I-131 iodine-metaiodobenzylguanidine (MIBG-iobenguan).
- It decays by emission of gamma radiations with photon energies of 364, 337, and 284 KeV and with beta radiation with the maximal energy of 0.61 MeV to stable Xe-131.

Principle:

After intracellular incorporation, the therapeutic effects of I-131 MIBG result from the emission of ionizing radiation from the decaying radionuclide. The beta particles have a tissue range of 0.5 mm and lead to the destruction of tumor cells which selectively uptake the I-131 MIBG; the extra-tumoral radiation is therefore reduced. The drug is excreted by urine in proportion of 55% within the first 24 h and up to 90% in 4 days.

Indications:

- Malignant pheochromocytoma
- Malignant paraganglioma
- Neuroblastoma stage III or IV
- Medullary thyroid carcinoma
- Metastatic, symptomatic carcinoid tumors

Patient preparation:

- Thyroid blockade: To protect the thyroid from free I-131, 100–200 mg potassium iodide is to be orally administered daily, starting 1 day prior to therapy and to be continued for 2 weeks. Perchlorate may be added to the thyroid blockade.
- To prevent the acute effects from the excess of catecholamines in the circulation during the therapy, the administration of alpha-blockers and beta-blockers may be indicated.
- Drug interactions: There are important interactions with some usual drugs from the patient's list of treatment which must be withdrawn at least 2 weeks before the therapy:
  - Labetalol
  - Reserpine
  - Calcium channel blockers
  - Tricyclic antidepressants
  - Ephedrine
  - Amphetamine
  - Dopamine
  - Guanethidine

Doses:

- A fixed dose of 3.7–11.1 GBq (100–300 mCi) I-131 MIBG with a specific activity of 1.48 GBq/mg is administered IV over 0.5–4 h through a lead-shielding infusion system.
- Treatment may be repeated only at 4–5 weeks interval.

Contraindications:

Absolute:

- Pregnancy
- Breastfeeding
- Myelosuppression
- Renal failure

Relative contraindication:

- Unstable condition

Side effects:

- Nausea and vomiting.
- Hematologic effects predominantly as an isolated thrombocytopenia.

- Rarely transient renal deterioration.
- Hypertensive crisis evoked by the release of catecholamines, requiring alpha blockade.
- Possible long-term effects are those of I-131 MIBG therapy in general, such as the hypothyroidism after an inadequate thyroid blockade and persistent hematological effects.

Further Reading

Bechereo A, Vierhapper H, Potzi C et al (2001) FDG-PET in adrenocortical carcinoma. Cancer Biother Radiopharm 16:289–295

Giammarile F, Chiti A, Lassmann M et al (2008) EANM procedure guidelines for 131I-meta-iodobenzylguanidine (131I-MIBG) therapy. Eur J Nucl Med Mol Imaging 35:1039–1047. doi:10.1007/s00259-008-0715-3

Gross MD, Shapiro B, Bui C et al (2003) Adrenal scintigraphy and metaiodobenzylguanidine therapy of neuroendocrine tumours. In: Sandler MP, Coleman RE, Patton JA, Wackers FJT, Gottschalk A (eds) Diagnostic nuclear medicine, 4th edn. Lippincott Williams & Wilkins, Philadelphia, pp 6715–6733

Ilias I, Yu J, Carrasquillo JA et al (2003) Superiority of 6-[18F] – fluorodopamine positron emission tomography versus [131I]-metaiodobenzylguanidine scintigraphy in the localization of metastatic pheochromocytoma. J Clin Endocrinol Metab 88:4083–4087

Martin WH, Sandler MP, Gross MD (2005) Thyroid, parathyroid and adrenal gland imaging. In Sharp FP, Gemmell HG, Murray AD eds. Practical nuclear medicine (3) Springer, London 264–271

Miskulin J, Shulkin BL, Doherty GM et al (2003) Is preoperative iodine 123 meta-iodobenzylguanidine scintigraphy routinely necessary before initial adrenalectomy for pheochromocytoma? Surgery 134:918–923

Mulatero P, Stowasser M, Loh K-C et al (2004) Increased diagnosis of primary aldosteronism, including surgically correctable forms, in centers from five continents. J Clin Endocrinol Metab 89:1045–1050

Shimizu A, Oriuchi N, Tsushima Y et al (2003) High [18F] 2-fluoro-2-deoxy-D-glucose (FDG) uptake of adrenocortical adenoma showing subclinical Cushing's syndrome. Ann Nucl Med 17:403–406

Neuroendocrine Tumors (NET) 10

"As the area of light expands, so does the perimeter of darkness"

A. Einstein

10.1 Overview

Neuroendocrine malignant tumors (NET), defined as epithelial neoplasms with predominant neuroendocrine differentiation, arise in most organs of the body. Some of the clinical and pathologic features of these tumors are characteristic of the organ of origin, but other attributes are shared by neuroendocrine neoplasms irrespective of their anatomic site. The multidisciplinary consensus group of experts (North American Neuroendocrine Tumor Society (NANETS), the College of American Pathologists (CAP), the European Neuroendocrine Tumor Society (ENETS)) in the field of NET has recommended a minimum pathology data set of features to be included in pathology reports. The system of classification and nomenclature is depending on the site of the tumor and also of the differentiation grade.

10.1.1 Systems of Nomenclature and Grading System for Neuroendocrine Tumors

10.1.1.1 Lung and Thymus NET (WHO)

Grade of differentiation:

- Low grade:
  - Carcinoid tumors
  - <2 mitoses/10 hpf (high-power field) and no necrosis
- Intermediate grade:
  - Atypical carcinoid tumors
  - 2–10 mitoses/10 hpf or foci of necrosis
- High grade:
  - Small cell carcinoma
  - Large cell neuroendocrine carcinoma
  - >10 mitoses/10 hpf

10.1.1.2 Gastroenteropancreatic (GEP) NET (WHO 2010, ESMO 2012)

Grade of differentiation:

- WHO 1-Low grade:
  - Neuroendocrine neoplasm, grade 1
  - <2 mitoses/10 hpf and <3% Ki 67 index
- WHO 2-Intermediate grade:
  - Neuroendocrine neoplasm, grade 2
  - 2–20 mitoses/10 hpf and 3–20% Ki 67 index
- WHO 3-High grade:
  - Neuroendocrine carcinoma, grade 3, small cell carcinoma
  - Neuroendocrine carcinoma, grade 3, large cell neuroendocrine carcinoma
  - >20 mitoses/10 hpf and >20% Ki 67 index
  - Mixed adenocarcinoma and neuroendocrine tumor
  - Tumorlike lesions

D. Piciu, *Nuclear Endocrinology*, DOI 10.1007/978-3-319-56582-8_10

Functionally active tumors:

- Functionally active NET present with clinical symptoms because of excessive hormone release from the tumor cell
- Examples of such events are:
  - Gastrinoma, excessive gastrin production, Zollinger–Ellison syndrome
  - Insulinoma, excessive insulin production, hypoglycemia syndrome
  - Glucagonoma, excessive glucagons production, glucagonoma syndrome
  - VIPoma, excessive production of vasoactive intestinal peptide (VIP), watery diarrhea-hypokalemia-achlorhydria syndrome
  - PPoma, excessive PP production (generally classified as nonfunctioning PETs)
  - Somatostatinoma, excessive somatostatin production
  - CRHoma, excessive corticotropin-releasing hormones production
  - Calcitoninoma, excessive calcitonin production
  - GHRHoma, excessive growth hormone-releasing hormone production
  - Neurotensinoma, excessive neurotensin production
  - ACTHoma, excessive production of adrenocorticotropic hormone
  - GRFoma, excessive production of growth hormone-releasing factor
  - Parathyroid hormone-related peptide tumor

Functionally inactive tumors:

- Functionally inactive NET are diagnosed in several ways:
  - During routine US performed for the investigation of unexplained upper abdominal complaints
  - In the case of large tumors of the pancreatic head because of the consequent extrahepatic jaundice
  - In the case of patients with relapsing abdominal cramps, as a result of intestinal pseudo-obstruction by a functionally inactive NET of the lower jejunum and ileum
  - As a result of tumor mass symptoms

Genetics:

- Non-sporadic NET arise as a result of syndromes caused by an autosomal dominant mutation

Symptoms:

- Insulinoma: hypoglycemia
- Gastrinoma: peptic ulcer disease
- VIPoma: diarrhea
- Glucagonoma: necrotic skin rush
- Somatostatinoma: mass effect
- Carcinoid: flush, rush, diarrhea, sweat
- Nonfunctional: mass effects

10.2 Nuclear Imaging of Neuroendocrine Tumors (NET)

Imaging studies for NET are generally performed for an initial evaluation of the extent of the disease and subsequent follow-up. The goals for the initial evaluation include the identification of the primary tumor, staging, and treatment planning. Subsequent follow-up imaging studies are performed for the surveillance after complete resection or during periods of stability and evaluation of response after the treatment.

Imaging modality commonly used includes the following:

- Small bowel series
- Computed tomography (CT)
- Magnetic resonance imaging (MRI)
- (In-111 DTPA) octreotide scintigraphy (OctreoScan)
- Metaiodobenzylguanidine (MIBG) scintigraphy
- Positron emission tomography (PET) and PET/CT

Imaging studies generally recommended at the time of the initial evaluation include plane film radiography of the chest, cross-sectional imaging (CT or MRI) of the abdomen and pelvis, and OctreoScan scintigraphy.

Among patients undergoing surveillance after complete resection, a chest radiography and periodic (every 6–12 months) cross-sectional imaging of the abdomen and pelvis are recommended. For patients having an advanced disease, it is important to evaluate if peptide receptor radionuclide therapy (PRRT) represents a good treatment option.

In-111- and Tc-99m Tektrotyd-labeled somatostatin analogues were developed for the scintigraphy of NET. It shares the receptor-binding profile of octreotide, which makes it a good radiopharmaceutical for imaging of somatostatin receptors 2 and 5.

Imaging is generally performed at 4–6 h and at 24 h. Imaging at 24 or even 48 h provides better contrast because of lower background activity. However, there is often physiological bowel activity that may produce false-positive results. SPECT/CT may be helpful in resolving the nature of indeterminate lesions found on CT and enhances the sensitivity and specificity of the study.

The scintigraphy can be performed for patients on long-acting octreotide but is best performed at the end of the dosing interval (3–6 weeks after the last dose).

For patients on octreotide delivered via a continuous infusion pump or those who received intermittent short-acting octreotide for rescue, it is recommended that these be stopped 48 h before and during testing if possible.

The In-111 octreotide scintigraphy is performed to evaluate the feasibility of PRRT as a scan with intense uptake at all known sites of disease, and it is associated with a higher response rate after radiotherapy with somatostatin receptor targeting.

I-123 MIBG molecular imaging has also been used for NET but has the greatest efficacy in patients with pheochromocytoma, paraganglioma, or neuroblastoma. Some tumors, negative on In-111 octreotide scintigraphy, can be better seen with I-123 MIBG.

Positron emission tomography F18-fluorodeoxyglucose (FDG) imaging, although successful for many solid tumors, has generally not provided additional information about the extent of the disease for well-differentiated NET because of their generally lower proliferative activity.

F18-FDG PET imaging may be used to characterize tumor aggressiveness with higher FDG uptake (expressed as SUV values) having a worse prognosis. This may be helpful when the tumor seems more aggressive than the histology indicates, and additional information for FDG imaging may result in changes of treatment.

Prior studies have shown C11-5-hydroxytryptophan (HTP) PET to be a promising imaging modality for the detection of NET. The serotonin precursor 5-HTP labeled with C-11 was used and showed an increased uptake and irreversible trapping of this tracer in NET. Other new PET imaging agents for NET include F18-DOPA, Ga-68 DOTATOC, Ga-68 DOTANOC, and F18-PGluc-TOCA. In addition, Tc-99m depreotide, which has a greater affinity to somatostatin receptor 3, has also been used for tumor imaging. Although these novel imaging techniques are promising, clinical experiences are limited.

As the latest ESMO guidelines (2012) recommend follow-up, investigations should include biochemical parameters and conventional imaging. In patients with R0/R1 resected NET G1/G2, it is recommended that imaging is performed every 3–6 months (CT or MRI) and, in NEC G3, every 2–3 months. Somatostatin receptor imaging, either OctreoScan or PET/CT using Ga-68 DOTATOC/NOC/TATE, should be included in the follow-up and is recommended after 18–24 months if expression of somatostatin receptor 2A has been proven on the tumor cells. In the case of rapid tumor progression or if imaging information is lacking, it may be necessary to re-biopsy liver metastases to reassess the proliferative activity.

10.2.1 NET Imaging with In-111 OctreoScan

Radiopharmaceutical:

- In-111 pentetreotide (OctreoScan)

Principle:

- OctreoScan is a radiolabeled analogue of somatostatin indicated for the scintigraphic localization of neuroendocrine tumors bearing somatostatin receptors.

Technique:

- Patient preparation:
  - Bowel preparation, especially for abdominal suspected lesions
  - Hydration and frequently voiding of the urinary bladder
  - Attention to diabetic patients where may cause paradoxical hypoglycemia
  - Temporarily withdrawal of octreotide therapy
  - Attention to breastfeeding and childbearing age patients (see Chap. 4)
- Dose: 3–6 mCi (11–220 MBq)/patient
- Injected I.V.
- It is necessary to wait 4–6 h after the injection for the first images. Delay images may be registered at 24 h or 48–72 h.
- Patient position: supine
- Gamma camera
  - Medium-energy general purpose (MEGP) collimator
- Acquisition:
  - The gamma camera is positioning anteriorly and next posteriorly or simultaneous in dual head camera.
  - Photon peaks at 172 and 245 keV and 20% windows.
  - 256 × 256 matrix or in whole body 256 × 1024.
  - Min 500,000 counts/image.
  - WBS speed 3 cm/min.
  - Also, spot images on the region of interest and lateral views of head/neck, chest, and abdomen may be obtained..
  - SPECT is usually recorded with 60 projections of 6° each or 90 projections of 4° each. Matrix 64 × 64..
  - 45–60 s/projection.
- Processing: There are special PC programs for image processing; additional analysis of counts in different region of interest (ROI) may be used.

Clinical applications:

- Diagnosis and management of receptor bearing gastroenteropancreatic (GEP) neuroendocrine tumors and carcinoid tumors; other non-GEP neuroendocrine tumors
- Diagnosis of carcinoid, islet cell carcinoma, gastrinoma, glucagonoma, insulinoma, VIPoma, motilinoma

Necessary additional examinations:

- CT, MRI
- Ultrasound
- Serologic tests of specific tumor markers
- Fine needle aspiration biopsy (FNAB)
- PET/CT with specific tracers

Comments:

- If there is no uptake of OctreoScan, the use of somatostatin analogues in the treatment is discouraged.
- SPECT/CT will add superior detection.

Reports:

- The report will include a description of the normal distribution and pathologic uptakes; the report should mention the correlation of nuclear findings with the morphological images.

10.2.2 NET Imaging with Tc-99m Tektrotyd

Radiopharmaceutical:

- Tc-99m Tektrotyd is a radiopharmaceutical indicated for diagnostics of pathological lesions in which somatostatin receptors are overexpressed (particularly subtype 2 and, to a lesser extent, subtypes 3 and 5) and which may be imaged by the labeled ligand.

Principle:

- OctreoScan is a radiolabeled analogue of somatostatin indicated for the scintigraphic localization of neuroendocrine tumors bearing somatostatin receptors.

Technique:

- Patient preparation:
  - Unless there are indications for other methods of the patient preparation, the patient is recommended to stay on light diet 1 day before examination. On the day of examination, the patient should fast until the end of the acquisition. If there is a need for examination after 24 h, it is recommended that a mild laxative be given to the patient starting the evening before. Method of patient preparation may depend on the applied examination protocol and the localization of imaged lesions. However, optimal imaging of abdominal cavity is obtained after the application of liquid diet 2 days before the examination and after administration of laxatives on the day before the examination.
  - Attention to breastfeeding and childbearing age patients (see Chap. 4).
- Dose: 370–925 MBq
- Tc-99m Tektrotyd is administered intravenously in a single dose after labeling of the kit using a sterile, oxidant-free sodium pertechnetate solution for injection. Technetium-99m in 1 ml of eluate of sodium pertechnetate Tc-99m solution for injection with activity of 740–1200 MBq (maximally 2200 MBq) may be used for labeling of one kit. This activity is sufficient for examinations of 1–2 adults. Radioactivity of administered dose should be always adjusted with respect to its diagnostic usefulness. The solution may be additionally diluted for more convenient administration.
- Patient position: supine
- Gamma camera
  - Low-energy high-resolution (LEHR) collimator
- Acquisition:
  - Acquisition should be carried out between 2 and 4 h after intravenous administration of the preparation. The examination may be complemented by acquisition after 10 min, 1 h, and 24 h after administration of the preparation. It is recommended to carry out the examinations using whole-body technique and SPECT of selected body areas. The gamma camera is positioning anteriorly and next posteriorly or simultaneous in dual head camera.
  - Photon peaks at 172 and 245 keV and 20% windows; WBS speed 3 cm/min.
  - Also, spot images on the region of interest and lateral views of head/neck, chest, and abdomen may be obtained.
  - SPECT is usually recorded with 60 projections of 6° each or 90 projections of 4° each. Matrix 64 × 64.
  - SPECT/CT should be applied whenever possible for better resolution and sensitivity.

Processing: There are special PC programs for image processing; additional analysis of counts in different region of interest (ROI) may be used.

Clinical applications:

- Gastroenteropancreatic neuroendocrine tumors (GEP-NET).
- Pituitary adenomas.
- Tumors originating in a sympathetic system.
- Pheochromocytoma, paraganglioma, neuroblastoma, ganglioneuroma, etc.
- Medullary thyroid carcinoma.

- The preparation may be potentially useful in the case of other tumors expressing somatostatin receptors of various intensities.
- Other tumors which may overexpress somatostatin receptors: breast cancer, melanoma, lymphomas, prostate cancer, NSCLC, sarcoma, renal cell carcinoma, differentiated thyroid carcinoma, astrocytoma according to WHO I–IV (including glioblastoma multiforme GBM), meningioma, and ovarian cancer.

Necessary additional examinations:
- CT, MRI
- Ultrasound
- Serologic tests of specific tumor markers
- Fine needle aspiration biopsy (FNAB)
- PET/CT with specific tracers

Comments:

If there is no uptake of Tc-99m Tektrotyd, the use of somatostatin analogues in the treatment is discouraged.

The studies published in the latest years showed comparable results with OctreoScan in NET detection but with lower irradiation, better dosimetry, and larger availability.

Reports:

The report will include a description of the normal distribution and pathologic uptakes; the report should mention the correlation of nuclear findings with the morphological images.

A synthetic presentation of diagnosis in NET is presented in Fig. 10.1, adapted from Bodei L (2015).

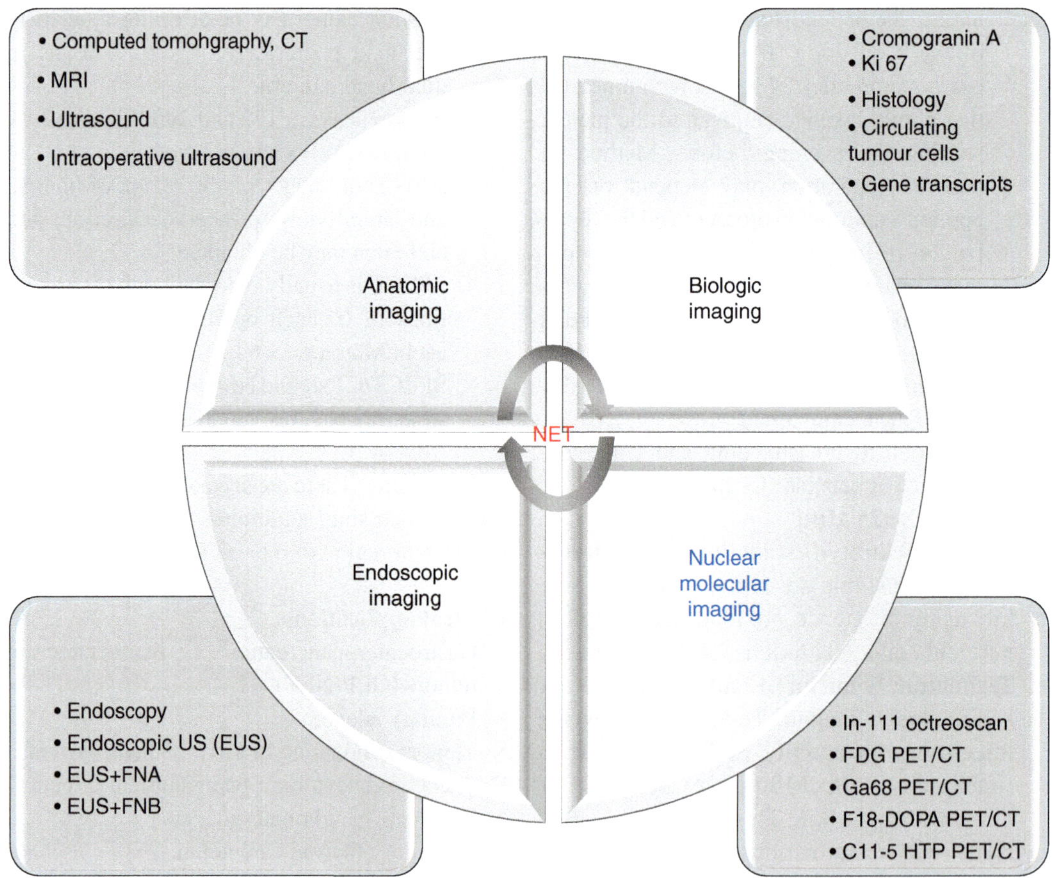

Fig. 10.1 Diagnosis methods used in neuroendocrine tumors, adapted from Bodei L (2015)

10.3 Nuclear Therapy of Neuroendocrine Tumors

The primary treatment of neuroendocrine tumors (NET), such as the carcinoid, is surgery with curative intent or with the intent to debulk the tumor mass. In 80% of patients with NET for whom this is impossible, alternatives such as external beam radiation therapy or chemotherapy are suboptimal because these well-differentiated tumors are relatively unresponsive. Most of these tumors express somatostatin receptors, especially subtype 2, in high abundance, which very rapidly bind and internalize targeted peptides. Somatostatin analogues, such as octreotide, can be used to treat carcinoid syndrome, and recent studies have also demonstrated substantial effects on tumor growth characteristics and modest prolongation of survival.

The rationale for using radiolabeled somatostatin analogues is based upon the evidence that they rapidly accumulate in the upregulated overexpressed somatostatin receptor-containing tumors. Somatostatin peptide analogues, coupled with a complexing moiety (DOTA), can be labeled with the beta emitters Y-90 or Lu-177. By targeting somatostatin receptor-positive tumors, they may deliver a tumoricidal radiation dose, and regression has been demonstrated after therapy with radiolabeled somatostatin analogues.

Somatostatin acts through interaction with receptors expressed on the surface of cells (in both normal and malignant tissues), named as somatostatin receptors. Six subtypes have been characterized and named somatostatin receptor subtypes 1–5 (SSTR1, 2A, 2B, 3, 4, and 5).

The **octreotide** is a somatostatin analogue with the structure:

$$\text{D-Phe}^1\text{-}\underbrace{\text{Cys}^2\text{-Phe}^3\text{-D-Trp}^4\text{-Lys}^5\text{-Thr}^6\text{-Cys}^7}\text{-Thr}^8\text{(ol)}$$

Researchers found that if Phe^3 is substituted with Tyr^3, it is possible to be labeled with radioiodine isotopes, both for diagnostic and for therapy.

$$\text{D-Phe}^1\text{-}\underbrace{\text{Cys}^2\text{-Tyr}^3\text{-D-Trp}^4\text{-Lys}^5\text{-Thr}^6\text{-Cys}^7}\text{-Thr}^8\text{(ol)}$$

Octreotide was derivatized with diethylenetriaminepentaacetic acid (DTPA) on the amine terminus. Attaching this chelate to the peptide allowed radiolabeling of the molecule with In-111.

Following that step, with the aim to find the best agent for PRRT, the chelating agent, DTPA (coupled to octreotide), was substituted with DOTA (tetraazacyclododecane-tetraacetic acid), which enabled the radiolabeling of this conjugate with Y-90, Lu-177, or other radionuclides.

DOTATOC: DOTA-Phe^1-Tyr^3-Octreotide

DOTANOC: DOTA-Nal^3-Octreotide (DOTA-naphthyl-alanine conjugate with octreotide)

Octreotate is another peptide analogue of somatostatin, which differs from octreotide where the C-terminal amino acid residue is threonine (instead of threoninol in octreotide).

DOTATATE: DOTA-Thy^3-Thre^8-Octreotide (Octreotate)

Lu-177 is a medium-energy beta emitter with a maximum tissue penetration of 1.6 mm and a physical half-life of 6.7 days. It also emits medium- and low-energy gamma radiation, which can be used for quantitative imaging and dosimetry. Binding of Lu-177 octreotate in NET expressing somatostatin receptor subtype 2 is nine times higher than that of the standard diagnostic imaging agent In-111 octreotide and seven times higher than that of the therapeutic agent Y-90 octreotide.

Tumor-targeted radiopeptide therapy is under investigational and clinical evaluation in European and Australian centers. Initial results with In-111 octreotide were disappointing, but more promising results were achieved with Y-90 octreotide and more recently with Lu-177 octreotate and Y-90 octreotate. Treatment of NET with Lu-177 octreotate results in impressive control of NET progression in a high percentage of patients, with little toxicity. However, virtually no malignancies have been cured using single-modality treatments. Multimodality treatment is required to control metastatic cancer. The synergistic combination of chemotherapy and radionuclides has the potential to enhance efficacy and minimize toxicity.

Radiation therapy of cancer, when combined with chemotherapy using either 5-fluorouracil (5-FU) or its prodrug capecitabine, has improved survival rates for a variety of tumor types when compared with radiation therapy alone.

Since the last edition of the book, in 2011, the progresses in this field were considerable. One of the most experimented scientists in peptide receptor radionuclide therapy (PRRT) is Lisa Bodei who published in 2016: "PRRT has been utilized for more than two decades and has been accepted as an effective therapeutic modality in the treatment of inoperable or metastatic gastroenteropancreatic neuroendocrine neoplasms (NENs) or neuroendocrine tumors (NETs). The two most commonly used radiopeptides for PRRT, Y-90-octreotide and Lu-177-octreotate, produce disease-control rates of 68–94%, with progression-free survival rates that compare favorably with chemotherapy, somatostatin analogues, and newer targeted therapies. In addition, biochemical and symptomatic responses are commonly observed. In general, PRRT is well tolerated with only low to moderate toxicity in most individuals."

Recently more clinical trials and strategies are developed including combinations with targeted therapies or chemotherapy, intra-arterial PRRT, and salvage treatments. Sophisticated molecular tools need to be incorporated into the management strategy to more effectively define therapeutic efficacy and for an early identification of adverse events. The strategy of randomized controlled trials is a key issue to standardize the treatment and establish the position of PRRT in the therapeutic algorithm of NENs.

10.3.1 Treatment Proposed Plan

- Lu-177 octreotate.
- Each patient receives an infusion of amino acids comprising 11.6 g/L lysine and 23 g/L arginine, at 250 mL/h for 4 h.
- At 30 min, 7.8 GBq [Lu-177 DOTA,Tyr^{3}] octreotate must be co-infused with the amino acids via a sideline over 10 min.
- Routine antiemetic therapy is given in the form of intravenous and oral 2 mg lorazepam.
- Chemotherapy with oral 1,650 mg/m^{2} capecitabine for 14 consecutive days was started on the morning of the radionuclide therapy.
- Cycles of capecitabine were repeated every 8 weeks at the time of each subsequent radiopeptide infusion.

A key concept emerging from targeted therapies is the recognition of the clinical importance of tumor stabilization in progressive malignancy.

10.3.2 Radiometabolic Therapeutic Approaches

In 2008, Modlin et al. reviewed the past decade of literature on neuroendocrine tumor treatment and summarized current therapeutic options. They remarked that the majority of tumors are diagnosed at a stage when radical surgical intervention, the only curative treatment, is no longer an option. Biotherapy with somatostatin analogues is currently the most efficient source of palliation. There may be a role for interferon agents in selected individuals, but substantial adverse events often limit their use. Conventional chemotherapy has minimal efficacy but may be of some use in undifferentiated or highly proliferating neuroendocrine carcinomas and pancreatic neuroendocrine tumors. Hepatic metastases, depending on size, location, and number, may be amenable to surgical resection, embolization, or radiofrequency ablation. PRRT (peptide receptor radionuclide therapy) may reduce tumor size, but in most circumstances has a tumor-stabilizing effect. Although various anti-angiogenesis and growth factor-targeted agents have been evaluated, so far, they fall short of expectations.

The somatostatin receptors, which are overexpressed in a majority of neuroendocrine tumors, are the first and best example of targets for radiopeptide-based imaging and radionuclide therapy.

The somatostatin analogue In-111 octreotide allows the localization and staging of neuroendocrine tumors that express the appropriate somatostatin receptors. Newer modified somatostatin analogues, including Tyr3 octreotide and Tyr3 octreotate, are successfully being used in tumor imaging and radionuclide therapy. Because there are few effective therapies for patients with inoperable or metastatic neuroendocrine tumors, this therapy emerges as a promising and novel option for these patients.

Forrer et al. stress the essential role of adequate dosimetry in effective and safe PRRT. Besides the kidneys, the bone marrow is a potentially dose-limiting organ. The radiation dose to the bone marrow is usually calculated using the MIRD model, according to which the accumulated radioactivity of the radiopharmaceutical in the bone marrow is worked out from that recorded in the blood.

The treatment of metastatic neuroendocrine tumors depends on the aggressiveness of the disease. Early diagnosis of metastatic spread of neuroendocrine tumors is hugely important, as the detection of distant metastases has a major impact on treatment choices. To date, however, no standard procedure was established for the early diagnosis of bone metastases from neuroendocrine tumors.

At present, there is a research interest in finding the best somatostatin (SST) analogue having the capability to link to all five isolated and characterized somatostatin receptors 1, 2, 3, 4, and 5 (SSTR1–5). In this way, it could be possible to increase the diagnostic sensitivity also in NET not expressing SSTR2 and SSTR5 (which are the main targets for octreotide), such as in insulinoma. As an alternative, a wider sensitivity can be achieved using other neuropeptides such as bombesin, vasoactive intestinal polypeptide (VIP), pituitary adenylate cyclase-activating polypeptide (PACAP), cholecystokinin (CCK), gastrin-releasing peptide (GRP), gastrin, neurotensin, neuropeptide Y (NPY), substance P, oxytocin, luteinizing hormone-releasing hormone (LH-RH), glucagon-like peptide 1 (GLP-1), calcitonin, endothelin, atrial natriuretic factor, and alpha-melanocyte-stimulating hormone (α-MSH).

Being at present more easily available and cheaper, DOTA peptides can be considered the first choice in NET, except for tumors not presenting a favorable SSTR expression, such as insulinoma. A wider experimental demonstration of a similar behavior between F-DOPA and I-131 MIBG could create an interesting perspective for the utilization of F-DOPA as a priori tracer for the therapeutic efficacy in patients with NET.

In general, since its first implementation by the Rotterdam group in 1994, only a few peer-reviewed papers have been published on PRRT in a larger cohort of patients over the last 15 years, even if there is an important number of abstracts, textbook articles, as well as review articles on PRRT by various groups that have been published worldwide over the last years.

Today, Y-90 and Lu-177 are the two radionuclides used for PRRT with SST analogues. In-111 pentetreotide was first pioneered for PRRT but was subsequently displaced by radiolabeled DOTA-TOC and DOTA-TATE derivates. This is due to the fact that In-111-labeled peptides are not ideal for PRRT because of the small particle range and thus a short tissue penetration.

The ENET Consensus Guidelines for the Standards of Care in NET tried to define the minimum requirements for patients eligible for PRRT, based on the fact that at the different centers, different SST analogues are being used, and their availability depends on national law and local permissions. Among these criteria, high uptake by the tumor lesions, inoperable disease, a Karnofsky score of >50%, and a life expectancy of at least 3–6 months are required. Contraindications are an impaired renal function (i.e., a creatinine clearance of <40–50 mL/min), an impaired hematological function, and severe hepatic and cardiac impairment.

In patients relapsing after PRRT with Y-90 DOTATOC, the Lu-177-labeled DOTATOC may be an alternative further treatment option that also was proven to be clinically safe and efficacious.

10.3.3 Combination Treatments

Long-acting octreotide (30 mg intramuscular every 4 weeks) has recently been shown to inhibit tumor progression in patients with metastasized well-differentiated midgut NET and may therefore have a potential role in the concomitant treatment of these patients.

Furthermore, a potential advantage of combined I-131 MIBG and Y-90 DOTATOC therapy was proposed by the researchers, suggesting that the response is optimal; the tumor dose for the combined agents may be achieved when the dose per activity, delivered to the tumor by Y-90 DOTATOC, is 2–3 times higher than that of I-131 MIBG.

Patients should always be evaluated by preceding SST scintigraphy and dosimetry, using respective octreotide or lanreotide analogues, preferably the Ga-68-labeled ones for PET. F18-fluorodeoxyglucose (F18-FDG) PET scanning shows a poor sensitivity to detect NET with a low metabolic activity and slow growth rate, while together with the Ga-68-labeled SST analogues, F18-FDG PET has clinical potential for the metabolic restaging of patients undergoing PRRT. The role of other PET radiopharmaceuticals, C-11-5-hydroxytryptophan (HTP) and F18-L-Dopa, for patients with NET, has to be comparatively assessed, and tumors may show an unbelievable variation.

In general, there is a need for randomized PRRT trials in order to establish which treatment scheme and which radiolabeled SST analogue, or combination of analogues, are optimal for PRRT.

Case 1: Suspicion of MEN I Syndrome *History*:
A 57-year-old male, with prolactin hypersecreting adenoma of the hypophysis, neuroendocrine tumor localized at the level of the duodenum and body of pancreas, surgically treated, bilateral suprarenal incidentaloma.

Clinical examination:

Symptoms: abdominal pain, unrelated with meals; diarrhea; fatigue; headache. The patient had important weight loss during the last 2 months; the presence of a postsurgical scar in the abdominal area. After the surgical treatment of the duodenal ulcer and pancreatic resection, he continues to express abdominal pain.

Examinations:

Serum level of PRL: 134 ng/mL (N.V. 1.8–17 ng/mL), increased.

Serum level of chromogranin A: 4551 ng/mL (N.V. 19.4–98.1 ng/mL), very increased.

Serum level of gastrin: 14,239 pg/mL (13–115 pg/mL), very increased.

Abdominal CT findings: low-density nodular lesion pre- and post-contrast localized at the level of pancreas body (23/19/28 mm); homogenous well-defined nodular lesion with a low uptake of I.V. contrast localized in the right suprarenal gland (23/13/22 mm); the same aspect in the left suprarenal gland (38/35/30 mm).

Cerebral MRI findings: nodular lesion localized at the level of hypophysis gland (10/12/13.5 mm).

Findings:

The scintigraphy with In-111 DTPA octreotide revealed in the early image at 4 h the pathologic uptake in the abdomen, related to the image described at CT in the pancreas (Fig. 10.2). The pathologic uptake was persistent at 24 h, confirmed on SPECT (Fig. 10.3).

Conclusion:

Pancreatic lesion with positive uptake of somatostatin analogue tracer.

Case 2: Inherited Pheochromocytoma-Paraganglioma *History*:
A 42-year-old male, with severe, uncontrolled high blood pressure and right adrenal incidentaloma. Retroperitoneal paraganglioma, lateral from urinary bladder, operated 6 years earlier, and thorax paraganglioma operated 1 year before the actual presentation.

Clinical examination:

Symptoms: fatigue, headache, sweating, and atrial fibrillation. The patient had mild weight loss during the last 2 months (4 kg).

Examinations:

Serum level of chromogranin A: 198 ng/mL (N.V. 19.4–98.1 ng/mL), increased.

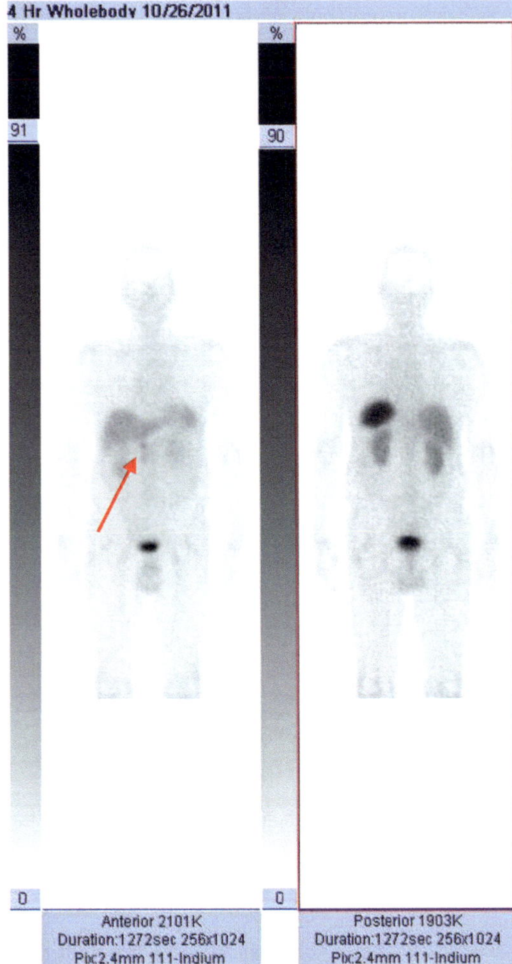

Fig. 10.2 In-111 octreotide scan at 4 h postinjection. Pathologic uptake in the area of the pancreas

Serum level of catecholamine: norepinephrine 1100 pg/mL (N.V. 70 750 pg/mL) and epinephrine <110 pg/mL.

Thorax and abdominal CT findings: low-density well-defined nodular lesion pre- and post-contrast localized in the right suprarenal gland (12/10/11 mm).

PGL4 germline mutation SDHB (succinate dehydrogenase B):

- 20–25% paraganglioma associated with pheochromocytoma.
- 50% thorax-abdominal paraganglioma.
- 20–30% head and neck paraganglioma.
- 20–25% are multifocal.
- 14% occurs as renal cancer.
- 30% might be malignant.

No pathologic findings on cerebral MRI.

Findings:

The scintigraphy with In-111 DTPA octreotide revealed in the early image at 2 h the pathologic uptake in the mediastinum and in pelvic area (Fig. 10.3). The pathologic uptakes were persistent at 4 h, with better visualization, but no other precise details about the localization (Fig. 10.4).

The SPECT/CT at 24 h (Figs. 10.5, 10.6, 10.7, and 10.8) reveals the intense uptake of the tracer at metastatic sites in the pelvic bones, thoracic spine, and sternum. No uptake in the adrenal gland.

Conclusion:

Syndrome pheochromocytoma-paraganglioma PGL4, SDHB.

Comments:

If hereditary PGL is known or strongly suspected in a patient presenting with an index tumor, then imaging from neck to pelvis should be performed to exclude synchronous lesions; Ga-68 DOTATATE PET imaging may be appropriate in this regard.

Case 3: Functionally Inactive NET of the Ileum *History*:

A 52-year-old male, with intermittent abdominal pain in the last 8 months, was admitted for the occurrence of an acute jaundice.

Clinical examination:

Symptoms: fatigue, headache, loss of appetite, weight loss of 6 kg in the last 6 months, and nausea. The patient had an acute episode of jaundice.

Examinations:

Serum level of chromogranin A: 78 ng/mL (N.V. 19.4–98.1 ng/mL), normal.

Serum level of catecholamine: norepinephrine and epinephrine, normal.

Urinary 5-HIAA 212 mg/24 h (N.V. 2–8 mg/24 h).

Thorax and abdominal CT findings: multiple hypodense masses in the liver (Fig. 10.9).

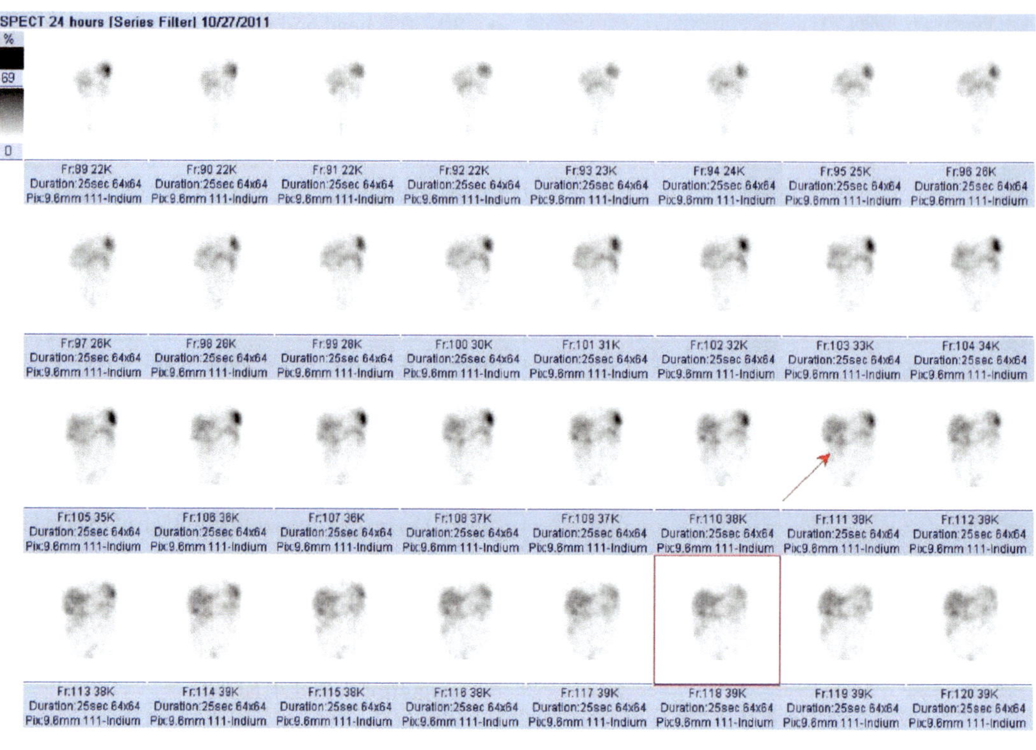

Fig. 10.3 In-111 octreotide scan at 24 h postinjection. Better visualization of the pathologic uptake in the area of the pancreas

Findings:

The scintigraphy with Tc-99m Tektrotyd revealed in the early image at 2 h the pathologic uptake in the multiple tumor masses of the liver (Fig. 10.10). No pathologic uptake visualized in the rest of the body.

The SPECT/CT at 24 h (Fig. 10.11) reveals the intense uptake of the tracer at metastatic sites in the liver and the primary tumor in the ileum.

Conclusion:

Ileum NET cu liver metastases expressing the receptor for somatostatin, with positive SSR scan.

Comments.

In the case of patients with relapsing abdominal pain, as a result of intestinal pseudo-obstruction by a functionally inactive NET of the lower jejunum and ileum, the clinician should note the possibility of NET tumors, and the evaluation in this direction should be carried on.

One of the most suggestive examples of theranostics, regarding the successful merging of diagnosis and therapy, is the selective, highly specific, and systemic role of nuclear tracers in NET. The positive image demonstrates the signature of the tumor in the spectrum of somatostatin receptors, fact that leads further to the use of those molecules targeted selectively for NET and linked with the therapeutic isotopes (Fig. 10.12).

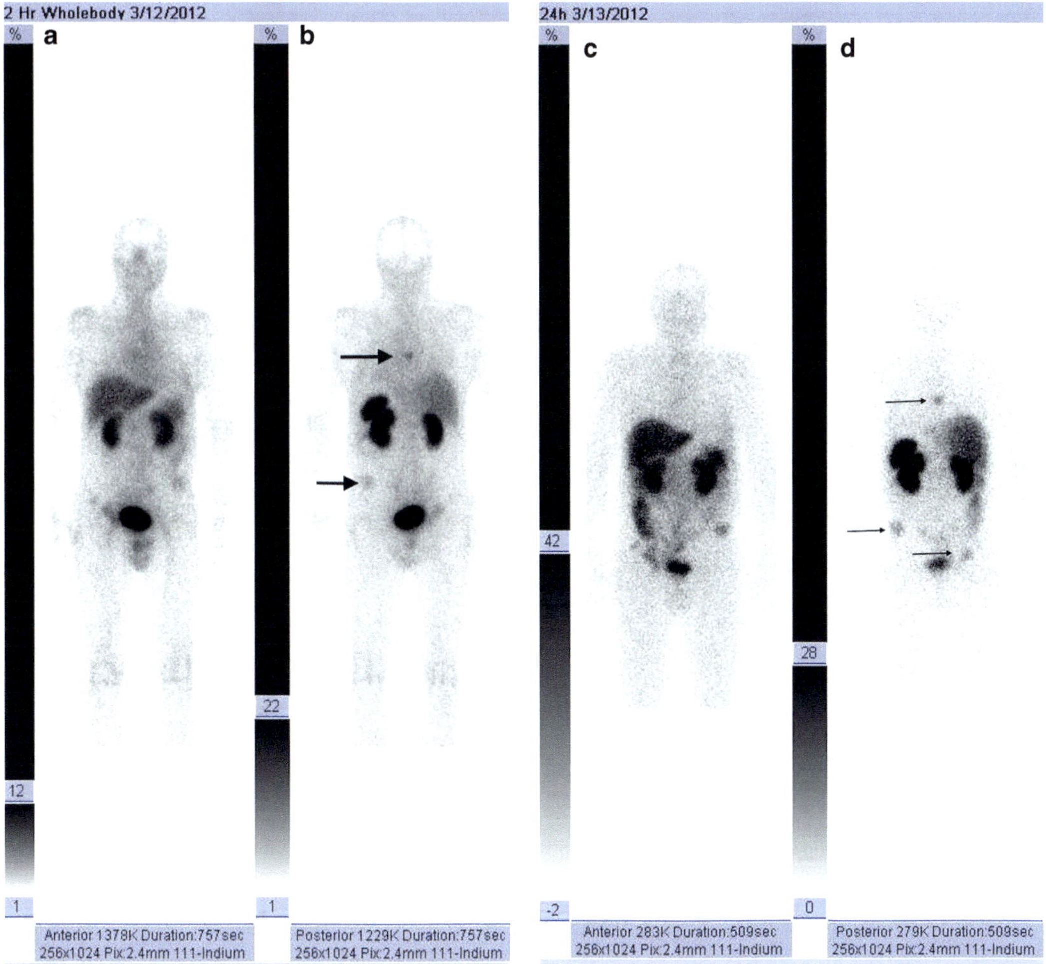

Fig. 10.4 In-111 octreotide scan at 2 h postinjection. Pathologic uptake in the mediastinum and pelvic area ((**a**) AP incidence and (**b**) PA incidence)

Fig. 10.5 In-111 octreotide scan at 24 h postinjection. Better visualization of the pathologic uptake in the mediastinum and pelvic area ((**c**) AP incidence and (**d**) PA incidence)

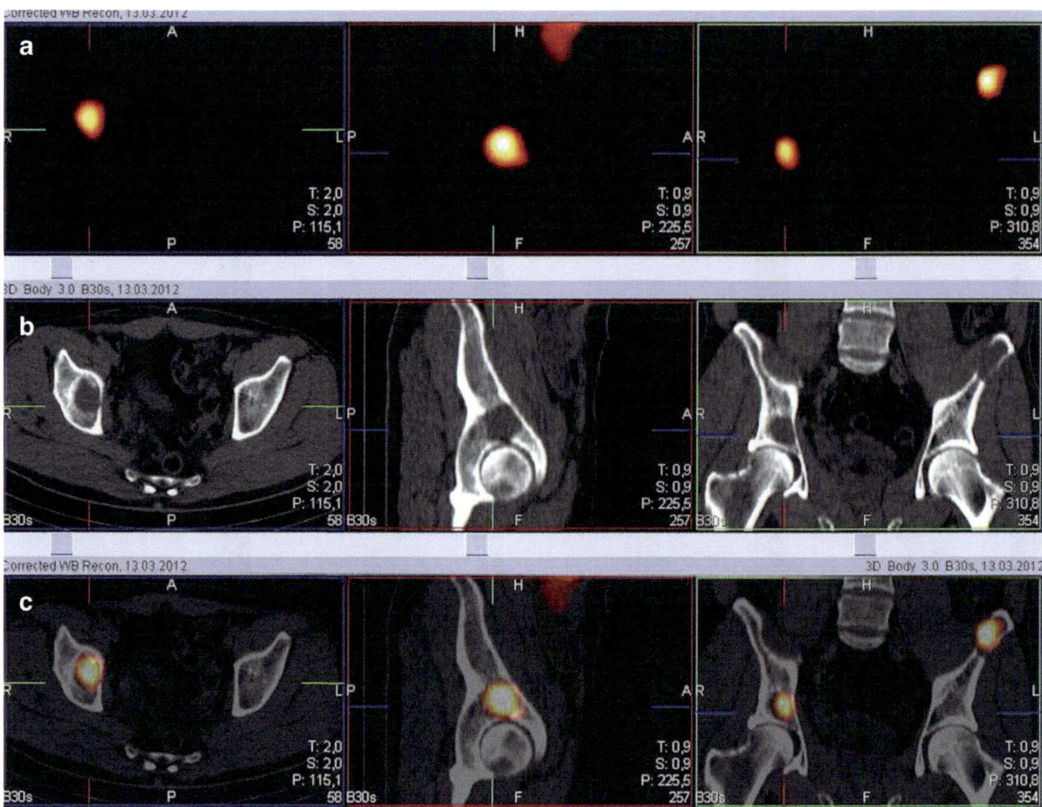

Fig. 10.6 In-111 octreotide scan SPECT/CT at 24 h postinjection. Pathologic uptake in the pelvic bones ((**a**) SPECT; (**b**) CT; (**c**) fused image SPECT/CT)

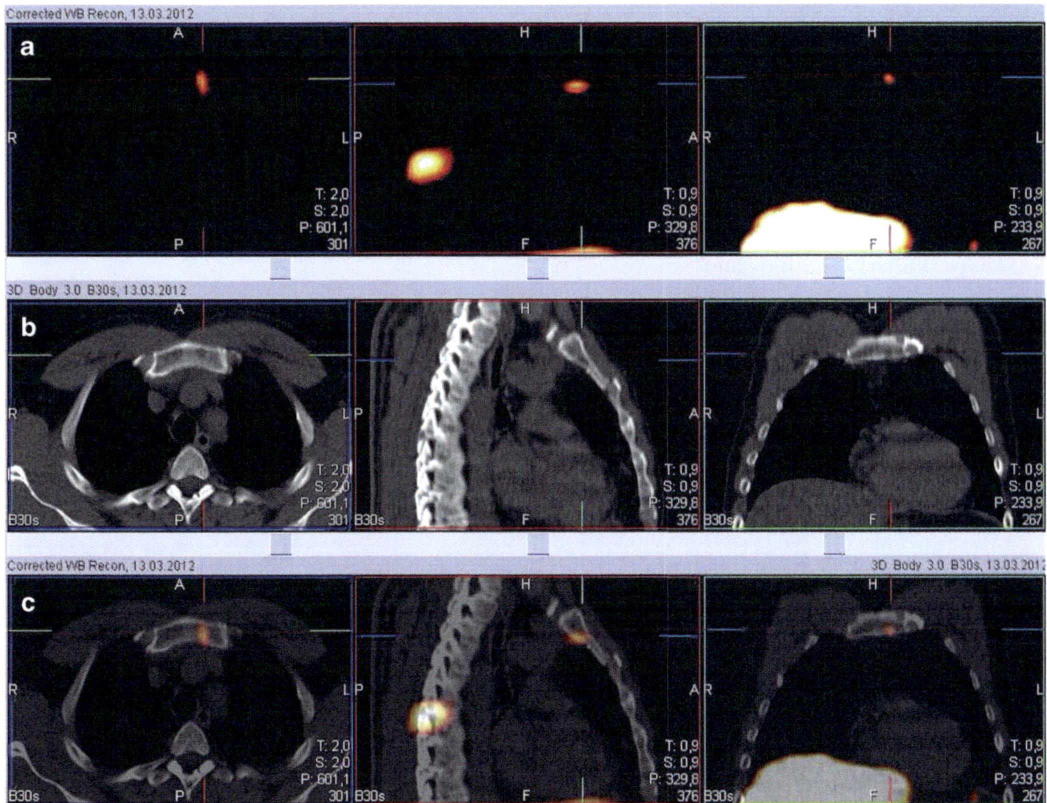

Fig. 10.7 In-111 octreotide scan at 24 h postinjection. Pathologic uptake in the thoracic spine and sternum ((**a**) SPECT; (**b**) CT; (**c**) fused image SPECT/CT)

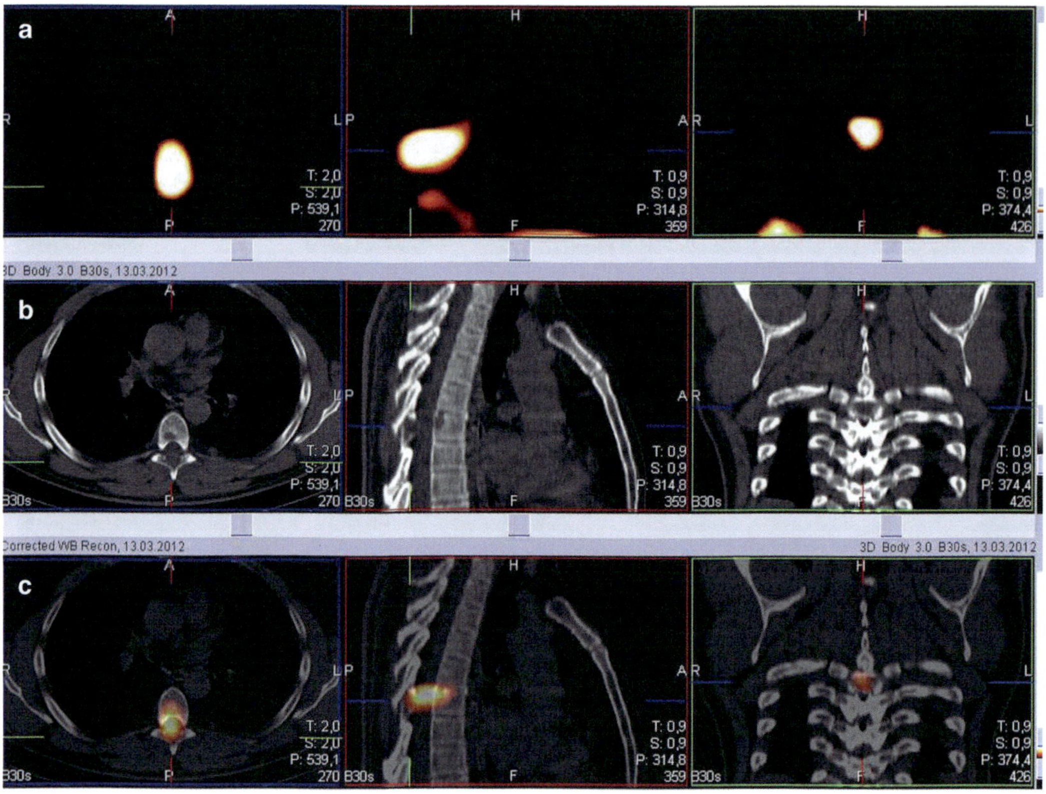

Fig. 10.8 In-111 octreotide scan at 24 h postinjection. Pathologic uptake in the thoracic spine ((**a**) SPECT; (**b**) CT; (**c**) fused image SPECT/CT)

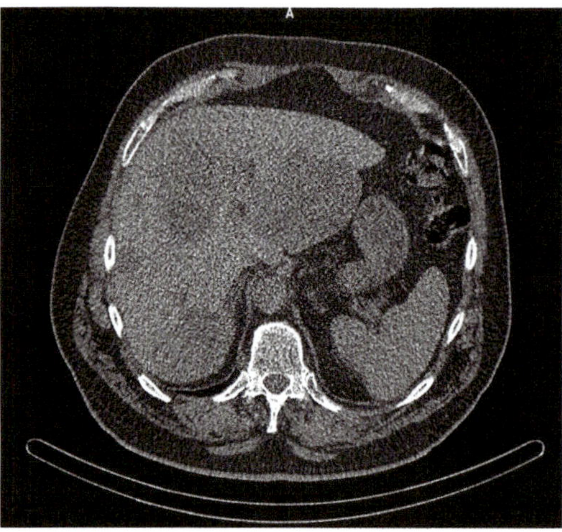

Fig. 10.9 CT image in transversal section showing multiple hypodense masses in liver, suggestive for metastases

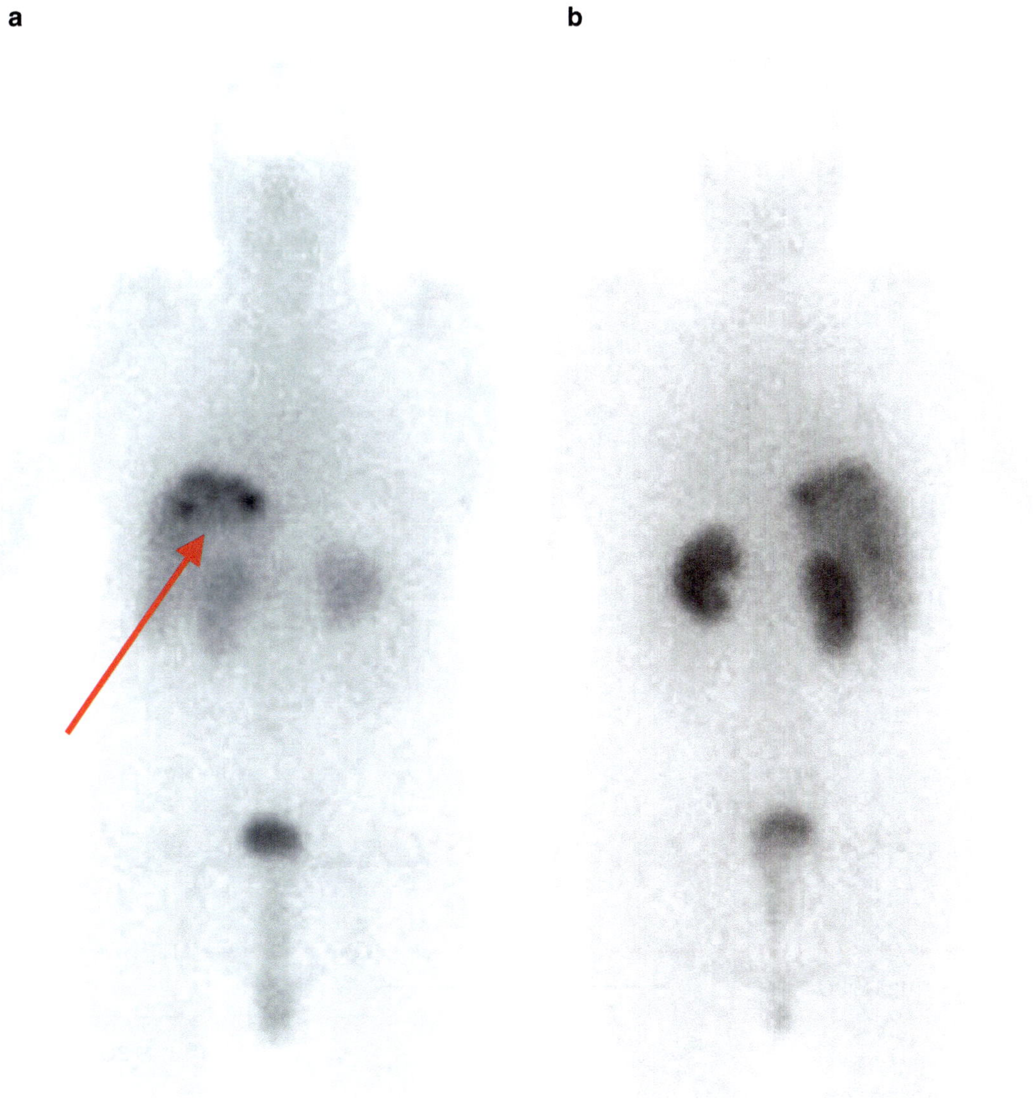

Fig. 10.10 Tc-99m Tekrotyd scan at 2 h postinjection. Pathologic uptake in the liver area, suggesting multiple metastases expressing SSR ((**a**) AP incidence and (**b**) PA incidence)

Fig. 10.11 Tc-99m Tekrotyd scan at 24 h post-injection, coronal section. The image reveals intense uptake of the tracer in the metastatic lesions of the liver and in the primary tumor in the ileum (fused image SPECT/CT)

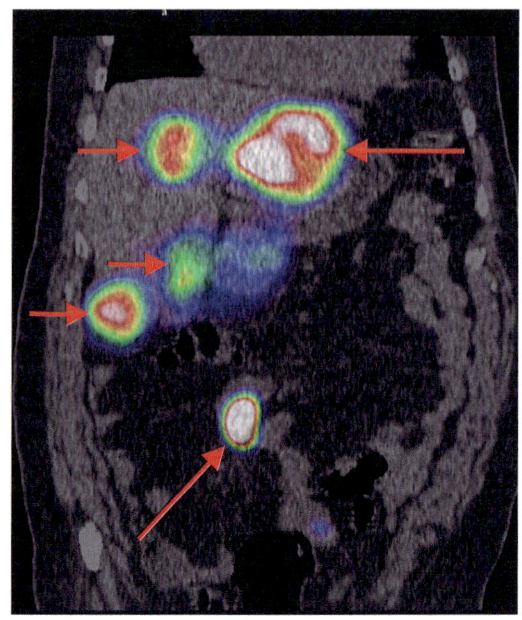

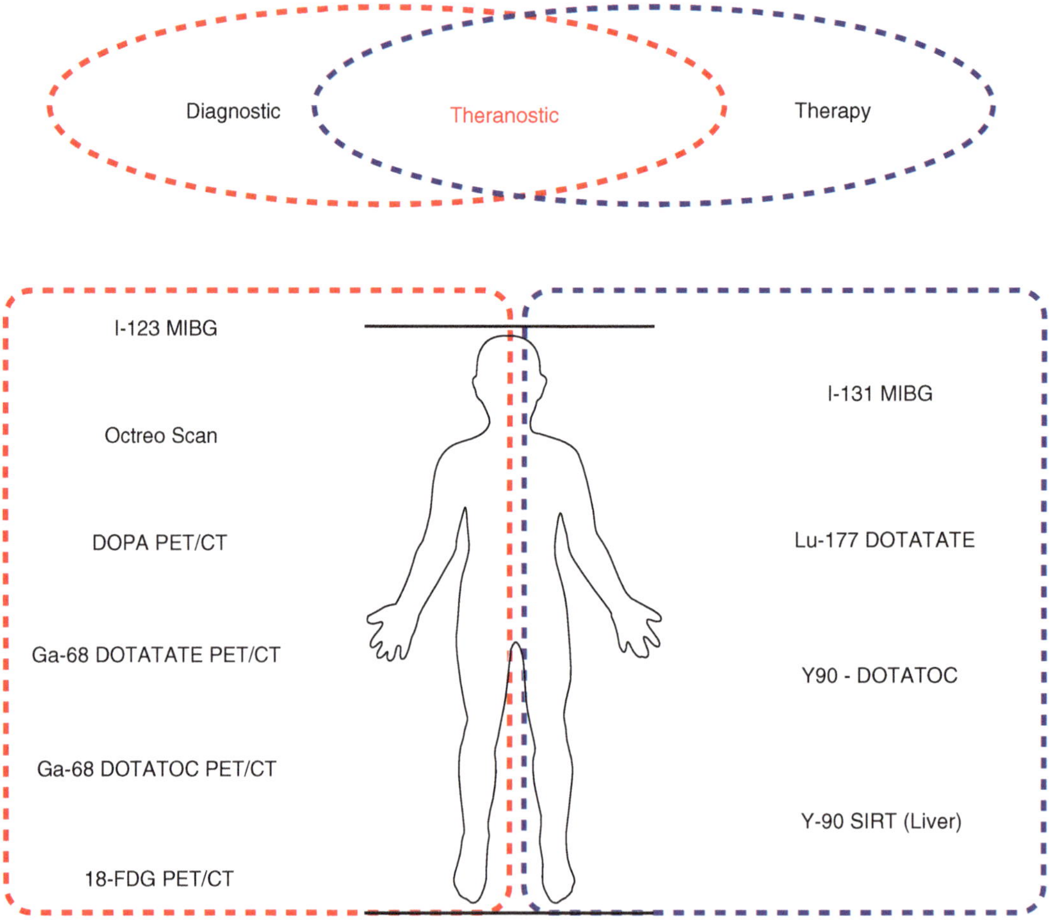

Fig. 10.12 The principle of theranostics in NET

Further Reading

Asnacios A, Courbon F, Rochaix P et al (2008) Indium-111-pentetreotide scintigraphy and somatostatin receptor subtype 2 expressions: new prognostic factors for malignant well-differentiated endocrine tumours. J Clin Oncol 26(6):963–970

Benn DE, Robinson BG, Clifton-Bligh RJ (2015) 15 years of paraganglioma: clinical manifestations of paraganglioma syndromes types 1–5. Endocr Relat Cancer, 22(4), T91–T103. http://doi.org/10.1530/ERC-15-0268

Bodei L, Kwekkeboom DJ, Kidd M et al (2016) Radiolabeled somatostatin analogue therapy of gastroenteropancreatic cancer. Semin Nucl Med 46(3):225–238

Bodei L, Kidd M, Paganelli G et al (2015) Long-term tolerability of PRRT in 807 patients with neuroendocrine tumours: the value and limitations of clinical factors. Eur J Nucl Med Mol Imaging 42(1):5–19.

Bodei L, Sundin A, Kidd M, et al (2015) The status of neuroendocrine tumor imaging: from darkness to light? Neuroendocrinology 101(1):1–17.

Bombardieri E, Ambrosini V, Aktolun C et al (2010) 111In-pentetreotide scintigraphy: procedure guidelines for tumour imaging. Eur J Nucl Med Mol Imaging 37:1441–1448. doi:10.1007/s00259-010-1473-6

Buchmann I, Henze M, Engelbrecht S (2007) Comparison of 68 Ga-DOTATOC PET and 111In-DTPAOC (Octreoscan) SPECT in patients with neuroendocrine tumours. Eur J Nucl Med Mol Imaging 34(10):1617–1626

Forrer F, Riedweg I, Maecke HR et al (2008) Radiolabeled DOTATOC in patients with advanced paraganglioma and pheochromocytoma. Q J Nucl Med Mol Imaging 52(4):334–340

Forrer F, Krenning EP, Kooij PP et al (2009) Bone marrow dosimetry in peptide receptor radionuclide therapy with [177Lu-DOTA(0), Tyr(3)]octreotate. Eur J Nucl Med Mol Imaging 36(7):1138–1146

Giammarile F, Chiti A, Lassmann M, Brans B, Flux G (2008) EANM procedure guidelines for 131I-meta iodobenzylguanidine (131I-mIBG) therapy. Eur J Nucl Med Mol Imaging 35:1039–1047. doi:10.1007/s00259-008-0715-3

Gibril F, Reynolds JC, Doppman JL et al (1996) Somatostatin receptor scintigraphy: its sensitivity compared with that of other imaging methods in detecting primary and metastatic gastrinomas. A prospective study. Ann Intern Med 125(1):26–34

Klimstra DS, Modlin IR, Coppola D et al (2010) The pathologic classification of neuroendocrine tumours: a review of nomenclature, grading, and staging systems. Pancreas doi:10.1097/MPA.0b013e3181ec124e

Kowalski J, Henze M, Schuhmacher J et al (2003) Evaluation of positron emission tomography imaging using [68Ga]-DOTA-D-Phe1-Tyr3-octreotide in comparison to [111In]-DTPAOC SPECT. First results in patients with neuroendocrine tumours. Mol Imaging Biol 5:42–48

Kwekkeboom DJ, Krenning EP, Bakker WH (1993) Somatostatin analogue scintigraphy in carcinoid tumours. Eur J Nucl Med 20(4):283–292

Kwekkeboom DJ, Krenning EP, Scheidhauer K et al (2009) ENETS consensus guidelines for the standards of care in neuroendocrine tumours: somatostatin receptor imaging with (111) In-pentetreotide. Neuroendocrinology 90:184–189

Modlin IM, Oberg K, Chung DC et al (2008) Gastroenteropancreatic neuroendocrine tumours. Lancet Oncol 9(1):61–72, Review. PubMed PMID: 18177818

Nicolas G, Giovacchini G, Müller-Brand J et al (2011) Targeted radiotherapy with radiolabeled somatostatin analogs. Endocrinol Metab Clin N Am 40(1):187–204, Review. PubMed PMID: 21349419

Olsen JO, Pozderac RV, Hinkle G et al (1995) Somatostatin receptor imaging of neuroendocrine tumours with Indium-111 pentetreotide (Octreoscan). Semin Nucl Med 25(3):251–261

Öberg K, Knigge U, Kwekkeboom D, Perren A on behalf of the ESMO Guidelines Working Group (2012) Neuroendocrine gastro-entero-pancreatic tumors: ESMO Clinical Practice Guidelines for diagnosis, treatment and follow-up. Ann Oncol 23 (suppl_7): vii124-vii130

Schmidt M, Scheidhauer K, Luyken C et al (1998) Somatostatin receptor imaging in intracranial tumours. Eur J Nucl Med 25(7):675–686

Vinik A, Woltering EA, Warner RRP et al (2010) NANETS consensus guidelines for the diagnosis of neuroendocrine tumour. Pancreas doi:10.1097/MPA.0b013e3181ebaffd

Virgolini I, Ambrosini V, Bomanji BJ et al (2010) Procedure guidelines for PET/CT tumour imaging with 68Ga-DOTA-conjugated peptides: 68Ga-DOTA-TOC, 68Ga-DOTA-NOC, 68Ga-DOTA-TATE. Eur J Nucl Med Mol Imaging 37:2004–2010

Wong KK, Cahill JM, Frey KA et al (2010) Incremental value of 111-In pentetreotide SPECT/CT fusion imaging of neuroendocrine tumours. Acad Radiol 17:291–297

11 Hybrid Positron Emission Tomography in Endocrinology

"The eye sees only what the mind is prepared to comprehend"
Henri Bergson (Nobel prize awarded 1859–1941)

11.1 Overview

Positron emission tomography (PET) is a tomographic technique that computes the three-dimensional distribution of radioactivity based on the annihilation photons that are emitted by positron emitter-labeled radiotracers. The use of PET/CT fusion scanners has been demonstrated to significantly increase accuracy of lesion detection, combining the high anatomical definition of CT with the high sensitivity of PET. Advanced functional MR imaging techniques such as DW imaging, MR spectroscopy, and perfusion-weighted imaging used with PET can further enhance detection and characterization of malignant lesions for prognosis assessment, biopsy and pretreatment planning, patient selection for certain therapeutic agents, and response prediction and assessment. PET allows noninvasive quantitative assessment of biochemical and functional processes. The most commonly used tracer at present is the glucose analogue F18-FDG (F18-fluoro-2-deoxy-d-glucose). F18-FDG accumulation in the tissue is proportional to the amount of glucose utilization. Increased consumption of glucose is a characteristic of most cancers and is in part related to the overexpression of the GLUT-1 glucose transporters and increased hexokinase activity. The PET radiotracer F18-FDG has obtained a large acceptance in clinical oncology due to its excellent diagnostic performance in many cancers such as lung, colorectal, lymphoma, melanoma, esophagus, pancreas, breast, ovary, and testicle. However, F18-FDG has reduced performance in some other cancers, less aggressive and most differentiated ones, such as prostate cancer or endocrine tumors. In these cancers, it is mandatory to perform PET with tracers "beyond F18-FDG," specific tracers with particular structure analogue with the examined organ or tumor.

The main indications of PET/CT examinations are:

1. Diagnosis of the primary site of the tumors:
   - Unknown primary malignancy
   - Differentiation of benign/malignant lesions, for example, a solitary lung nodule
2. Staging on presentation: non-small-cell lung cancer, esophageal cancer, Hodgkin disease, non-Hodgkin lymphoma, locally advanced cervical cancer, neuroendocrine tumors with risk factors, and locally advanced breast cancer
3. Response evaluation to treatment
4. Restaging in the event of potentially curable relapse (for F18-FDG avid tumors)
5. Establishing and localizing disease sites as a cause for elevated serum markers (e.g., colorectal, thyroid, ovarian, cervix, melanoma, breast, and germ cell tumors)
6. Image-guided biopsy (e.g., brain tumors) and radiotherapy planning

D. Piciu, *Nuclear Endocrinology*, DOI 10.1007/978-3-319-56582-8_11

The most important differences of SPECT-PET might be summarized as follows:

- SPECT has a lower resolution and sensitivity.
- Different radiotracers are used in PET, which are positron emitters.
- The presence of collimators in SPECT reduces significantly the efficiency of the detection.

Both techniques by fusing with CT increase the effective dose of the body, due to irradiation. The CT component contributes 54–81% of the total combined dose, a fact that leads to a new concept of low-dose CT or so-called localization CT. In this case the parameters used during the CT acquisition are modulated to the lowest efficient level, the aim being for localization of the metabolic process detected by PET and not the highly sensitive diagnosis. It was demonstrated that by decreasing one CT parameter (kV) from 140 to 80 kV, the total measured dose is reduced with 67% (Fahy 2009).

The latest years brought impressive achievements in the field of hybrid imaging. The results of multicenter trials and studies were published in the last 2–3 years, and after 15 years, since the method was introduced in the clinical practice, the impact of PET/CT is considered essential:

- PET/CT changes from an *intended nontreatment to a treatment plan*, in 28.3% of cases.
- 8.2% of cases changed *from treatment to nontreatment*.
- *A major change in intended management* occurred in 30.3–39.7% depending on the indication.
- Overall, physicians *changed their intended treatment plan in 36.5%* of cases after PET/CT.

In the present chapter, the focus will be mainly on PET/CT; the new technique of PET/MRI is still not on large, and routine availability and the indication in endocrinology are limited. Table 11.1 is presenting the main advantages and disadvantages of one method over the other one.

In the majority of endocrine diseases, except pituitary pathology, MRI is better than CT imaging, but PET/MR seems to be equal to PET/CT, all lesions seen on PET are also seen on MR, and information is redundant. Great strides have been made to solve technical inadequacies of PET/MR in the last 5 years, and the task is to define reasonable PET/MR imaging protocols mainly in oncology, "rule out metastases" protocols (brain, liver), and neurology "rule out other pathologies" protocols (Gustav K. von Schulthess, Zurich).

With respect to endocrine pathologies, the role of PET/MR is still undefined, limited experience being achieved all around the world, considering that the first commercial whole-body system used in humans was in 2010. The following

Table 11.1 PET/CT and PET/MRI strengths and weaknesses

	PET/CT	PET/MRI
Strengths	• Lung and compact bone imaging • Attenuation correction	• Brain and bone marrow imaging • Excellent soft tissue contrast • Lesser radiation dose from MRI • Simultaneous multimodality preclinical imaging • Plenty of tracers available for PET • Enables good visualization, quantification, and translational studies
Weaknesses	• Brain and soft tissue imaging • Metal artifacts • Higher radiation dose due to CT	• Lung and compact bone imaging • Attenuation correction • It requires high initial capital cost • There is lack of protocol and standardization due to huge variations in MR protocols • No combined reporting of PET and MR components • Limited flexibility of combined PET/MR systems • High acquisition times of up to 60 min

chapter will focus on PET/CT imaging, based on authors' experience in this field.

The main indications of PET/CT in endocrinology are as follows:

- Detection of radiological occult lesion
- Characterization of the functional, metabolic behavior of the detected lesion
- Staging
- Evaluation of treatment response
- Evaluation of prognosis in endocrine malignant diseases

11.2 PET/CT F18-FDG

Radiopharmaceutical:

- F18-fluorodeoxyglucose (F18-FDG)

Principle:

- F18-FDG accumulation in tissue is proportional to the amount of glucose utilization. The malignant tissues are highly glucose consuming. F18-FDG is proportionally trapped with the intensity of the glucose metabolism and vascularization, so it is an excellent imaging marker of the aggressiveness of the disease.

Technique:

- Patient preparation: the main purpose of the patient preparation is the reduction of tracer uptake in normal tissue (kidneys, bladder, skeletal muscle, myocardium, brown fat, digestive tract) while maintaining and optimizing tracer uptake in the target structures (tumor tissue).
  - Patients are not allowed to consume any food or sugar for at least 6 h prior to the start of the PET study.
  - Medication can be taken as prescribed.
  - Adequate prehydration is important to ensure a sufficiently low FDG concentration in urine and for radiation safety reasons.
  - Parental nutrition and intravenous fluids containing glucose should be discontinued at least 4 h before the PET/CT examination. In addition, the infusion used to administer intravenous prehydration must not contain any glucose.
  - During the injection of FDG and the subsequent uptake phase, the patient should remain seated or recumbent and silent to minimize FDG uptake in muscles.
  - The patient should be kept warm starting at 30–60 min before the injection of FDG and throughout the following uptake period and PET examination to minimize FDG accumulation in the brown fat (especially relevant if the room is air-conditioned). Moreover, all patients must avoid (extreme) exercise for at least 6 h before the PET study.
  - Patients with diabetes mellitus type II (controlled by oral medication) should take their medication and be in fasting condition. Special condition is metformin that should be changed 2–4 days prior to the examination in order to avoid its high uptake in the bowel.
  - In patients having type I diabetes mellitus and insulin-dependent type II diabetes mellitus, ideally, an attempt should be made to achieve normal glycemic values prior to the PET study.
  - The blood glucose level of the patient is checked before starting any procedure.
  - Essential information should be given prior to scheduling the test: last surgical intervention, recent radiotherapy, chemotherapy, administration of growth factors, etc. (minimum of 10 days after the last cycle).
- Dose: the dose is calculated depending on the weight of the patient and the type of the instrument used and the protocol:
  - 5 MBq/kg body weight dose, which may vary according to the mentioned data
- Dose calibration.
- Injected I.V.
- It is necessary to wait 60 min after injection.
- Patient position: supine.
- Acquisition: specific parameters of PET and CT according to producers.

  - The CT parameters should be adjusted for every patient, in order to achieve the maximum benefit from a low-dose CT with minimum irradiation (decrease accordingly the kV and mA).
- Processing:
  - Both uncorrected and attenuation-corrected images need to be assessed in order to identify any artifacts caused by contrast agents, metal implants, and/or patient motion.
  - Criteria for visual analysis must be defined for each study protocol.
  - SUV is a measurement of the uptake in a tumor normalized on the basis of a distribution volume.
  - It is calculated as follows:
  - SUV = activity in tumor volume (MBq/mL)/activity administered (MBq/body weight); there are a multitude of other types of SUV considering the glucose level, the body surface, min, mean, max, etc.

Necessary additional examinations:
- Clinical examination: remember to discuss and to examine the patient before the injection in order to limit the hazardous radiation exposure.
- Because this examination occurs frequently after performing the conventional imaging tests, it is important to have the results for data corroboration.
- Comparison with previous examinations should be part of the PET/CT report. PET/CT examinations are more valuable if they are interpreted in the context of results of other imaging examinations (e.g., CT, PET, PET/CT, MRI) and relevant clinical data. If a PET/CT examination is performed in the context of the assessment of response to a therapy, the extent and the intensity of the FDG uptake should be documented. The European Organization for Research and Treatment of Cancer (EORTC) has published the criteria for the assessment of therapy response with FDG as metabolic marker. At present, relative changes in SUV under therapy represent the most robust parameter.

Comments:
- The place of PET/CT in the assessment of malignant diseases is well established by the international algorithms of diagnostic and treatment in order to obtain the maximum benefit with reduced risks.

Reports:
- The reports respect the general format of the department with all the identification data of the patient, the institution, and the physician.
- The description of the localization, the extent, and the intensity of pathologic FDG accumulations related to normal tissue, the description of relevant findings in CT, and their relation to pathologic FDG accumulations.
- FDG accumulation should be reported as mild, moderate, or intense and compared to the background uptake. However, the criteria for visual interpretation must be defined for each study protocol and/or type of cancer because they may differ for different tumor locations and types.
- If possible, a definite diagnosis should be stated whenever possible. Alternatively, an estimate of the probability of a diagnosis should be given.
- If relevant, differential diagnoses should be discussed.
- If appropriate, repeat examinations and/or additional examinations should be recommended to clarify or confirm findings.

11.3 PET/CT F18-FCH

Radiopharmaceutical:
- F18-fluorocholine (F18-FCH)

Principle:
- F18-choline is an essential component for the formation of new cell membrane components, and the current understanding is that malignancy-induced upregulation of choline kinase leads to the incorporation and trapping of choline in the tumor cell membrane.

Technique:
- Patient preparation: no special requirements
- Dose: the dose is calculated depending on the weight of the patient and the type of the PET/CT equipment used and the protocol:
  - FCH 3 MBq/kg of body mass, which may vary according to the mentioned data

- Dose calibration
- Injected I.V.
- Low-dose CT (100–120 kV, 30–50–80 mA) acquired first.
- Subsequently, with the patient staying inside the tunnel of the PET/CT camera, the FCH dose is administrated intravenously in an infusion line connected to saline.
- Immediately after injection, PET dynamic acquisition is performed during 10 min with the detector ring centered on the neck, immediately followed by a "static" PET acquisition (2 min per bed position) ranging from the skull to mid-thighs for men (in order not to miss potential prostate foci) and to the lower limit of the liver for women.
- Dynamic images may be reframed by summing up images from the second to the eighth minute to facilitate interpretation.
- Processing:
  - Both uncorrected and attenuation-corrected images need to be assessed in order to identify any artifacts caused by contrast agents, metal implants, and/or patient motion.
  - Criteria for visual analysis must be defined for each study protocol.
  - SUV is a measurement of the uptake in a tumor normalized on the basis of a distribution volume. The type of SUV should be defined and reported by the laboratory (SUVbsa, lbm, bw, min, max, mean, etc.).

Necessary additional examinations:
- Clinical examination: remember to discuss and to examine the patient before the injection in order to limit the hazardous radiation exposure.
- The positive diagnosis frequently refers to the recurrence of the hyperparathyroidism and to the surgical options. Comparison with previous examinations should be part of the PET/CT report. PET/CT examinations are more valuable if they are interpreted in the context of results of other imaging examinations (US, Tc-99m MIBI scan, etc.) and relevant clinical data.

Comments:
- The examination is not the first-line option, all studies trying to compare the results with the gold standard method of Tc-99m MIBI.

Reports:
- The reports respect the general format of the department with all the identification data of the patient, the institution, and the physician.
- The description of the localization of parathyroid adenoma, if it is in normal or ectopic position, its relation to thyroid, and previous surgery.
- The quantification of uptake in case of F18-FCH used for HPT is less important.

11.4 PET/CT Ga-68 DOTATOC/DOTANOC/DOTATATE (Ga-68 SSTR)

Radiopharmaceutical:
DOTA (tetraazacyclododecane-tetraacetic acid):

- Ga-68 DOTATOC: Ga-68 DOTA-Phe^1-Tyr^3-Octreotide
- Ga-68 DOTANOC: Ga-68 DOTA-Nal^3-Octreotide
- Ga-68 DOTATATE: Ga-68 DOTA-Thy^3-Thre^8-Octreotide (octreotate)

Principle:
- Ga-68 SSTR F18-choline is an essential component for the formation of new cell membrane components, and the current understanding is that malignancy-induced upregulation of choline kinase leads to the incorporation and trapping of choline in the tumor cell membrane.

Technique:
- Patient preparation:
  - Discontinuation of somatostatin analogue treatment before PET/CT is desired but not mandatory and has been shown not to influence results.
  - Fasting is not required.
- Dose:
  - The recommended dose of Ga-68 SSTR is usually 132–222 MBq (4–6 mCi), but should not be less than 100 MBq.
- Dose calibration.
- Injected I.V.

- Acquisition:
  - CT is acquired first using low-dose CT protocol (120 kV, 30–50–80 mA).
  - PET/CT is acquired 45–60 min postinjection, with the general consensus that best images are obtained at 60 min.
  - Images are acquired from the skull (must include the pituitary gland) to mid-thigh.
  - Additional views can be taken as and when required.
  - Use of intravenous contrast during CT part of PET/CT is controversial, with few studies advocating their use.
- Processing:
  - The images are reconstructed using iterative reconstruction using standard protocols.
  - Both uncorrected and attenuation-corrected images need to be assessed in order to identify any artifacts caused by contrast agents, metal implants, and/or patient motion.
  - Criteria for visual analysis must be defined for each study protocol.
  - SUV is a measurement of the uptake in a tumor normalized on the basis of a distribution volume.

Necessary additional examinations:

- Clinical examination: remember to discuss and to examine the patient before the injection in order to limit the hazardous radiation exposure.
- Frequently, these examinations are not in the first line, so patients already have CT, MRI, and even other functional tests, like I-123/I-131 MIBG, SRS, and F18-FDG PET/CT. The positive diagnosis refers to staging and affinity for these tracers; during follow-up, if PRRT is done, the results should mention the assessment of therapy response.

Comments:

- Despite different affinities, there is currently no evidence of a clinical impact of these differences in SSTR binding affinity, and therefore no preferential use of one compound over the others can be advised.

Reports:

- The reports respect the general format of the department with all the identification data of the patient, the institution, and the physician.
- The description of the localization of pathologic uptake.
- The quantification of uptake should be done and reported.

11.5 PET/CT and PET/MR in Pituitary Gland Pathology

Pituitary tumors are the most common pituitary disorder. However, they are not, in the great majority of cases, life-threatening. Pituitary tumors can disrupt the gland's normal ability to release hormones and also, by local invasion, produce cerebral effects. There are two types of pituitary tumors—secretory and nonsecretory. These hormonal imbalances can cause problems in many different areas of the body. The "gold standard" of diagnosis is pituitary MRI. Nowadays, by increasing the indication of PET/CT in different oncology areas, the incidental pathological findings in the pituitary gland became more frequent.

Incidental pituitary uptake on whole-body F18-FDG PET/CT was studied in a multicenter study, published by Jeong et al. in 2010. Focally increased pituitary F18-FDG uptake on PET/CT was found in 30 of 40,967 patients, accounting for an incidence of 0.073%. The conclusion of the study was that incidental pituitary F18-FDG uptake was a *very rare finding*. Cases with incidental pituitary F18-FDG uptake were diagnosed primarily with clinically nonfunctioning adenomas, and there were also a few functioning adenomas. Further evaluations, including hormone assays and pituitary MRI, are warranted when pituitary uptake is found on F18-FDG PET/CT.

The most frequent diseases that might affect pituitary gland in their evolution are breast and lung cancers, colonic cancer, less common non-Hodgkin lymphoma and malignant melanoma, or thyroid carcinoma. The most common symptom seems to be diabetes insipidus, reflecting a predominance of metastasis to the posterior lobe. Komninos et al. (2004) cited in their review a study of 40 symptomatic cases, where diabetes insipidus occurred in 70%, whereas only 15% had one or more anterior pituitary deficiencies.

The role of PET/CT F18-FDG in pituitary gland is related to a correct assessment of the primary tumor, knowing and considering that this gland might be affected during the metastatic process (Fig. 11.1).

PET/MR has a special role in the diagnosis and evaluation of pituitary gland, mainly in malignant metastatic diseases, due to its better sensitivity and lesser radiation dose, with brain and cardiology being until now the main indications of this hybrid imaging. Figure 11.2 is presenting a case of pituitary adenoma visualized in PET/MR with somatostatin analogue tracer (Ga-68 DOTATOC).

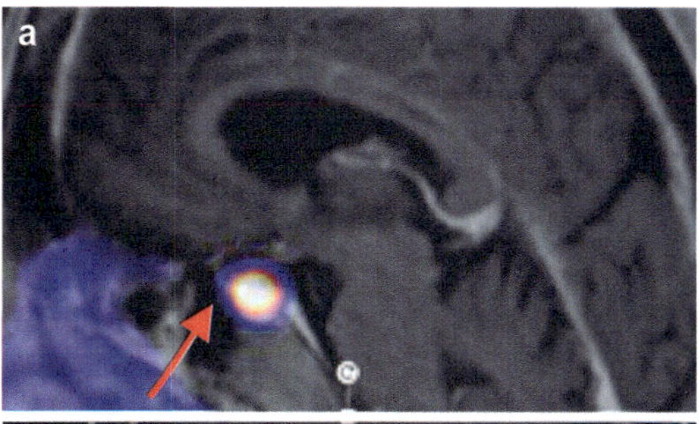

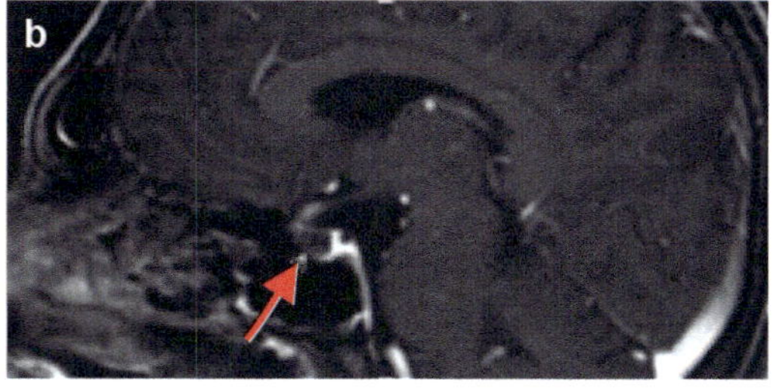

Fig. 11.2 PET/MR Ga-68 DOTATOC ((**a**) sagittal slice) and MR ((**b**) sagittal slice) showing an increased uptake in the pituitary gland, normally being visualized due to its somatostatin receptors; in this case is a pituitary adenoma

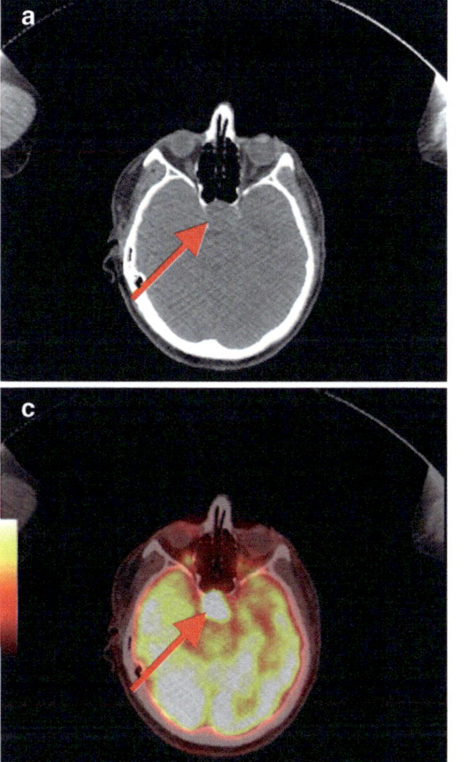

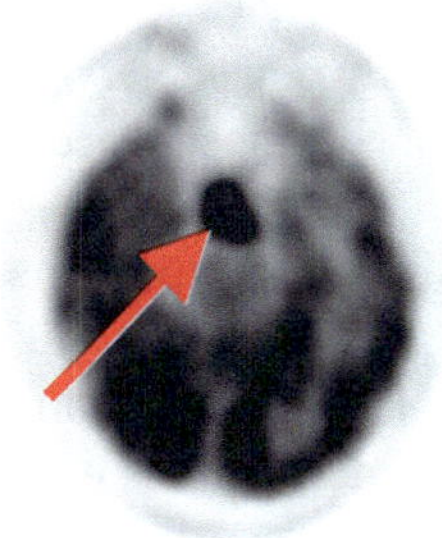

Fig. 11.1 PET/CT F18-FDG (**a**) transversal slice of CT, (**b**) transversal slice of PET and (**c**) transversal slice of fused PET/CT showing an increased, pathologic uptake in the pituitary gland, in a case of metastatic breast cancer

11.6 PET/CT in Parathyroid Gland Pathology

The place of parathyroid scintigraphy in the assessment of hyperparathyroidism is being largely presented in Chap. 8; the use of SPECT/CT improved specificity, but unfortunately could not improve importantly sensitivity. The most challenging clinical issue is the association of multinodular goiter with primary hyperparathyroidism due to parathyroid adenoma; researchers worldwide trying to find one modality were able to depict optimally the two entities. Many studies were carried on trying to find the best imaging method and protocol, but until now, beyond Tc-99m MIBI scan, all other methods need to be compared with it.

In this light, PET/CT introduced, in the last years, a new tracer: F18-fluorocholine (F18-FCH), with some promising results (Fig. 11.3). First description of F18-fluorocholine uptake in hyperfunctioning parathyroid glands was in 2013. The indications of the method consist in:

- Diagnosis of primary HPT
- Indication for parathyroid surgery
- US and SPECT nondiagnostic/inconclusive

Some pilot studies already published that in patients with hyperparathyroidism and with discordant or equivocal results on scintigraphy or on ultrasonography, adenomatous or hyperplastic parathyroid glands can be localized by F18-FCH PET/CT with good accuracy. One pilot study (Michaud et al. 2014) confirmed that F18-FCH PET/CT is an adequate imaging tool in patients with primary or secondary hyperparathyroidism, since both adenomas and hyperplastic parathyroid glands can be detected. The authors underlined that the sensitivity of F18-FCH PET/CT was better than that of US and similar to that of dual-phase dual-isotope I-123/Tc-99m scintigraphy. Unfortunately, the study involved a limited number of patients, 12 patients, so the conclusions are not strong enough to affirm the method. Considering Tc-99m MIBI scan as "gold standard," further studies should evaluate whether F18-FCH could replace this one as the functional agent for parathyroid imaging (Michaud et al. 2015).

Similar, the introduction of F18-FCH PET/MRI should bring better data, especially in case of HPT associated with multinodular goiter.

11.7 PET/CT in Thyroid Pathology

Among all the endocrine malignancies, the thyroid carcinoma is the most frequent, accounting for about 5% of thyroid nodules and being responsible for the mortality caused by cancer in 0.12–1.2% of cases. The differentiated thyroid cancer forms represent about 80–90% of all thyroid cancers, with a good prognosis and with a very specific treatment strategy based on surgery and radioiodine therapy.

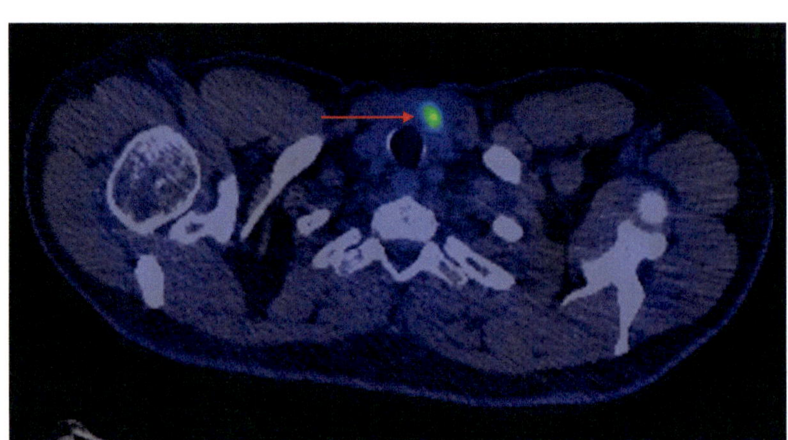

Fig. 11.3 PET/CT F18-FCH (transversal slice) showing an increased, pathologic uptake in a right parathyroid adenoma

In the last decade, more aggressive natural history of this cancer was reported, and new investigation methods were developed. The metabolic F18-fluoro-2-deoxy-d-glucose has already been accepted as an essential tool in staging, restaging, and therapy response assessment of many tumors.

The PET/CT investigation in the thyroid pathology is related to three major subjects:

1. The evaluation of thyroid nodules
2. The role of PET/CT in different forms of thyroid carcinoma
3. The diagnosis of other malignancies associated with thyroid carcinomas

11.7.1 PET/CT in the Differential Diagnosis of Benign Thyroid Nodules and Malignant Thyroid Nodules

Normally, there is no significant F18-fluoro-2-deoxy-d-glucose uptake in the thyroid bed. The presence of this radiotracer in the area of the thyroid in a PET/CT examination indicated for another type of pathology is described in literature as "metabolom." If focal F18-FDG uptake is described on a PET/CT image, it is important to refer the patient to the endocrinologist in order to make a clinical examination, thyroid function tests, and thyroid ultrasound.

The study of Seong et al. published in September 2009 regarding the incidental thyroid lesions detected by F18-FDG PET/CT demonstrated that prevalence and risk of thyroid cancer in these lesions are very low. F18-FDG PET/CT was performed on 3379 patients for evaluation of suspected or known cancer or cancer screening without any history of thyroid cancer. Among them, 285 patients (8.4%) were identified to have F18-FDG uptake on thyroid area, 99 patients with focal or diffuse F18-FDG uptake underwent further evaluation, and 22 patients were diagnosed with thyroid cancer. The cancer risk of incidentally found thyroid lesions on F18-FDG PET/CT was 0.65% (22/3379), a fact that underlines that this examination is not recommended as screening of thyroid carcinoma.

Regarding the differential diagnosis between the benign and malignant nodules, there is a factor that may play a role in the decision of further thyroid evaluation after the discovery of a "metabolom": there is a significant difference in the standardized uptake value (SUV) between the benign and malignant nodules (3.35 ± 1.69 vs 6.64 ± 4.12). If SUV maximum is suspicious, an examination in the endocrinology department is indicated.

Soelberg et al. published in 2012 a very important and consistent study referring to the evaluation of thyroid carcinomas discovered incidentally in patients or healthy volunteers by F18-FDG PET systematically searched in the PubMed database from 2000 to 2011. There were 22 studies comprising a total of 125,754 subjects. Of these, 1994 (1.6%) had unexpected focal hypermetabolic activity; a diagnosis was assigned in 1051 of the 1994 patients with a focal uptake, 366 of whom (34.8%) had thyroid malignancy. In the eight studies reporting individual maximum SUV, the mean SUV(max) was 4.8 ± 3.1 in benign lesions and 6.9 ± 4.7 in malignant lesions.

Considering the above studies, a cutoff value of SUVmax of 6 is highly suspicious for malignancy in a case of focal thyroid F18-FDG uptake in PET/CT (Fig. 11.4).

In case of diffuse thyroid uptake, the malignancy is less probable and the diagnosis of thyroiditis should be mentioned (Fig. 11.5).

The evaluation of thyroid gland in case of F18-FDG PET/CT performed for other oncological clinical cases is important to be mentioned, both with respect to possible synchronous neoplasia and in order to exclude possible metastases in thyroid.

A nodular goiter with no F18-FDG uptake discovered in a patient with a primary known cancer is essential to be pointed. Figure 11.6 is presenting a case of breast cancer with incidental nodular goiter discovered at PET/CT with no F18-FDG uptake, being highly probable to be a benign thyroid pathology, with no impact in the assessment of the primary cancer (Fig. 11.6).

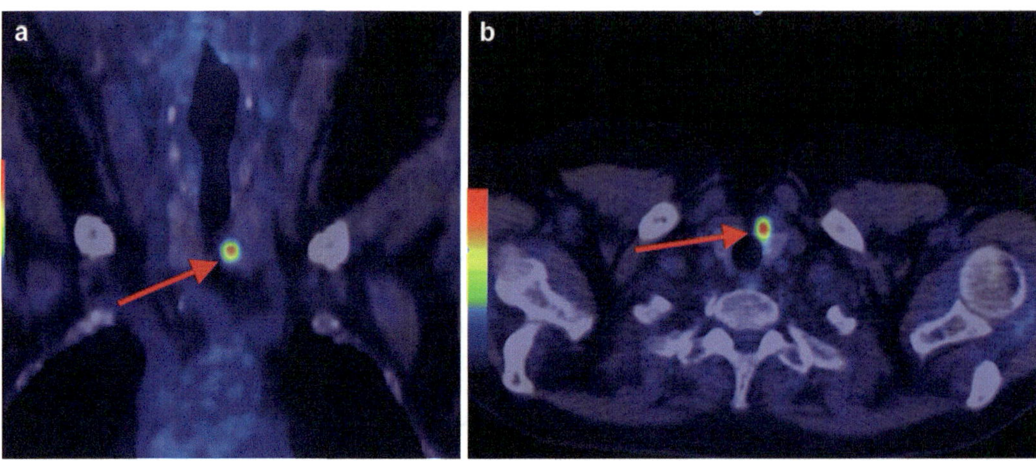

Fig. 11.4 F18-FDG PET/CT showing incidental focal uptake in the left thyroid lobe, in a patient performing the examination during the monitoring protocol for a malignant melanoma ((**a**) coronal slice; (**b**) transversal slice). The patient was operated and the histological specimen confirmed a papillary thyroid carcinoma

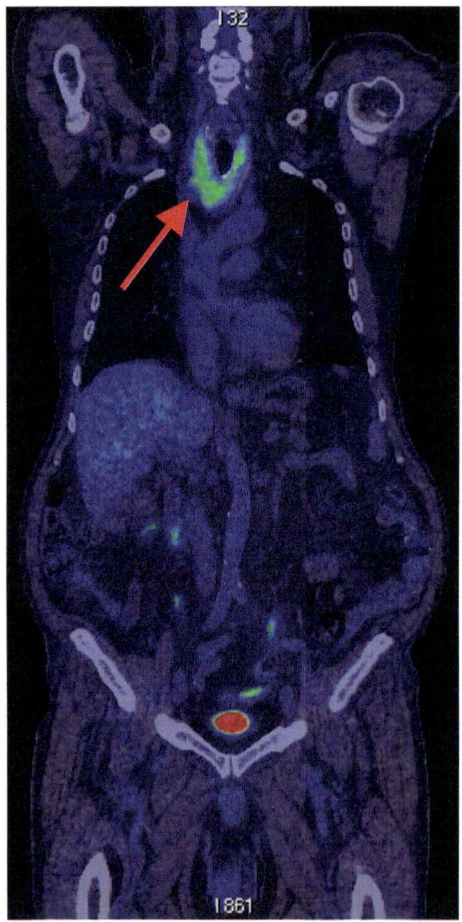

Fig. 11.5 F18-FDG PET/CT showing incidental diffuse uptake in the thyroid gland, in a patient performing the examination for a restaging of a colon cancer (coronal slice); the image is highly suggestive for chronic Hashimoto's thyroiditis

Similarly, in a case of colon cancer, with nodular goiter, without FDG uptake in PET/CT is presented in Fig. 11.7.

Thyroid incidentaloma is commonly defined as a thyroid uptake incidentally and newly detected by imaging techniques performed for an unrelated and non-thyroid purpose. Its management is challenging for referring clinicians and for nuclear medicine physicians because it needs further investigation to clarify its nature. The overall reported incidence of F18-FDG PET or PET/CT thyroid incidentalomas varies from 0.2 to 8.9%, whereas the prevalence of thyroid cancer in these incidental lesions ranges from 8 to 64%, and the most significant conclusions regarding this issue are summarized as follows (Bertagna et al. 2012):

1. Thyroid incidentalomas are relatively frequent, ranging from 0.2 to 8.9%, and the pooled incidence is 2.46%.
2. Diffuse uptakes are commonly benign.
3. Most focal uptakes are benign, but about one-third of focal uptakes are malignant.
4. All thyroid incidentalomas need further investigation and clinical evaluation.
5. The most frequent malignant histological type responsible for F18-FDG PET/CT thyroid incidentaloma is PTC.
6. There is no safe SUV cutoff over which it is certain or reasonably safe to suspect or rule out malignancies.

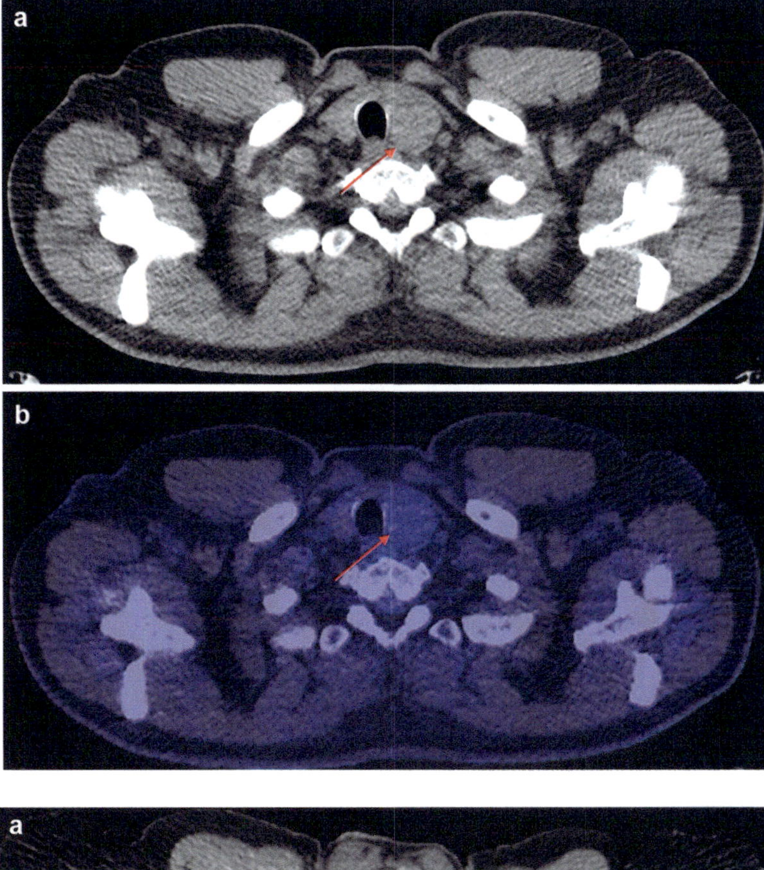

Fig. 11.6 F18-FDG PET/CT in a patient with breast cancer showing incidental nodule in the left lobe of the thyroid gland, with no F18-FDG uptake, being highly probable to be a benign nodule ((**a**) CT transversal slice; (**b**) PET/CT transversal slice)

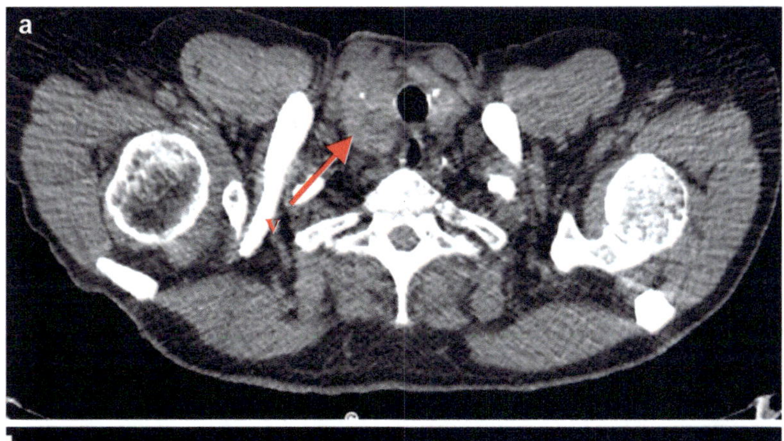

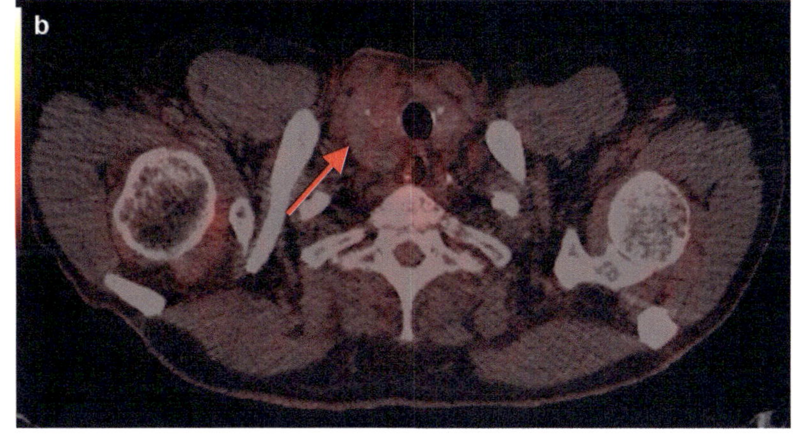

Fig. 11.7 F18-FDG PET/CT in a patient with colon cancer showing multinodular goiter, with no pathologic F18-FDG uptake, being highly probable to be a benign macronodular goiter ((**a**) CT transversal slice; (**b**) PET/CT transversal slice)

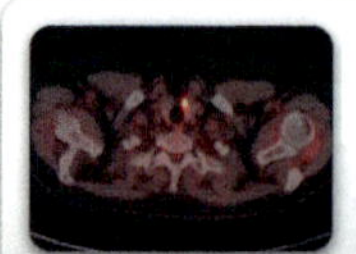

Thyroid nodule without F18-FDG uptake
• Highly probable benign nodules
• To be mentioned in the raport, without inpact in the assesment of the primary tumor

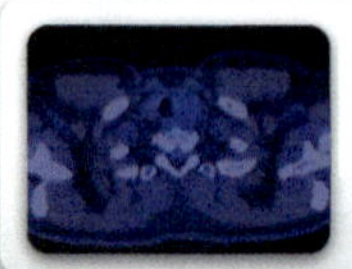

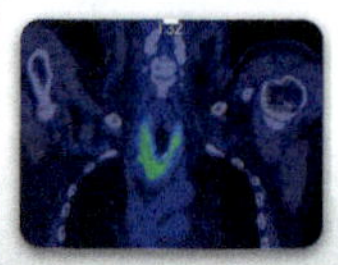

Fig. 11.8 The workup for an increased thyroid uptake of F18-FDG in PET/CT

The workup for an incidentally increased thyroid uptake of F18-FDG in PET/CT is presented in Fig. 11.8.

11.7.2 PET/CT in the Follow-Up of Thyroid Carcinoma

In case of thyroid carcinoma, the experience regarding the use of hybrid imaging shows an increasing role and a very well-defined place of PET/CT. The changes in the behavior and aggressiveness of thyroid cancer represent an important indication for F18-FDG PET/CT. The most important situations, where the hybrid method brings essential information, are:

- Biochemical evolution of the disease, with no clinical and imaging signs
- Increasing serological tumor markers, negative WBS I-131
- Radioiodine-refractory differentiated thyroid cancer (DTC)
- Aggressive course of the disease
- Progressive disease in medullary thyroid cancer (MTC)
- Anaplastic thyroid cancer (ATC)
- Thyroid lymphoma
- Association with other malignancies

11.7.2.1 PET/CT in the Follow-Up of Differentiated Thyroid Carcinoma (DTC)

DTC is not one of the types of cancers where PET/CT is a standard indication or is included in the guidelines of diagnosis and treatment. Despite that, there is a very well-defined situation where PET/CT plays a major role, so-called TENIS (Tg elevated and negative I-131 scan) syndrome:

- Confirmed DTC with radical treatment
- Detectable serum Tg or dynamic rising of Tg and/or anti-Tg
- WBS I-131 negative

The American Thyroid Association affirms in the guidelines of thyroid cancer in 2009 (ATA 2009): "if after an empiric dose of 100–200 mCi, I-131 WBS fails to localize the tumor, especially in patients with unstimulated serum Tg level of 10–20 ng/mL, F18-FDG-PET should be considered."

The same recommendation is given by the National Comprehensive Cancer Network (NCCN 2016) on thyroid cancer guidelines in 2011. From 2003, the insurance system (Medicare) from the USA pays for this condition of thyroid cancer patients who have the indication for this examination and also in most of the European countries.

The recent guidelines (ATA 2015; BTA 2014; ETA/ESMO and NCCN 2016) introduced precisely the indication and the place of PET/CT in the management of thyroid cancers.

ATA (2015)

Recommendation 68

- A, strong recommendation
  - F18-FDG PET scanning should be considered in high-risk DTC patients with elevated serum Tg (generally >10 ng/mL) with negative WBS I-131 imaging; according to multiple studies published recently, the sensitivity of the method was 83% (ranging from 50% to 100%), and the specificity was 84% (ranging from 42% to 100%) in non-131I-avid DTC.
- B, weak recommendation
  - A part of initial staging in poorly differentiated thyroid cancers and invasive Hurthle cell carcinomas, especially those with other evidence of disease on imaging or because of elevated serum Tg levels
  - A prognostic tool in patients with metastatic disease to identify lesions and patients at highest risk for rapid disease progression and disease-specific mortality
  - An evaluation of posttreatment response following systemic or local therapy of metastatic or locally invasive disease

BTA (2014)

In case of TENIS syndrome, BTA guidelines recommend:

- Chest CT without contrast.
- F18-FDG PET/CT.
- Neck MRI.
- CT.
- Spine MRI.
- Bone scan.
- I-131 WBS.
- Very occasionally In-11 octreotide or Ga-68 DOTATATE PET/CT may be positive.

Positive F18-FDG PET/CT indicates histologic transformation from low- to high-risk poor prognosis tumors, as F18-FDG uptake reflects dedifferentiation.

Patients with positive F18-FDG PET/CT scan have been shown to have a markedly reduced 3-year survival compared with F18-FDG PET/CT scan-negative patients. If PET imaging is positive, I-131 imaging is typically negative and the patient is I-131 refractory.

The most frequent situation of indication for F18-FDG PET/CT in DTC consisted in:

- Radical treatment of DTC: surgery, radioiodine therapy, and suppressive hormonal treatment
- No clinical signs of disease
- Dynamic rising of serum level of Tg or/and anti-Tg
- WBS I-131 negative
- Neck ultrasound negative or doubtful
- Conventional imaging negative (thorax radiographies, cervical and mediastinum computed tomography)
- No other acute or chronic severe diseases that may lower life expectancy under 1 year
- Financial support available, where the examination is not reimbursed by national health insurances

The F18-FDG PET/CT is indicated with respect to a minimum level of serum Tg above 2 ng/mL if all previous mentioned criteria are fulfilled; also it is important to have demonstrated that in the same conditions of sample analysis, in two consecutive determinations at 6-month interval, there was a significant dynamic rising of the value of Tg.

Regarding the F18-FDG PET/CT in DTC, there is a special detail that is important to be stressed: the role of TSH in the F18-FDG uptake. The elevated TSH serum level (withdrawal of thyroid hormonal treatment or using the rhTSH) influences the F18-FDG uptake. Petrich et al. published in 2002 that the sensitivity of FDG

PET was 53% during TSH suppression and 87% following rhTSH stimulation. Other authors showed that there is no influence of TSH in F18-FDG uptake, but the higher sensitivity is seen on Tg value >20 ng/mL.

Iagaru A et al. (2007) published that F18-FDG PET/CT had excellent sensitivity (88.6%) and specificity (89.3%) in this patient population. Metastatic lesions were reliably identified but were less F18-FDG avid than recurrence/residual disease in the thyroid bed. TSH levels at the time of PET/CT did not appear to impact the FDG uptake in the lesions or have the ability to detect disease. In the setting of high or rising levels of Tg, their study confirms that it is indicated to include PET/CT in the management of patients with differentiated thyroid cancer; ATA 2015 set the cutoff value at 10 ng/mL.

According to BTA 2014, thyroid hormone withdrawal (THW) or recombinant human TSH (rhTSH) administration has been shown to increase the sensitivity of F18-FDG PET/CT scan; this issue recently was amended by other authors, being clearly demonstrated that is related to the level of Tg. So, the level of Tg, no matter if in understimulated condition or not, is recommended to be >10 ng/mL in order to have the maximum sensitivity of PET/CT F18-FDG in DTC.

If in the previous edition of this book, this issue was debatable, to date, *there is no evidence that TSH stimulation improves the prognostic value of F18-FDG PET imaging.* Singh et al. published in 2017 the results of their study, and they underline a significant association of SUV with thyroglobulin (Tg) level ($P = 0.035$) but not with thyroid-stimulating hormone (TSH) level ($P = 0.85$).

As a commentary, from the personal experience of the author, the level of Tg is less important than the aggressiveness of the histology: very low detectable levels of Tg, even <5 ng/mL, may lead to a severe positive scan in F18-FDG PET/CT, if the course of the disease is highly aggressive (see examples in the clinical cases presented below).

Iodine 124 emits positrons, allowing PET/CT imaging in DTC patients. It is used as a dosimetric and also as a diagnostic tool to localize disease. I-124 PET/CT permits an accurate measurement of the volume and uptake in positive lesions on the scan, allowing a reliable individual dosimetric assessment for each neoplastic focus.

The sensitivity of I-124 PET for the detection of residual thyroid tissue and/or metastatic DTC was reported to be higher than that of a diagnostic I-131 planar WBS, but is not yet widely available for clinical use and is primarily a research tool at this time.

11.7.2.2 PET/CT in the Follow-Up of Medullary Thyroid Carcinoma (MTC)

As in DTC situation in MTC, there is a strict place of F18-FDG PET/CT: radical treatment, serum calcitonin level rising, and conventional imagery negative. The overall sensitivity of F18-FDG PET/CT is less than 75%, but the new radiotracers such as F18-dihydroxyphenylalanine, F18-DOPA, and Ga-68-labeled somatostatin analogues give optimistic horizons. As is known in literature, in MTC, there is a lack of sensitivity of many investigations: F18-fluoro-2-deoxy-d-glucose PET/CT, 78%; pentavalent Tc-99m dimercaptosuccinic acid (DMSA), 33%; Tc-99m sestamibi (MIBI), 25%; indium-111 pentetreotide, 25%; CT, 50%; and MRI, 82%. Even if the specificity may raise to 100% (MIBI), these low rates of sensitivity justify the efforts to develop new radiotracers for PET. Recent studies (Giraudet et al. 2016) established that PET/CT using F18-FDOPA is the most sensitive radiopharmaceutical for localizing persistent/recurrent MTC, its sensitivity being related to a threshold value serum calcitonin of around 150 pg/mL. The authors recommend F18-FDG PET/CT in MTC when there is a short calcitonin or CEA doubling time; this underlines the aggressiveness of the disease (Fig. 11.9). Same results were published also by Archier et al. in 2016: F18-DOPA PET/CT enables early diagnosis of a significant number of patients with distant metastases. It has a limited sensitivity in the detection of

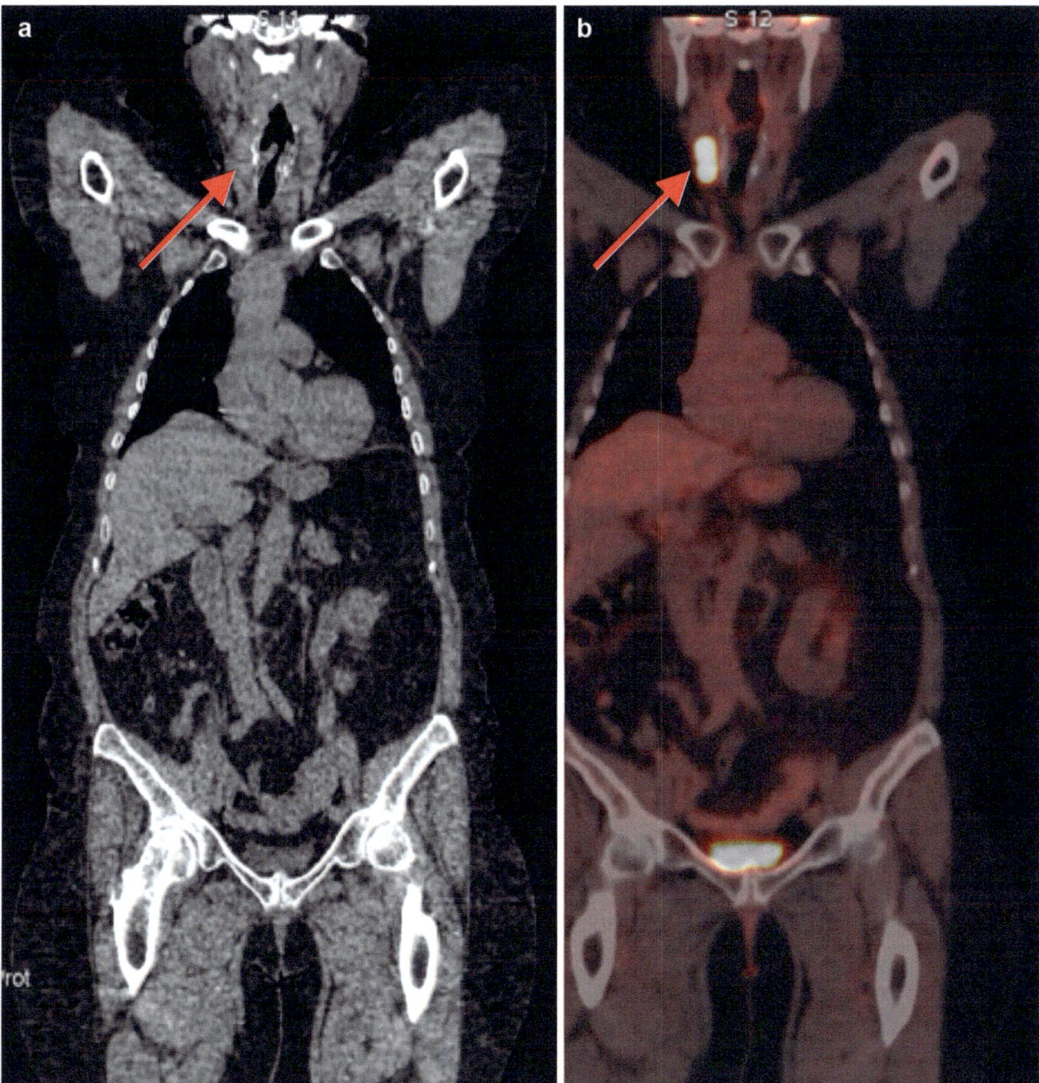

Fig. 11.9 F18-FDG PET/CT coronal slice (**a**) CT and (**b**) PET/CT in a patient with aggressive medullary thyroid cancer, with rapid progression of lymph node metastases

residual disease but provides high performance for regional analysis.

Considering that metastatic MTC is an incurable disease, the management aims are to provide locoregional disease control; palliate symptoms of hormonal excess, pain, or bone fracture; and control metastases that threaten life. In this light, all efforts should be done to find the best imaging tool able to visualize earlier the persistent, recurrent, or metastatic disease.

11.7.2.3 PET/CT in the Follow-Up of Anaplastic Thyroid Carcinoma (ATC)

Unfortunately, this examination does not have significant importance in this case because of the very aggressive natural history of the disease, of the rapid local evolution, and of the often-limited medical intervention. Frequently, CT and MRI are able to establish the extension of the disease.

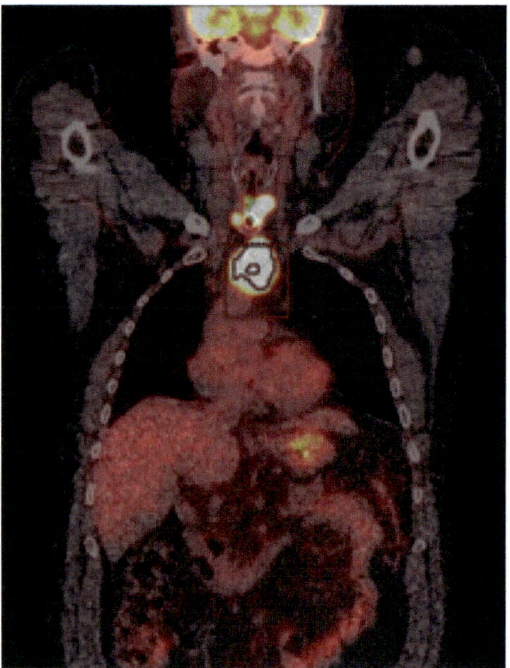

Fig. 11.10 F18-FDG PET/CT coronal slice in a patient with aggressive anaplastic thyroid cancer, with tracheostomy

If disease is controllable, consider F18-FDG PET/CT 3–6 months after initial therapy (NCCN 2016). The aggressiveness of the disease makes anaplastic thyroid cancer very sensitive to F18-FDG PET/CT, lesions presenting high FDG uptake (Figs. 11.10 and 11.11).

Scintigraphy with radiolabeled somatostatin analogues (SRS) has proven useful in diagnosing somatostatin receptor-positive tumors (SSTRs). Recently, PET-SSTR analogues with Ga-68 have been successfully introduced. The content of SSTR is important for the success of SSTR therapy with or without radiolabeling. There are some studies about the SSTR status of thyroid cancer patients (DTC radioiodine non-avid, MTC, ATC) comparing the recently described radiopharmaceutical Ga-68 DOTA-LAN and established Ga-68 DOTATOC by PET imaging for patient selection for peptide receptor radionuclide therapy (PRRT).

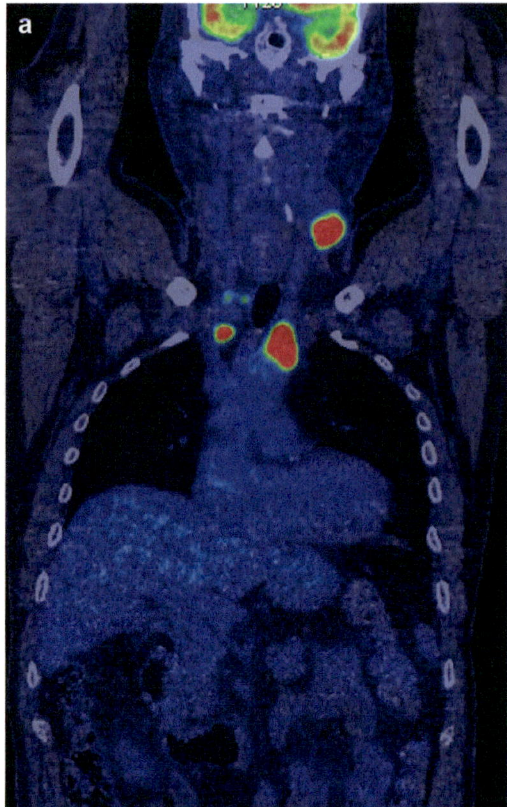

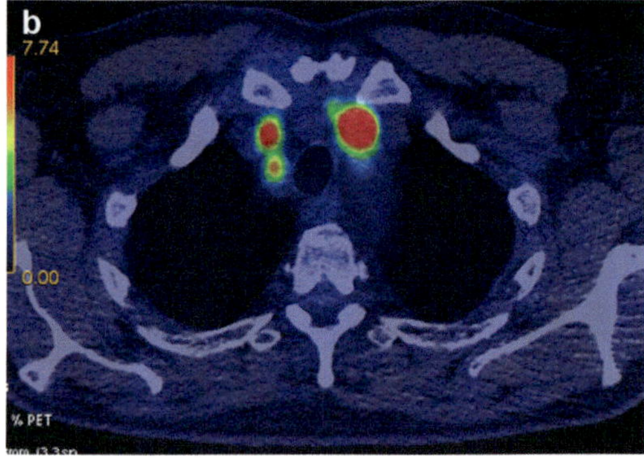

Fig. 11.11 F18-FDG PET/CT coronal slice (**a**) and transversal slice (**b**) in a patient with aggressive anaplastic thyroid cancer of the left lobe and lymph node metastases

11.7.3 The Role of PET/CT in Other Malignancies Associated with Thyroid Carcinoma

In the situation of second malignancies, PET/CT gives the chance of a better prognosis to patients, so synchronic or metachronic cancers benefit from early detection. A multicenter study performed in 13 medical centers in Europe, Canada, Australia, and Singapore showed a 30% increased risk of second primary cancer after thyroid cancer and increased risks of thyroid cancer after various primary cancers. Also, North American researchers published similar results.

The author (Piciu et al. 2016) published from the personal database that second primary malignancies occurred after DTC in 1990 patients treated between 1970 and 2003. The mean long-term follow-up period was 182 months. The relative risk of development of second malignancy in DTC patients was increased ($p < 0.0001$) for breast, uterine, and ovarian cancers compared with the general population. The overall risk concerning the development of second primary malignancies was related to the presence of DTC, but not to exposure to the low and medium activities of radioiodine administered as adjuvant therapy.

The oncologists published the relation between disorders in the thyroid and breast leading to carcinomas, so in both cancers there is a special attention given to screening. The PET/CT has an important role in these situations.

A special attention should be given to thyroid lymphoma, where the pathology is treated as a hematological disease, and the diagnosis and monitoring protocols are those established by the specific committees. A standard place is reserved to F18-FDG PET/CT, due to its importance in the algorithm of follow-up. The intensity of F18-FDG uptake expressed by SUV is considered an essential tool in the treatment response assessment. The Deauville criteria (the five-point scale) introduced for the assessment of response to therapy might be also applied in particularly affected thyroid gland.

The German authors published (Baras et al. 2017) that the increased risk of subsequent primary malignancies (SPM) in survivors of adult-onset Hodgkin lymphoma (HL) and non-Hodgkin lymphoma (NHL) in 128, 587 patients registered during more than 20 years was significantly increased over twofold for HL survivors and 1.5-fold for NHL survivors compared with the general German population. These cancers consisted in lip/oral cavity, colon/rectum, lung, skin melanoma, breast, kidney, and thyroid. Significantly increased SIRs for esophagus, stomach, liver, pancreas, testis, prostate, and brain/central nervous system were observed following NHL only.

Considering these data, the consistent screening by PET/CT in lymphoma should be essential in early diagnosis and correct assessment of both diseases.

Some clinical examples will be detailed in this chapter, keeping in mind that:

- Thyroid cancer might be associated with other malignancies, so during PET/CT performed for the specific indication of TC, these pathologies are discovered.
- Thyroid might be the host for metastases from other cancer, mainly renal, breast, lung, and melanoma.
- Other malignancies during their monitoring protocols by PET/CT might be associated with thyroid cancer, expressed by increased focal uptake in the thyroid.

Case 1: Papillary Thyroid Carcinoma and Colon Cancer

History:

A 62-year-old male, with the diagnosis of papillary thyroid carcinoma operated 2 years before with total thyroidectomy and selective lymph node dissection, was irradiated with 100 mCi (3.7 GBq) I-131. He was examined in the follow-up.

T3N1aM0—stage III.

Clinical examination:

The patient was under L-thyroxin 150 μg/daily, in normal thyroid status; he had no signs of thyroid dysfunction.

The neck examination revealed a post-thyroidectomy scar, without any palpable tumor mass or lymph nodes in the cervical area. No other signs or symptoms to be mentioned.

Examinations:

Ultrasound—no thyroid tissue remnant, no lymph nodes.

TSH 0.07 mIU/L (N.V. 0.4–4.5 mIU/L)—suppressed under therapy.

Tg 1.8 μg/L (N.V. < 0.1 μg/L)—detectable under thyroxin suppression.

Anti-Tg <10 kIU/L (N.V. < 115 kIU/L)—normal.

rhTSH administered I.M. 2 × 0.9 mg for two consecutive days raised the TSH at >100 mIU/L and Tg at 7.8 μg/L.

A high EBR 64 mm/h (N.V. < 15 mm/h) is to be mentioned.

Findings:

The patient received 5 mCi (185 MBq) I-131.

The diagnosis WBS I-131 showed no pathologic uptake in the body (Fig. 11.12).

The PET/CT FDG revealed no pathologic thyroid mass but showed the presence of a colon tumor with liver metastases.

The patient was reevaluated, and the diagnosis of colon cancer with liver metastases was confirmed by the pathology of the tumor surgically removed both from the colon and liver (Fig. 11.13).

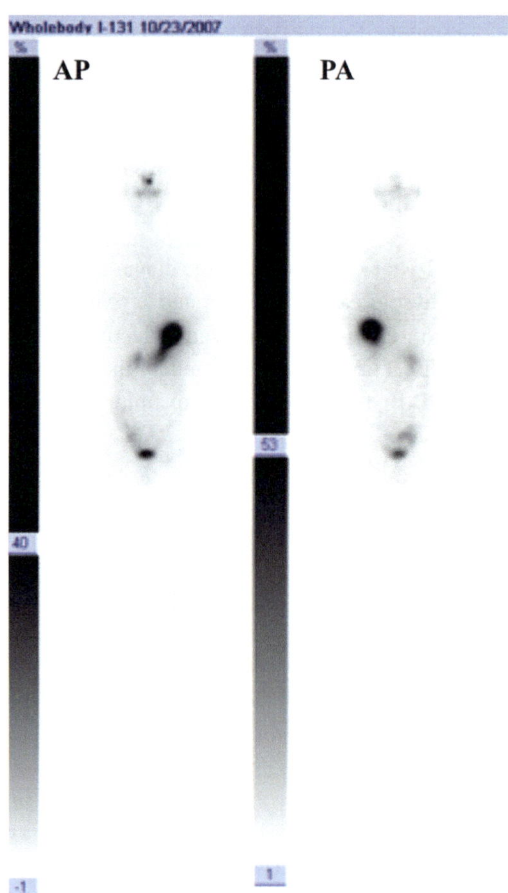

Fig. 11.12 WBS I-131 at 48 after diagnosis dose of 5 mCi I-131. Negative scan

Conclusion:

The diagnosis was papillary thyroid carcinoma and colon carcinoma with liver metastases; synchronic cancers.

Key Points

- The discrepancy between the Tg values in suppressed condition and discrete increasing during stimulation is unusual; even after FDG examination, the site of Tg origin was not discovered. A "black shot" dose of radioiodine is recommended in such circumstances.
- The PET/CT examination with the purpose of discovering a digestive cancer in this particular case was hurried because of the previous existence of thyroid cancer and screening during its follow-up.
- The liver metastases frequently sent the patient to PET/CT, intending to find the primary tumor.
- The liver metastases of papillary thyroid cancer are almost improbable, fact that suggests the search for another tumor origin.

Case 2: Papillary Thyroid Carcinoma and Breast Cancer

History:

A 51-year-old female, with the diagnosis of papillary thyroid carcinoma operated 3 years before with total thyroidectomy and selective lymph node dissection, was irradiated with 70 mCi (2.59 GBq) I-131. She was examined during the follow-up.

T2N0M0—stage II.

Clinical examination:

The patient was under L-thyroxin 150 μg/daily, in normal thyroidal status; she had no signs of thyroid dysfunction.

The neck examination revealed post-thyroidectomy scar, without any palpable tumor mass or lymph nodes in the cervical area. No other signs or symptoms to be mentioned.

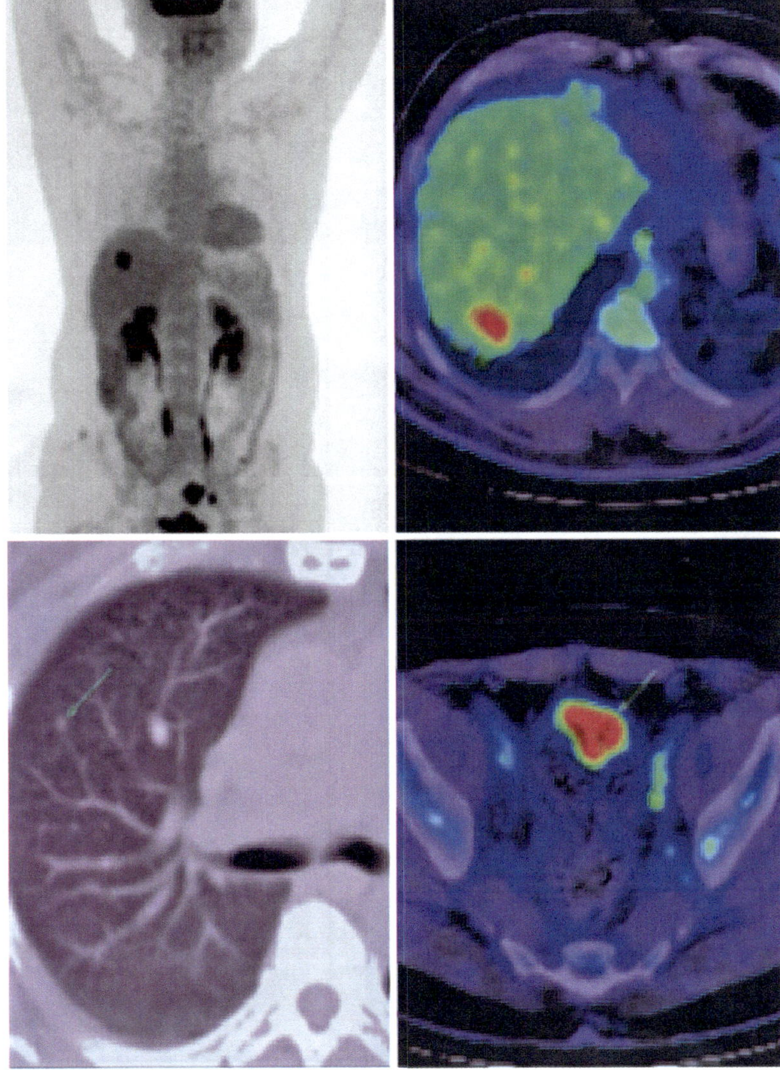

Fig. 11.13 PET/CT FDG—colon cancer with liver metastases (with courtesy of Prof. Galuska László and Lajos Szabados. SCANOMED Ltd.; University of Debrecen, Dept. of Nuclear Medicine)

Examinations:

The ultrasound revealed no thyroid tissue remnant and no pathological lymph nodes.

TSH 55.1 mIU/L (N.V. 0.4–4.5 mIU/L) after 4 weeks of hormonal withdrawal.

Tg 17.39 μg/L (N.V. < 0.1 μg/L)—detectable.

Anti-Tg 1405 kIU/L (N.V. < 115 kIU/L)—increased.

Findings:

The diagnosis WBS I-131 showed no pathologic uptake in the body.

Due to dynamic evolution of anti-Tg, the PET/CT FDG was done; the test revealed no pathologic thyroid mass but showed the presence of a left breast tumor with axillary metastatic suspicious lymph nodes.

The patient was surgically evaluated, and the diagnosis of minimal invasive breast carcinoma with axillary metastases was confirmed (Fig. 11.14).

During follow-up after 9 years of complete remission, at a new PET/CT, the image revealed recurrence of the disease with metastatic lymph node in the left subpectoralis area (Fig. 11.15).

Conclusion:

The diagnosis was papillary thyroid carcinoma and breast carcinoma with axillary metastases; synchronic cancers.

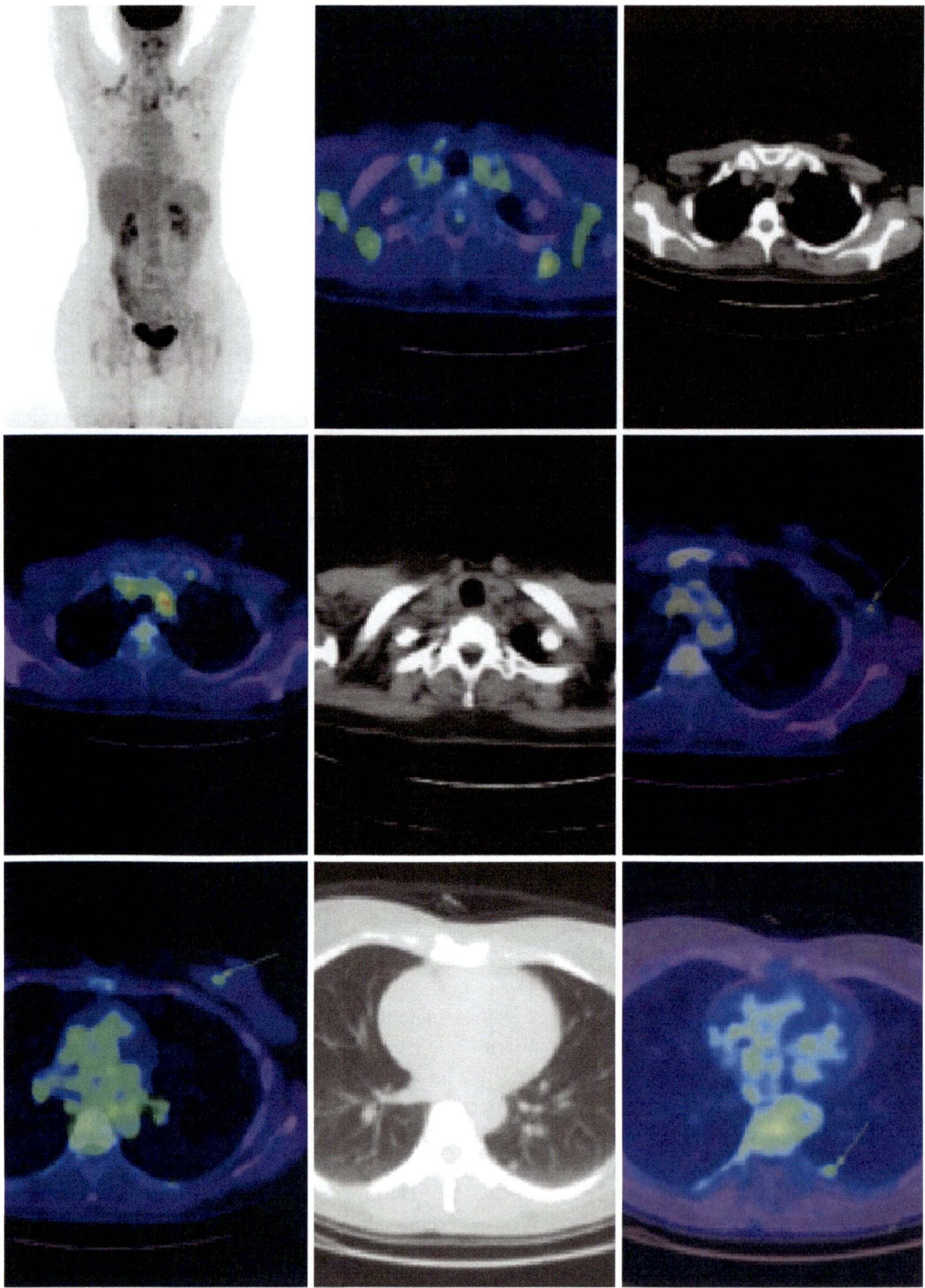

Fig. 11.14 PET/CT FDG—left breast carcinoma with axillary metastases (with courtesy of Prof. Galuska László and Lajos Szabados. SCANOMED Ltd.; University of Debrecen, Dept. of Nuclear Medicine)

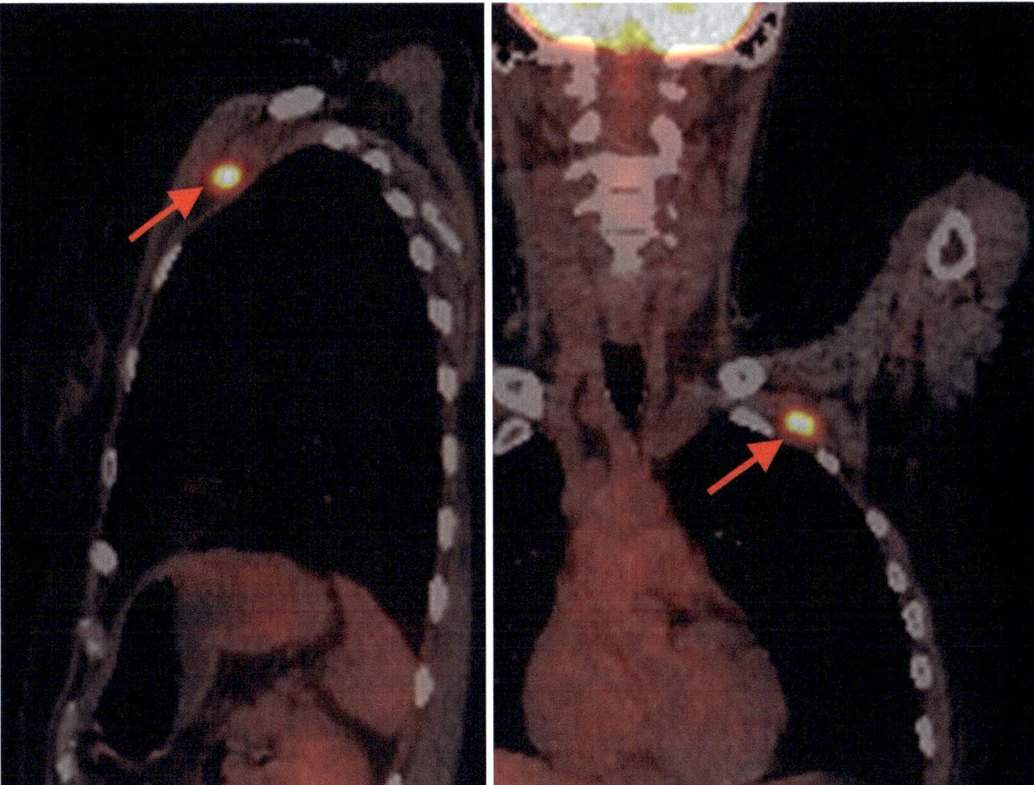

Fig. 11.15 PET/CT FDG—left subpectoralis metastatic lymph node in a patient with thyroid cancer and breast cancer in her history; relapse after 9 years of complete remission

Key Points

- The high incidence of thyroid carcinoma in female patients comparing with male brings the women to periodic medical control; this fact permits the screening in a systematic manner of the most important oncologic pathologies that might affect them: genital and breast carcinomas.
- Despite an explanation related to the addressability, there are studies that note a gene relation between the two cancers, fact that requests examination of both pathologies.

Case 3: Follicular Thyroid Carcinoma and Prostate Cancer

History:

A 76-year-old male with the diagnostic of follicular thyroid carcinoma with lymph node metastases and pulmonary metastases treated with a total dose of 420.31 mCi I-131in five fractions is referred to F18-FDG PET/CT scan.

TSH 62.9 mIU/L (N.V. 0.4–4.5 mIU/L) after 4 weeks of hormonal withdrawal.

Tg 2280 μg/L (N.V. < 0.1 μg/L)—very increased.

Anti-Tg 21 kIU/L (N.V. < 115 kIU/L)—increased.

WBS I-131 after therapy was positive for lymph node and lung metastases (Fig. 11.16); after

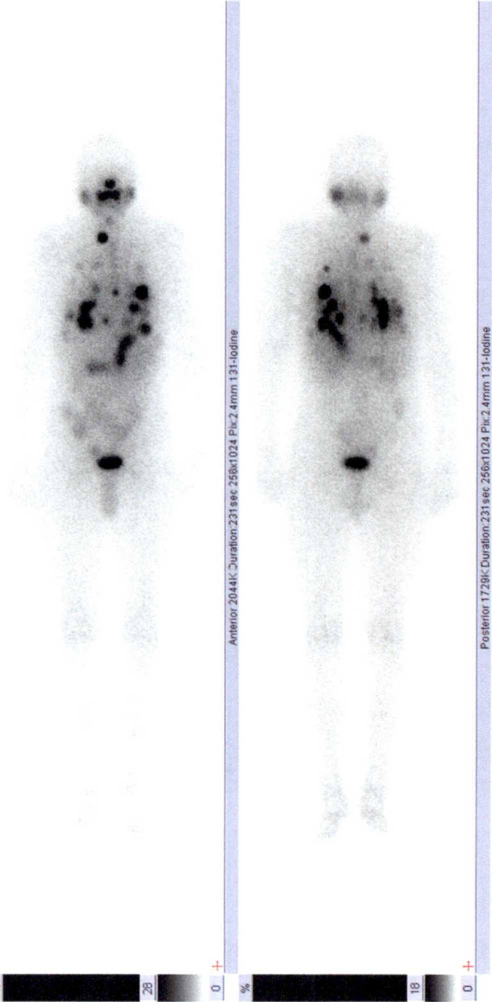

Fig. 11.16 WBS I-131 posttherapy which revealed pathologic uptake of radioiodine in mediastinum lymph node and lung metastases

two cures of I-131, the scan became negative.

F18-FDG PET/CT scan revealed discretely increased FDG uptake in mediastinum lymph nodes, lung metastases, and pathological focal uptake of FDG with SUV Ibm max of 7.13 in the prostate area. Radical prostatectomy with pelvic lymphadenectomy was performed, and the histopathology revealed prostate cancer with a Gleason score of 7 (Fig. 11.17).

Beyond the clinical cases presented above, there are several hypothesis regarding the possible indications and results of PET/CT F18-FDG in DTC, which are summarized below:

1. *F18-FDG PET/CT might be positive* in the follow-up of DTC:
   - US negative, WBS I-131 negative and detectable, but low levels of stimulated Tg < 10 µg/L, negative anti-Tg
   - US negative, WBS I-131 negative and detectable, high levels of stimulated Tg >10 µg/mL, negative anti-Tg
   - US negative, WBS I-131 negative and detectable, very high levels of Tg either on suppressed or stimulated conditions, negative anti-Tg
   - US negative, WBS I-131 negative, and increased level of anti-Tg, with either positive or negative Tg
   - US negative, WBS I-131 negative and undetectable Tg both on suppressed and stimulated conditions, and negative anti-Tg; PET/CT positive due to other pathologies
2. *F18-FDG PET/CT might be negative* in the follow-up of DTC:
   - US negative, WBS I-131 negative and any detectable levels of Tg, negative anti-Tg
   - US negative, WBS I-131 negative, and undetectable levels of Tg, but increased anti-Tg
   - Complete remission, all mentioned parameters being negative

The following clinical cases will cover the mentioned situations.

Case 4: Papillary Thyroid Carcinoma
History:

A 48-year-old male, with the diagnosis of papillary thyroid carcinoma operated 11 years before by total thyroidectomy and selective lymph node dissection, was irradiated with 100 mCi (3.7 GBq) I-131. He was examined in the follow-up.

T2N1bM0—stage III.

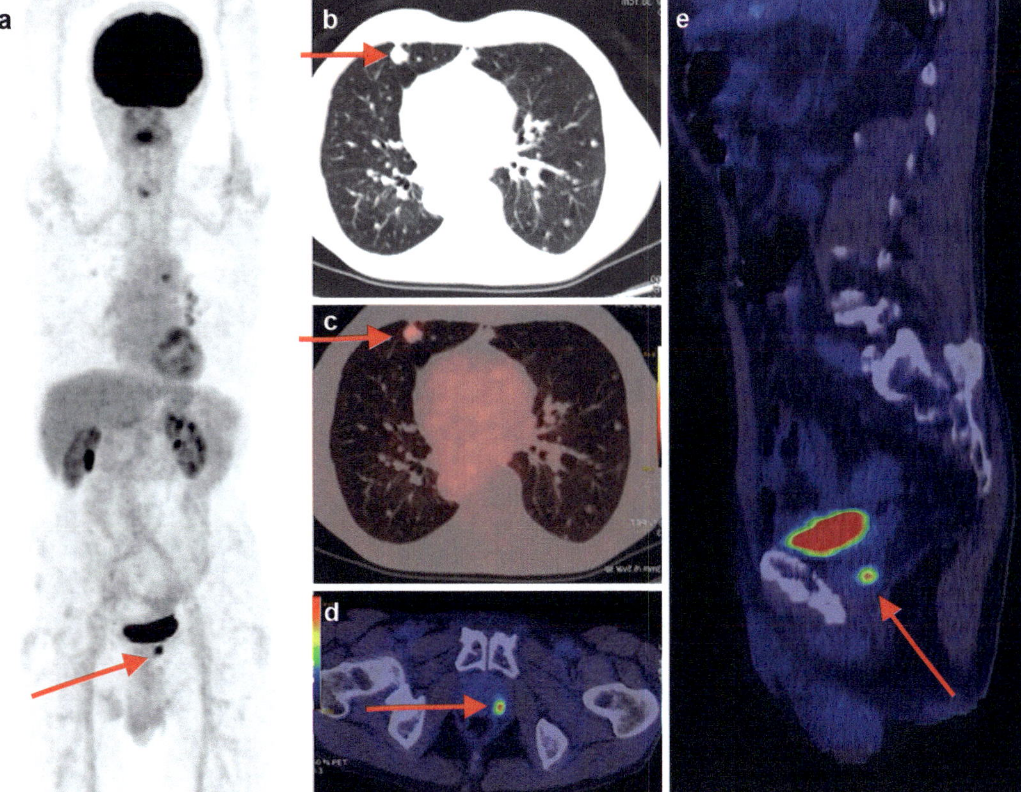

Fig. 11.17 PET/CT FDG in mediastinum lymph node and lung metastases ((**a**) MIP PET; (**b**) thorax transversal slice CT; (**c**) thorax axial PET/CT) and pathological focal uptake of FDG with SUV lbm max of 7.13 in the prostate area ((**d**) axial pelvic PET/CT; (**e**) sagittal thorax PET/CT)

Clinical examination:

The patient was under L-thyroxin 125 μg/daily, in normal thyroidal status; he had no signs of thyroid dysfunction.

The neck examination revealed a post-thyroidectomy scar, without any palpable tumor mass or lymph nodes in the cervical area. No other signs or symptoms to be mentioned.

Examinations:

Ultrasound—no thyroid tissue remnant, no lymph nodes.

rhTSH administered I.M. 2 × 0.9 mg for two consecutive days increased the TSH at 87.28 mIU/L (N.V. 0.4–4.5 mIU/L).

Tg 2.76 μg/L (N.V. < 0.1 μg/L)—detectable.

Anti-Tg 20.02 kIU/L (N.V. < 115 kIU/L)—normal.

It is to be mentioned that the patient had a period of 10 years of disease-free with Tg < 0.1 μg/L in stimulated conditions and a constant dynamic increasing of Tg during the last year.

Findings:

The diagnosis WBS I-131 showed no pathologic uptake in the body.

The PET/CT FDG revealed no pathologic thyroid mass but showed the presence of left lateral lymph nodes with metastases.

The patient was surgically reevaluated, and the diagnosis of papillary thyroid metastases was confirmed (Fig. 11.18).

Conclusion:

The diagnosis was recurrent lymph node metastases of papillary thyroid carcinoma.

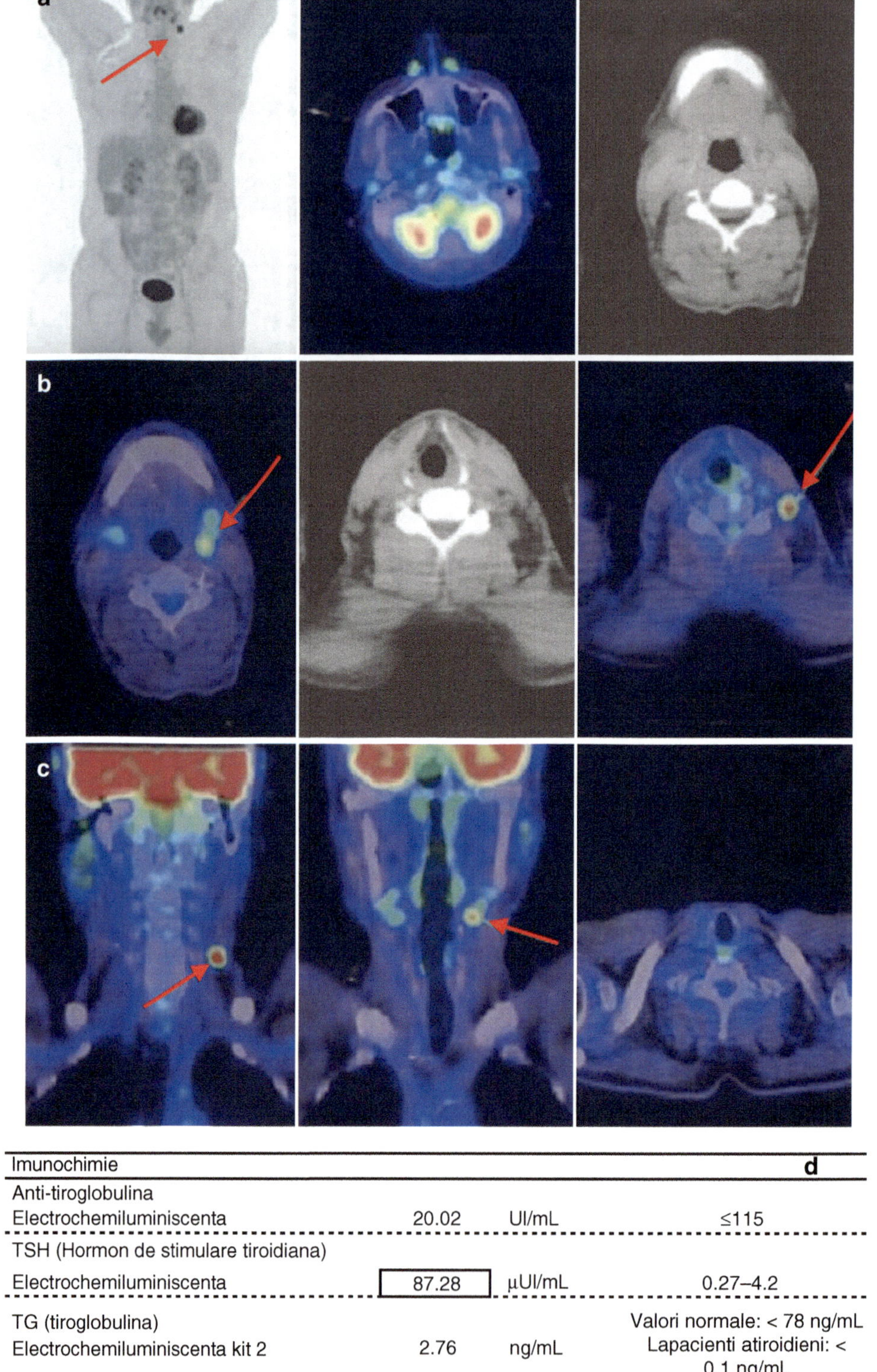

Imunochimie			
Anti-tiroglobulina Electrochemiluminiscenta	20.02	UI/mL	≤115
TSH (Hormon de stimulare tiroidiana) Electrochemiluminiscenta	87.28	µUI/mL	0.27–4.2
TG (tiroglobulina) Electrochemiluminiscenta kit 2	2.76	ng/mL	Valori normale: < 78 ng/mL Lapacienti atiroidieni: < 0.1 ng/mL

Fig. 11.18 PET/CT FDG—left cervical metastases; (**a**) MIP and transversal CT and PET/CT slices; (**b**) transversal slices MIP, CT, and PET/CT; (**c**) coronal and transversal PET/CT slices; (**d**) serum tumor markers in stimulated condition (with courtesy of Prof. Galuska László and Lajos Szabados. SCANOMED Ltd.; University of Debrecen, Dept. of Nuclear Medicine)

Key Points

- The long evolution of natural history of thyroid cancer calls for lifelong monitoring and follow-up.
- The high rate of recurrence in this pathology underlines the need for attentive evaluation of patients even after many years, especially in a high-risk group.
- An inappropriate suppression and forward substitutive therapy may accelerate the recurrence.
- The cutoff value of Tg that might have significance for recurrent disease and calls for PET/CT evaluation is set at 2 µg/L in TSH suppression condition, but the most accurate value is that of dynamic progressive increasing of Tg values.

Case 5: Papillary Thyroid Carcinoma

History:

A 63-year-old female, with the diagnosis of papillary thyroid carcinoma operated 12 years before with total thyroidectomy, was irradiated with 210 mCi (7.76 GBq) I-131, in two different doses. She was examined during the follow-up.

T4aN0M0—stage III.

Clinical examination:

The patient was under L-thyroxin 200 µg/daily, in discrete clinical hyperthyroidism; she had basal high heart rate (110/min), insomnia, and sporadic diarrhea.

The neck examination revealed a post-thyroidectomy scar, without any palpable tumor mass or lymph nodes in the cervical area. No other signs or symptoms to be mentioned.

Examinations:

The thyroid ultrasounds revealed no thyroid tissue remnant and no lymph nodes; these examinations were made twice per year and no abnormality was found.

- TSH 0.002 mIU/L (N.V. 0.4–4.5 mIU/L) during the suppressive therapy.
- TSH >100 mIU/L (N.V. 0.4–4.5 mIU/L) after 4 weeks of hormonal withdrawal.
- Tg 41.9 µg/L (N.V. < 0.1 µg/L)—increased.

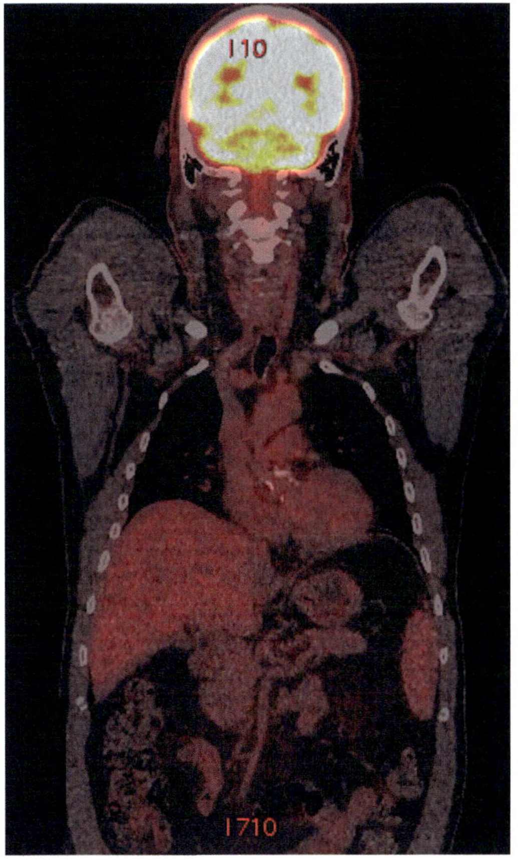

Fig. 11.19 PET/CT FDG—no pathologic FDG uptake in the entire body

- Anti-Tg 12 kIU/L (N.V. < 115 kIU/L).
- WBS I-131 was repeated as diagnosis test and after therapy was several times negative.

Findings:

The diagnosis WBS I-131 showed no pathologic uptake in the body.

The PET/CT FDG revealed no pathologic thyroid mass, no lymph nodes with pathologic uptake, and no other pathologies to be mentioned (Fig. 11.19).

The thyroid ultrasound performed 3 months later revealed a pathologic lateral-cervical lymph node, which was consistent for a metastatic lesion (Fig. 11.20).

Conclusion:

PET/CT FDG negative; the examination failed to detect the source of serum Tg pathologic level.

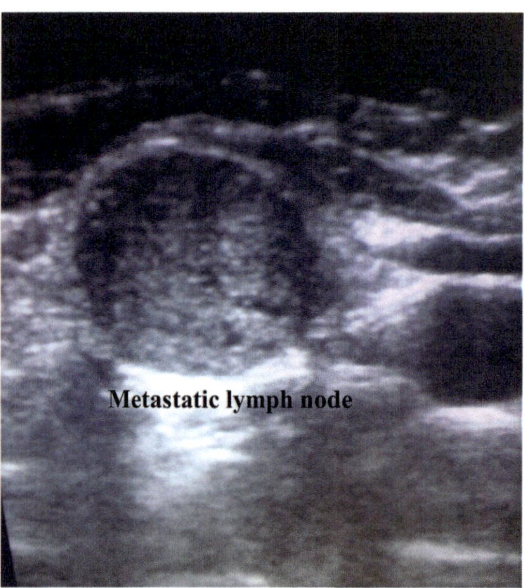

Fig. 11.20 Thyroid ultrasound. Pathologic right lateral-cervical lymph nodes

> **Key Points**
>
> - In this particular case presented, the simple thyroid ultrasound succeeds to identify the metastatic lymph nodes, which confirmed the presence of metastases at pathology after surgical removal; US is the method of choice in the follow-up of thyroid carcinoma.
> - The PET/CT FDG examination in thyroid carcinoma is not a first-line test and is reserved to special situations, which are covered in this chapter.

Case 6: Aggressive Papillary Thyroid Carcinoma

History:

A 63-year-old female with no family history of thyroid carcinoma was diagnosed with papillary thyroid carcinoma after total thyroidectomy for nodular goiter.

T3N0Mx, stage III.

Clinical examination:

The patient was evaluated at 6 weeks after surgery in the absence of thyroid hormone replacement. Mild myxedema was observed and no palpable tumor mass or cervical lymph nodes.

Examinations:

Ultrasound—no thyroid tissue and no pathologic lymph nodes.

TSH >100 mIU/L (N.V. 0.4–4.5 mIU/L) after 4 weeks of hormonal withdrawal.

Tg 0.712 μg/L (N.V. < 0.1 μg/L)—low but detectable, considered at that moment as normal.

Anti-Tg 71 kIU/L (N.V. < 115 kIU/L). A 100 mCi I-131 was administered.

After 2 years from initial surgery, the patient underwent a CT scan which revealed tumor recurrence in the cervical area. The patient underwent selective lymphadenectomy, and the lymph node metastases were confirmed.

There were four cures of I-131, total activity 303 mCi (11.2 GBq).

TSH >100 mIU/L (N.V. 0.4–4.5 mIU/L) after 4 weeks of hormonal withdrawal

Tg 14.22 μg/L (N.V. < 0.1 μg/L)—detectable and in dynamic rising.

Anti-Tg 19 kIU/L (N.V. < 115 kIU/L). A 100 mCi I-131 (3.7 GBq) was administered.

WBS I-131 negative and the patient underwent F18-FDG PET/CT scan which revealed bilateral cervical lymph nodes with very intense FDG uptake, with SUV lbm max 31.74 (Fig. 11.21).

It was indicated that selective lymphadenectomy and the histopathology show lymph node metastases and after surgery in stimulated conditions, Tg– 1.23 (N.V. <0. 04 ng/mL).

Conclusion:

We suspected an undifferentiated neoplastic component (radioiodine refractory tumor) which explains the intense FDG uptake at a low value of Tg even in unsuppressed conditions.

The medical team decided to initiate the external radiation therapy and the systemic TKI therapy.

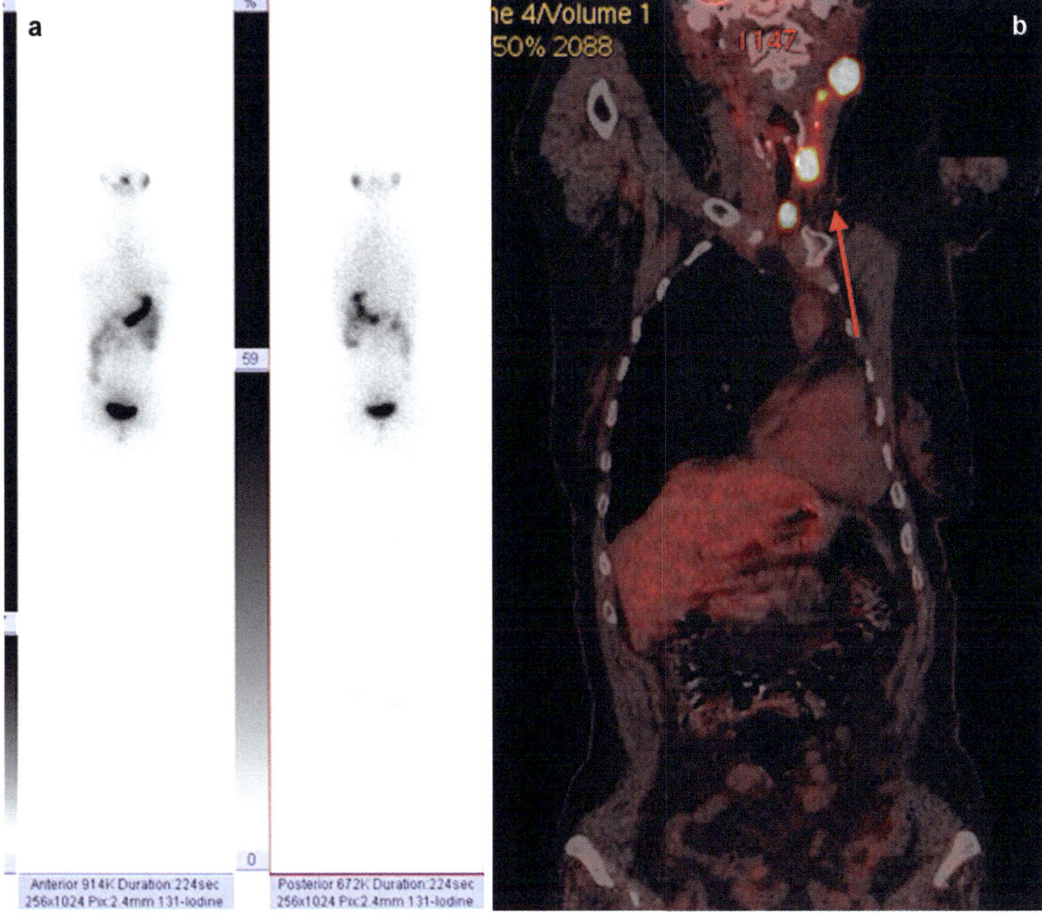

Fig. 11.21 I-131 WBS (**a**) negative, no pathologic radioiodine uptake; PET/CT FDG coronal slice (**b**), which reveals multiple lateral-cervical lymph nodes with increased FDG uptake, confirmed to be thyroid carcinoma metastases

Key Points

- In this particular case, we would like to underline the importance of a comprehensive view of this pathology; the most important relation would be not only with the levels of Tg or anti-Tg but firstly with the details of the histology.
- There is no recommended cutoff value for Tg, as we demonstrated in this case, there might be distant metastases even at levels of <2 μg/L of unsuppressed Tg.
- The PET/CT FDG examination in thyroid carcinoma is a marker of the aggressiveness of the tumor.

Case 7: Papillary Thyroid Carcinoma

History:

A 70-year-old male with the diagnosis of papillary thyroid cancer and lymph node metastases with total thyroidectomy and selective lymphadenectomy.

T3N1b (2/7 +) Mx—stage IV A.

Clinical examination:

The patient was evaluated after total thyroidectomy; in the absence of the thyroid hormone replacement, moderate signs of myxedema were observed. Post-thyroidectomy scar was identified in the anterior cervical area.

Examinations:

Cervical ultrasonography revealed no tumor mass or lymph nodes in the area.

The initial blood test TSH stimulation:

Anti-Tg 16 kIU/L (N.V. <115 kIU/L)—normal.
TSH 48.71 mIU/L (N.V. 0.4–4.5 mIU/L)—increased.
Tg 9.84 μg/L (N.V. < 0.04 μg/L)—increased.

The patient underwent a 70 mCi (2.5GBq) I-131 dose ablation for the remnant tissue.

After 6 months he came for the oncological control in unsuppressed TSH. The level of Tg increased at 27.32 μg/L with US signs of lymph node involvement; the medical team decided to perform the selective lymphadenectomy.

Despite the two surgeries, and repetitive radioiodine therapy reaching a total dose of 399.15 mCi (14.8 GBq) in four fractions, the Tg level continued to increase with negative WBS I-131.

The patient was referred for the F18-FDG PET/CT scan.

Blood test before PET/CT scan:

Anti-Tg 10 kIU/L (N.V. <115 kIU/L)—normal.
TSH 19.9 mIU/L (N.V. 0.4–4.5 mIU/L)—increased.
Tg 322.7 μg/L (N.V. < 0.04 μg/L)—increased.

F18-FDG PET/CT revealed persistent disease in the right lobe thyroid area with mediastinum lymph node involvement (Fig. 11.22).

After the PET/CT, the patient was referred for the TKI (tyrosine kinase inhibitor) treatment.

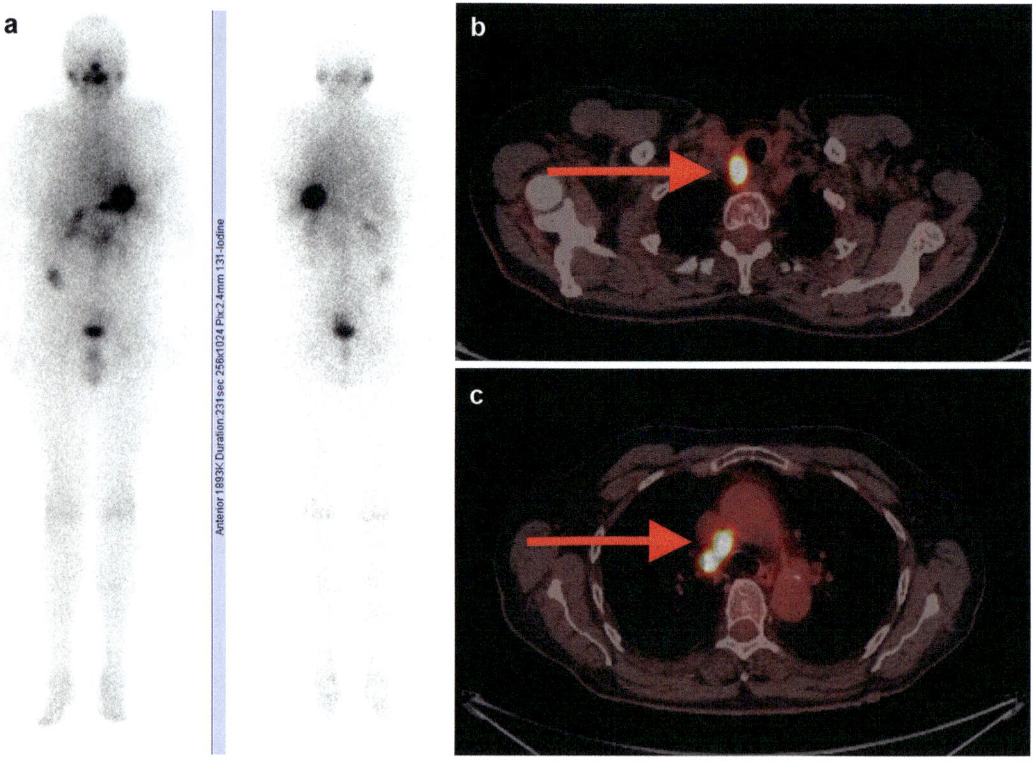

Fig. 11.22 I-131 WBS (**a**) negative, no pathologic radioiodine uptake; PET/CT FDG transversal slice cervical level (**b**), which reveals right paratracheal tumor with increased FDG uptake; transversal slice mediastinum level (**c**), which reveals lymph nodes with increased FDG uptake in thyroid carcinoma metastases

Key Points:

- Despite the predominant papillary thyroid cancer histology, there were some areas of solid and trabecular type with high aggressiveness.
- The dynamic velocity of Tg was more important than the absolute value.
- The multiple foci metastases identified by PET/CT scan with high SUV lbm Max values indicated a very aggressive disease stage with no response to the radioiodine therapy; dedifferentiation of the thyroid cancer might be the explanation of this situation.
- The indication for tyrosine kinase inhibitors was established according to the PET/CT result, the increasing thyroglobulin levels, and the lack of response to the radioiodine therapy.

Case 8: Follicular Thyroid Carcinoma

History:

A 78-year-old female diagnosed in 2013 with follicular thyroid cancer, trabecular variant, operated by total thyroidectomy was referred for radioiodine therapy.

T4N1M1—stage IV C.

Clinical examination:

The examination took place at 6 weeks postsurgery.

The neck examination revealed the post-thyroidectomy scar and no palpable tumor mass or cervical lymph nodes.

Examination:

Ultrasound—no thyroid tissue remnant, no pathologic lymph nodes.

Anti-Tg 61 kIU/L (N.V. <115 kIU/L)—normal.
TSH >100 mIU/L (N.V. 0.4–4.5 mIU/L)—very increased.
Tg 7137 µg/L (N.V. < 0.04 µg/L)—very increased.

The high level of thyroglobulin level indicates that there are distant metastases. In order to perform the radioiodine evaluation and to exclude cerebral lesions, the patient underwent a native cerebral CT scan with negative result for cerebral lesions.

Findings:

Postoperative radioiodine scan was performed with 138.85 mCi (5.1 GBq) in order to evaluate the patient.

I-131 WBS revealed lung metastases.

The patient underwent a total I-131 dose of 505.9 mCi (18.6 GBq) in six fractions with curative intention, but despite this, the patient had persistent biochemical disease and the WBS I-131 turned negative (Fig. 11.23).

Blood tests before PET/CT scan:

Anti-Tg 30 kIU/L (N.V. <115 kIU/L)—normal.
TSH 82.06 mIU/L (N.V. 0.4–4.5 mIU/L)—very increased.
Tg 3836 µg/L (N.V. < 0.04 µg/L)—very increased.

At this moment, the patient was referred for the F18-FDG PET/CT evaluation which identified right cervical lymph node metastases, multiple lung metastases, and left hilar lymphadenopathy (Fig. 11.24).

Key Points:

It is well known that follicular thyroid cancer spreads via hematological pathway to the lungs, liver, and bones.

A very high level of postoperative thyroglobulin with no thyroid tissue identified by ultrasound in the cervical area indicates an advanced stage of the disease with distant metastases.

The PET/CT result correlates with the high thyroglobulin level in this patient and increased SUV lbm Max values.

Despite the intense uptake on FDG PET/CT scan, the medical team decided to continue the radioiodine therapy, and the patient was not referred to other therapies, due to the patient's age and the risk of worsening the QoL (quality of life); Tg continues to decrease and the metastases stable.

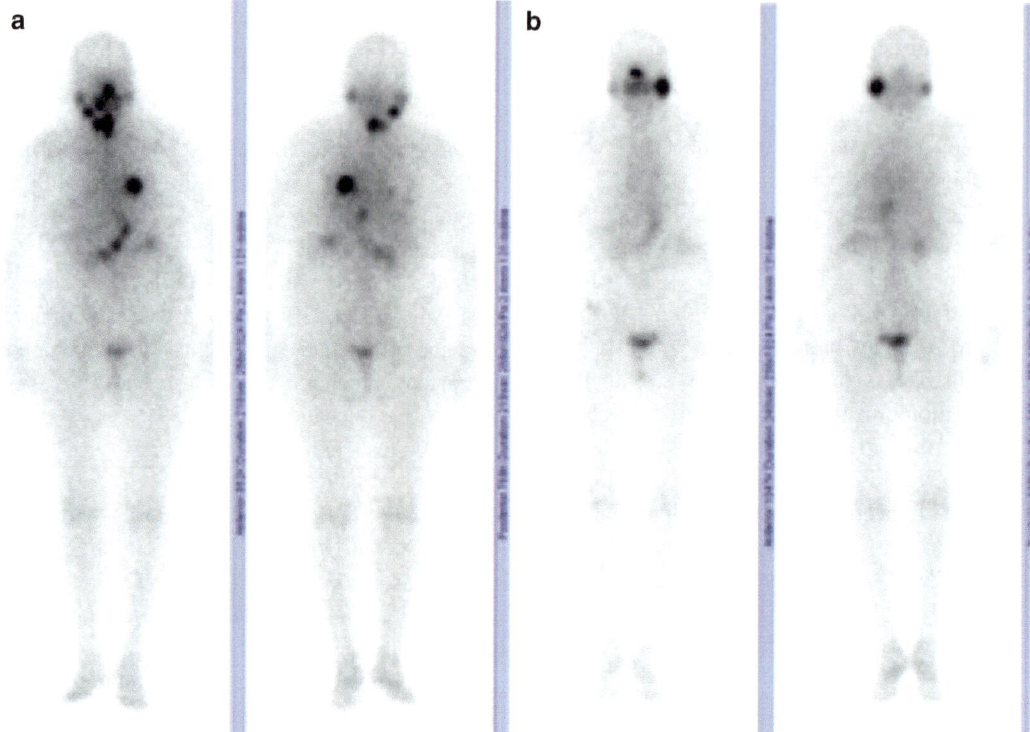

Fig. 11.23 I-131 WBS-positive posttherapy revealed multiple pathologic I-131 uptake foci, in cervical area and lung metastases (**a**); WBS negative, no pathologic radioiodine uptake (**b**)

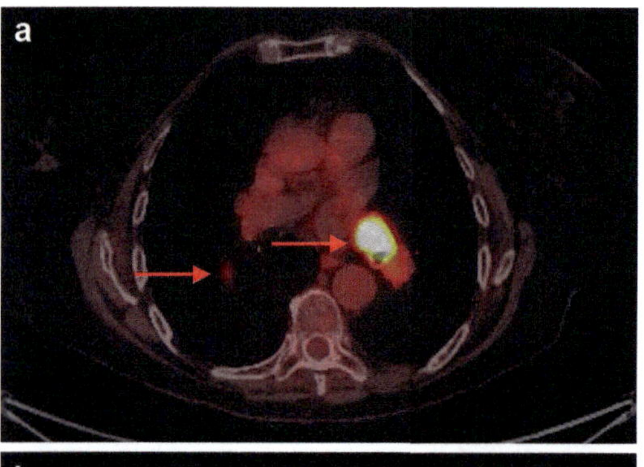

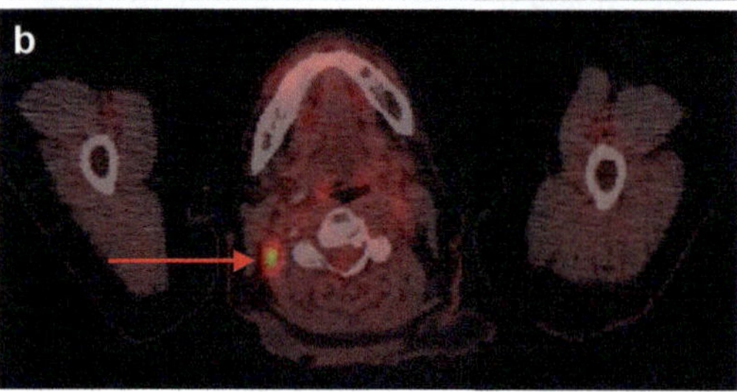

Fig. 11.24 PET/CT FDG transversal slice cervical level (**a**), which reveals right lateral-cervical lymph node with increased FDG uptake; transversal slice thorax level (**b**), which reveals lymph nodes with increased FDG uptake in the left mediastinum and lung thyroid carcinoma metastases

Case 9: Highly Aggressive Hurthle Cell Follicular Thyroid Carcinoma

History:

A 51-year-old male was referred with the diagnosis of thyroid tumor mass with disseminated bone metastases.

Clinical examination:

The anterior cervical area was modified by a left thyroid tumor with multiple bilateral lymph nodes.

Examinations:

Ultrasound identifies no nodules in the right lobe and large tumor mass on the left thyroid lobe about 60/49 mm with intra- and peri-nodular Doppler signal, intranodular calcifications, and bilateral lymph nodes.

The patient was operated with total thyroidectomy with the histopathological result of Hurthle cell follicular thyroid carcinoma T3NxMx—stage III.

Postsurgical blood test evaluation after 3 weeks of stimulated conditions:

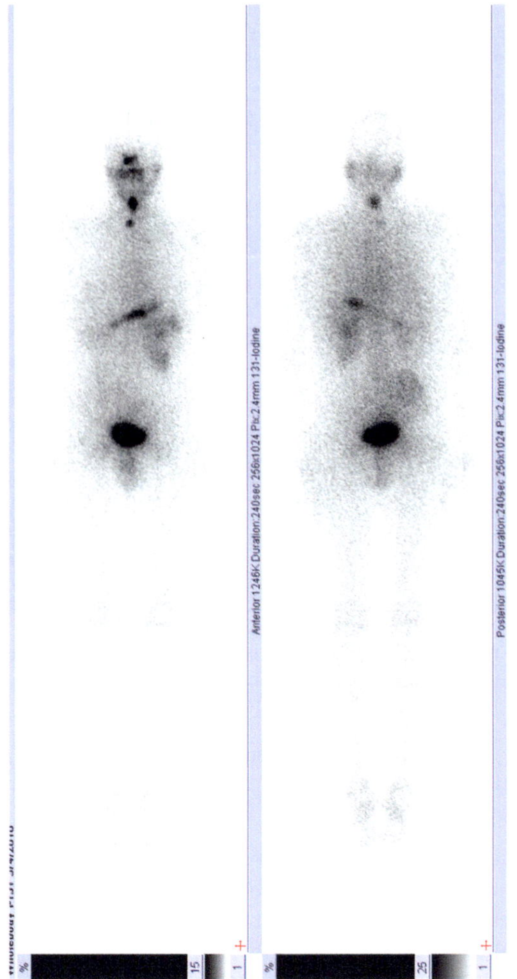

Fig. 11.25 I-131 WBS-positive posttherapy revealed pathologic I-131 uptake in the cervical area and no other radioiodine uptake, discordant with the high level of Tg

Anti-Tg 252 kIU/L (N.V. <115 kIU/L)—increased.
TSH 74.81 mIU/L (N.V. 0.4–4.5 mIU/L)—very increased.
Tg 32,727 μg/L (N.V. < 0.04 μg/L)—very increased suggesting distant metastases.

He received 150 mCi (5.5 GBq) I-131 in order to evaluate distant lesions.

Findings:

WBS post-therapeutic minimal uptake in the thyroid bed, discordant with the very high level of thyroglobulin (Fig. 11.25).

The patient was sent to perform F18-FDG PET/CT scan, and the result was multiple disseminated bone lesions with D8-D9 medullar compression syndrome; the SUV lbm Max of 27.05 indicates very aggressive disease (Fig. 11.26).

A similar case of Hurthle cell follicular thyroid carcinoma, with very aggressive and rapid evolution, with discrepancy between the relatively not very high value of Tg and the dramatic image on F18-FDG PET/CT, is presented in Fig. 11.27.

Case 10: Follicular Thyroid Carcinoma

History:

A 59-year-old female diagnosed in July 2015 with oncocytic type of follicular thyroid carcinoma with solid and trabecular pattern was referred for evaluation and radioiodine therapy.

T3NxMx—stage III.

Clinical examination:

The patient was evaluated after total thyroidectomy on stimulated TSH conditions.

Post-thyroidectomy scar was identified in the anterior cervical area, no other findings to be mentioned.

Examinations:

The initial blood test after 2 weeks of thyroid hormone withdrawal:

Anti-Tg 15 kIU/L (N.V. <115 kIU/L)—normal.
TSH 59.74 mIU/L (N.V. 0.4–4.5 mIU/L).
Tg 8.84 μg/L (N.V. < 0.04 μg/L)—increased.

The patient received 96.3 mCi (3.55 GBq) of radioactive iodine.

Findings:

After the second radioiodine dose, the WBS scan turned negative, and the patient was sent for PET/CT examination because of the persistent biochemical disease.

Before PET/CT blood test results:

Anti-Tg <10 kIU/L (N.V. <115 kIU/L)—normal.
TSH 27.35 mIU/L (N.V. 0.4–4.5 mIU/L).
Tg 7.23 μg/L (N.V. < 0.04 μg/L)—increased.

F18-FDG PET/CT findings: multiple lung metastases disseminated with intense uptake with

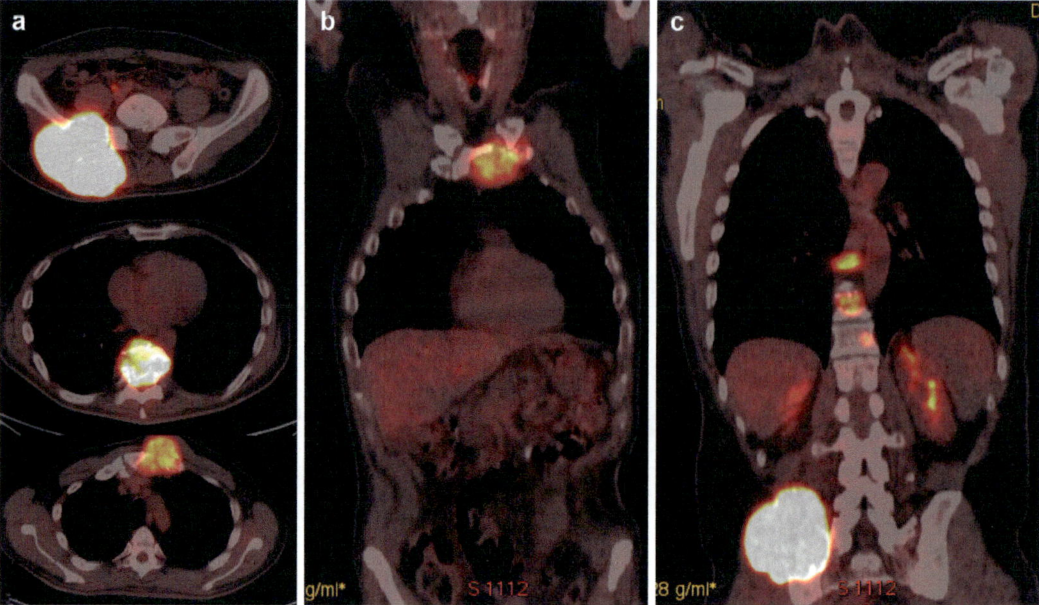

Fig. 11.26 PET/CT FDG transversal slices at the pelvic and thorax levels (**a**), which revealed large metastases in the pelvic bones, spine, and sternum with very increased FDG uptake; coronal slice at the thorax level (**b** and **c**)

SUV lbm Max of 5.3. Despite the low level of persistent blood thyroglobulin level which does not necessary traduce metastases, the PET/CT result identified a progressive disease (Fig. 11.28).

Case 11: Folliculo-Papillary Thyroid Carcinoma with NRAS Gene Mutation

History:

A 45-year-old female diagnosed with folliculo-papillary thyroid carcinoma operated by total thyroidectomy was referred for evaluation and radioiodine therapy.

T3N1bMx—stage IV A.

Clinical examination:

The patient was evaluated after total thyroidectomy and 3 weeks of thyroid hormone withdrawal. Post-thyroidectomy scar was identified in the anterior cervical area, no palpable lymph nodes.

Examinations:

No evidence of lateral-cervical lymph nodes and no tumor mass in the anterior cervical.

Anti-Tg 13 kIU/L (N.V. <115 kIU/L)—normal.
TSH > 100 mIU (N.V. 0.4–4.5 mIU/L)—very increased.
Tg 765.6 μg/L (N.V. < 0.04 μg/L)—very increased.

The patient underwent a 120 mCi (4.4 GBq) I-131 dose ablation.

Findings:

WBS posttherapy was slightly positive in the neck area, and after two doses of radioiodine therapy, the WBS turned negative, but the Tg blood level remains very increased. The patient was referred for the F18-FDG PET/CT examination in March 2014 which showed a unique lesion on vertebral C2 with SUV lbm Max of 2.48. The medical team indicated a neurosurgical consult in order to perform the lesion ablation. The MRI failed to localize the lesion and the surgery was canceled.

She came back for the oncological control, and the blood test after 2 weeks of thyroid hormone withdrawal showed biochemical progressive disease:

Anti-Tg 10 kIU/L (N.V. <115 kIU/L)—normal.
TSH 23.38 mIU (N.V. 0.4–4.5 mIU/L)—very increased.
Tg 496 μg/L (N.V. < 0.04 μg/L)—very increased.

The patient performed another PET/CT scan in February 2015 which showed progressive disease with multiple disseminated bone

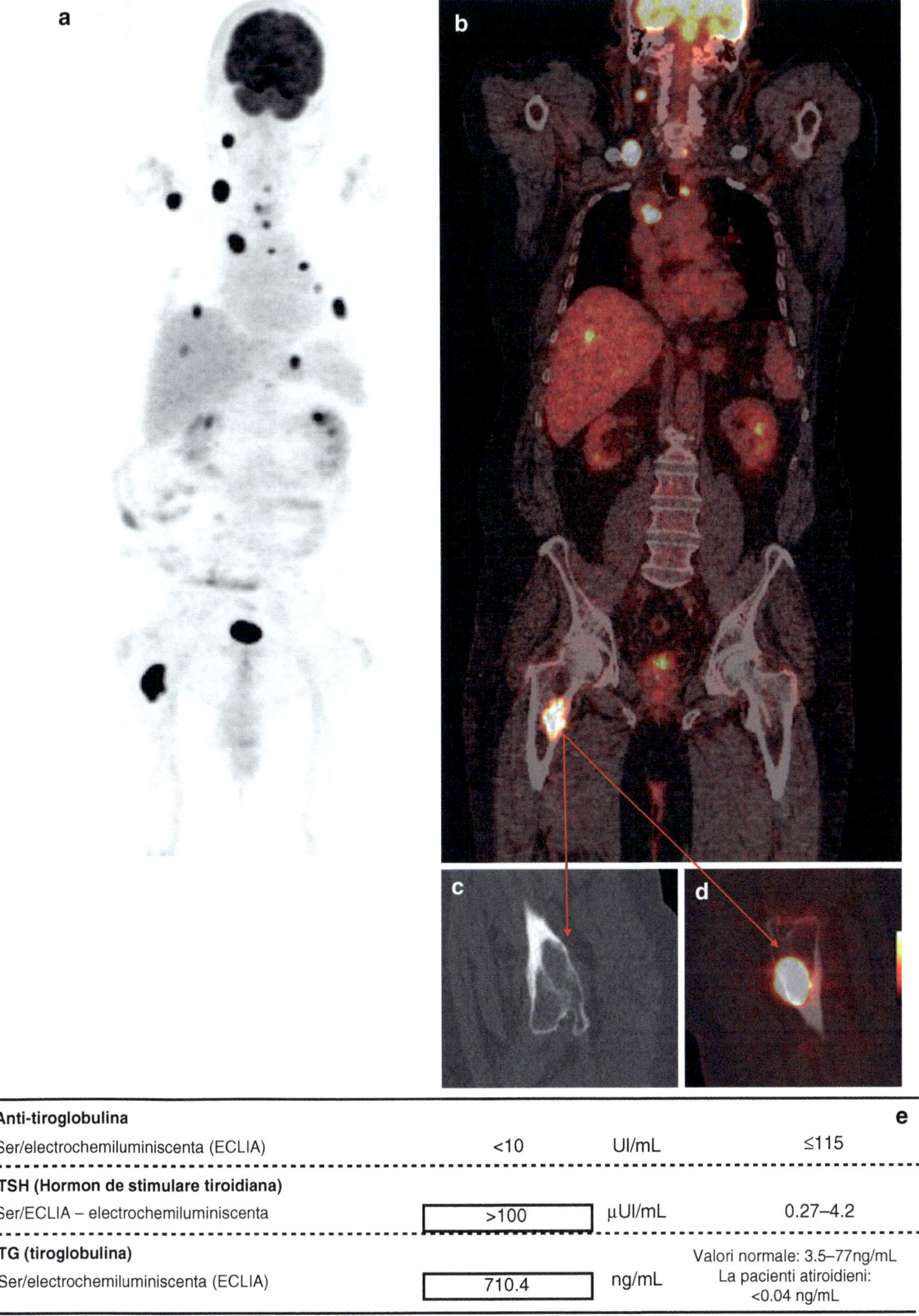

Anti-tiroglobulina			
Ser/electrochemiluminiscenta (ECLIA)	<10	UI/mL	≤115
TSH (Hormon de stimulare tiroidiana)			
Ser/ECLIA – electrochemiluminiscenta	>100	μUI/mL	0.27–4.2
TG (tiroglobulina)			Valori normale: 3.5–77ng/mL
Ser/electrochemiluminiscenta (ECLIA)	710.4	ng/mL	La pacienti atiroidieni: <0.04 ng/mL

Fig. 11.27 PET/CT FDG coronal slices MIP (**a**), PET/CT (**b**), femoral CT (**c**), PET/CT (**d**), and serologic results (**e**) which revealed large metastases in cervical lymph nodes, lungs, liver, and bones with very increased FDG uptake

metastases and compressive lesion in C2 vertebra, with loss of function and numbness in the arms. In March 2015, she was operated in the neurosurgery department in order to reduce the medullar compression syndrome (Fig. 11.29).

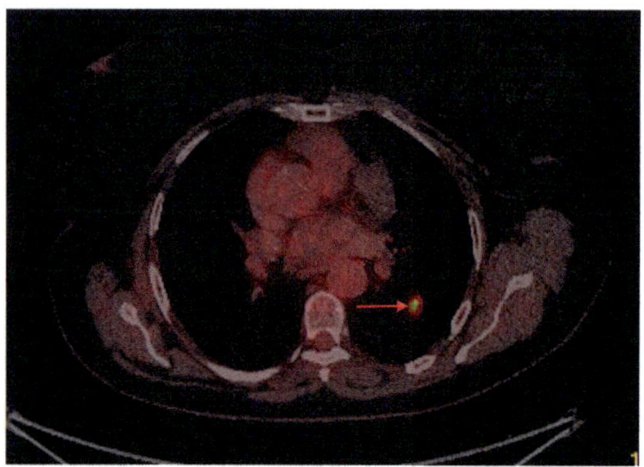

Fig. 11.28 PET/CT FDG thorax transversal slice which reveals left lung metastases with increased FDG uptake

The patient is currently under systemic treatment, having performed also the genetic test. She was investigated on TruSight tumor 15 panel (AKT1, BRAF, EGFR, ERBB2, FOXL2, GNA11, GNAQ, KIT, KRAS, MET, NRAS, PDGFRA, PIK3K, RET, TP53), and the results were consistent for the following gene mutation: NRAS missense, p.Lys117Asn; c.351G > T; and transcript ENST00000369535; all other genes were normal. Few studies have examined the role of *NRAS* mutation as a prognostic factor in PTC, but the results showed that these cases were associated significantly with the presence of a distant metastasis.

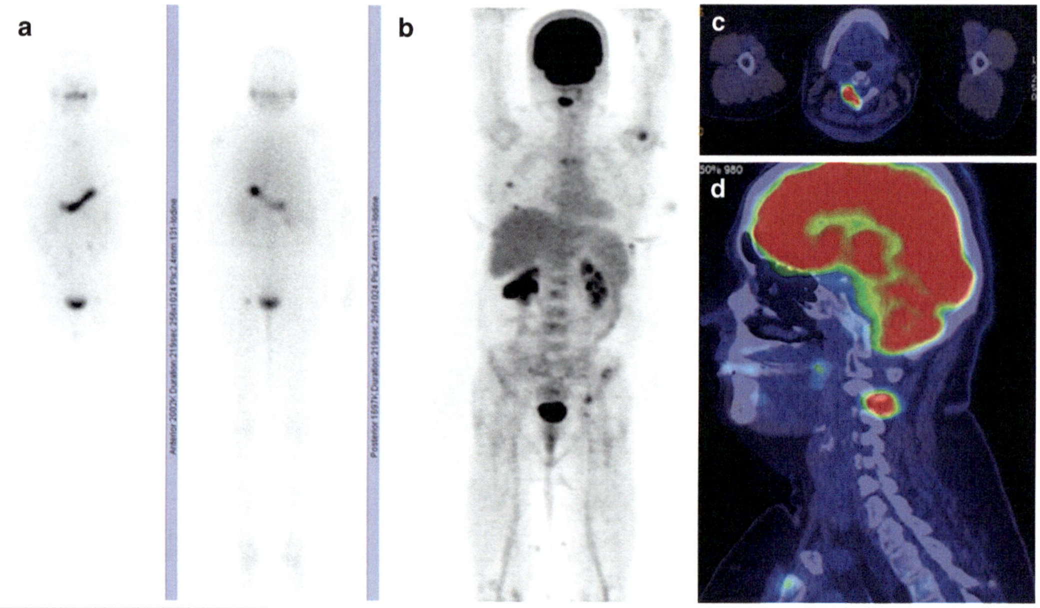

e

Anti-tiroglobulina			
Ser/electrochemiluminiscenta (ECLIA)	10	UI/mL	≤115
TSH (Hormon de stimulare tiroidiana)			
Ser/ECLIA – electrochemiluminiscenta	23.38	μUI/mL	0.27–4.2
TG (tiroglobulina)			
Ser/electrochemiluminiscenta (ECLIA)	496	ng/mL	Valori normale: 3.5–77ng/mL Lapacienti atiroidieni: <0.04 ng/mL

Fig. 11.29 WBS I-131 showing just a slight uptake in the left ischium bone (**a**); F18-FDG PET/CT showing multiple pathologic uptake in the spine, lung, pelvis, and left humeral bone (**b**); transversal slice (**c**) and sagittal slice (**d**) PET/CT which reveals cervical C2 metastasis with increased FDG uptake; blood test results (**e**) showing the high level of Tg

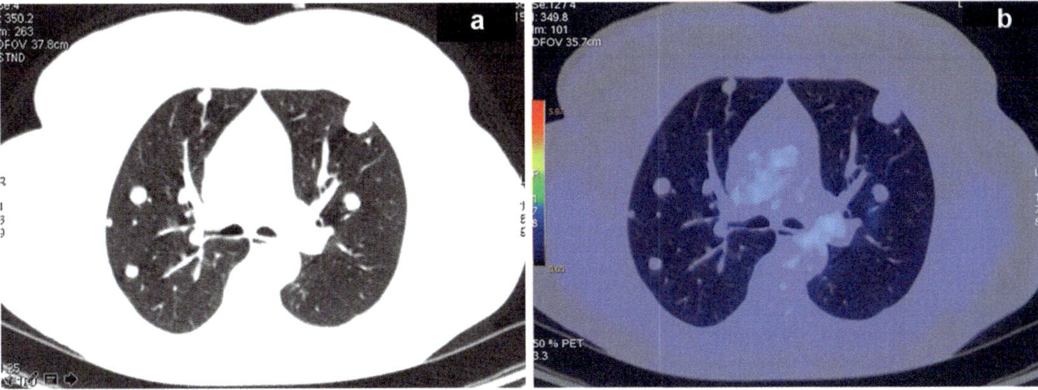

Fig. 11.30 PET/CT FDG thorax transversal slices ((**a**) CT; (**b**) PET/CT) which reveal multiple lung metastases without FDG uptake, suggesting a complete remission of the disease, after radioiodine therapy

Case 12: Follicular Thyroid Carcinoma and Lung Metastases Complete Remission on PET/CT

History:

A 44-year-old female with follicular thyroid carcinoma operated by total thyroidectomy and selective lymphadenectomy and with radioiodine therapy, with multiple lung metastases detected on thorax CT, was referred for F18-FDG PET/CT scan.

T3N1bM1—stage II.

Clinical examination:

The neck examination revealed the post-thyroidectomy scar and no palpable tumor mass or cervical lymph nodes. She was associated with type II diabetes and heart disease.

Examinations:

The initial postsurgical evaluation after 3 weeks of hormonal withdrawal showed:

Anti Tg-121 kIU/L (N.V. <115 kIU/L)—increased.
TSH >100 mIU/L (N.V. 0.4–4.5 mIU/L)—very increased.
Tg 1303 μg/L (N.V. < 0.04 μg/L)—very increased.

She received a 108.85 mCi (3.9 GBq) I-131.

Findings:

She received a total activity of I-131305.8 mCi in four fractions.

The last oncological control showed persistent biochemical disease with negative WBS.

Anti-Tg 17 kIU/L (N.V. <115 kIU/L)—normal.
TSH >100 mIU/L (N.V. 0.4–4.5 mIU/L)—very increased.
Tg < 0.04 (N.V. < 0.04 μg/L)—undetectable.

The patient was referred for PET/CT scan which showed multiple lung metastases without uptake of FDG, and the patient was declared in complete remission (Fig. 11.30).

11.8 PET/CT in Adrenal Pathology

The adrenal imaging comprises patients with:

- Adrenal tumors incidentally detected by imaging (CT, MRI) performed for other reasons than adrenal disease. PET/CT with F18-FDG is useful for establishing the extent of the disease, to differ benign from malignant incidentalomas, and can be helpful in the imaging of pheochromocytoma and adrenocortical cancer.
- Known adrenal tumors that must be characterized and selected for a specific treatment; scintigraphy with I-123/I-131 MIBG remains the mainstay for molecular imaging of pheochromocytoma and is mandatory in patients for whom I-131 MIBG therapy is considered. In the diagnostic and follow-up of pheochromocytoma and neuroblastoma patients, as these NETs can show high expression of somatostatin receptors (SSR), radiolabeled octreotide is less sensitive than I-123/I-131 MIBG, suggesting that SSR scintigraphy

should be the first choice for use in negative MIBG cases.
- Adrenalitis.

The tracers used in this pathology are in the majority introduced recently and large cohort of patients not yet available.

- C11-metomidate PET/CT can differentiate adrenocortical from nonadrenocortical tumors.
- A PET tracer for the imaging of pheochromocytoma is the norepinephrine analogue C11-hydroxyephedrine, used mainly in the diagnosis of recurrent malignant disease.
- Other specialized PET tracers for the imaging of pheochromocytoma are F18-fluorodihydroxyphenylalanine (F18-DOPA) and F18-fluorodopamine.
- The octreotide derivative 4,7,10-tetraazacyclododecane-*N,N′,N′′,N′′′*-tetraacetic-acid-d-Phe1-Tyr3-octreotide (DOTATOC) has recently been labeled with gallium-68, which has led to a dramatic improvement in sensitivity and specificity for imaging NETs, using PET/CT. Thus, this technique has proven to be superior to In-111-octreotide, both planar scintigraphy and SPECT imaging in NET, and also to I-123 MIBG.

Kroiss et al. (2011) revealed in their study that Ga-68 DOTATOC PET may be superior to I-123 MIBG gamma-scintigraphy and even to the reference CT/MRI technique in providing particularly valuable information for pretherapeutic staging of pheochromocytoma and neuroblastoma.

- F18-DOPA PET is a useful tool in the detection and staging of NET lesions. Compared to Ga-68 DOTATOC, the initial results allow the conclusion that Ga-68 DOTATOC PET may have a stronger clinical impact in NET patients, as it does not only offer diagnostic information but is decisive for the further treatment management, i. e., PRRT, as well (Putzer 2010).
- Ga-68 DOTATATE and F18-FDG have similar results in detecting lesions in pheochromocytoma and paraganglioma (96.2% vs 91.4%); I-123/I-124 MIBG detected fewer lesions (30.4%). Overall, Ga-68 DOTATATE PET/CT detected similar number but has significantly greater lesion-to-background contrast compared to F18-FDG PET/CT. Depending on DOTATATE findings and the clinical question, FDG and MIBG remain useful and, in selected cases, may provide more accurate staging and disease characterization and guide treatment choices (Chang 2016).

Due to its lack of availability, Ga-68 DOTATOC is not considering, at least for the moment, the imaging of choice in known adrenal tumors; moreover, in case of the possibility of selective I-131 MIBG therapy, the usefulness of this one should be confirmed on positive imaging.

F18-FDG remains a marker of aggressiveness and should be used whenever the course of the disease imposes it.

The next clinical cases will target the following situations:

1. Adrenal adenomas incidentally discovered during F18-FDG PET/CT examination for other pathologies
2. Adrenal metastases discovered during F18-FDG PET/CT examination for other primary cancers
3. Adrenal malignant primary tumor
4. Adrenalitis postchemotherapy in malignant melanoma

Case 1: Adrenal Adenoma Incidentally Discovered During F18-FDG PET/CT Examination for Other Pathology

History:

A 51-year-old male, with the diagnosis of non-small cell lung adenocarcinoma operated 1 year before with left upper lung lobectomy, was irradiated and undergone chemotherapy. He was examined in the follow-up.

Clinical examination:

The patient had no signs of respiratory dysfunction.

The thorax examination revealed a postsurgery scar, without any palpable tumor mass or lymph nodes in the cervical and axillary area. No other signs or symptoms to be mentioned.

Examinations:

Chest CT—except the surgery—nothing to be mentioned.

Abdominal CT—tumor mass in the left adrenal gland, raising the suspicion of adrenal metastases.

Findings:

The PET/CT FDG revealed no pathologic adrenal uptake and normal activity in an adrenal mass of21/19 mm, suggestive for adrenal adenoma, not for malignant metastases from lung cancer.

The patient was reevaluated, and the diagnosis of complete remission was established (Fig. 11.31).

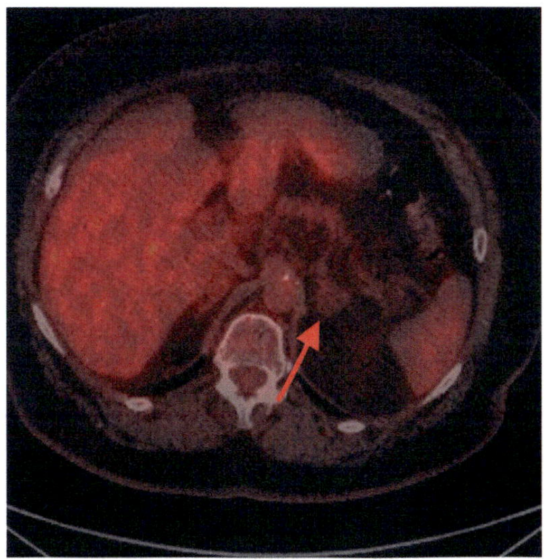

Fig. 11.31 PET/CT F18-FDG transversal slice of fused image, showing a left adrenal tumor mass, without pathologic uptake of FDG, in a patient with lung cancer, suggestive for left adrenal adenoma

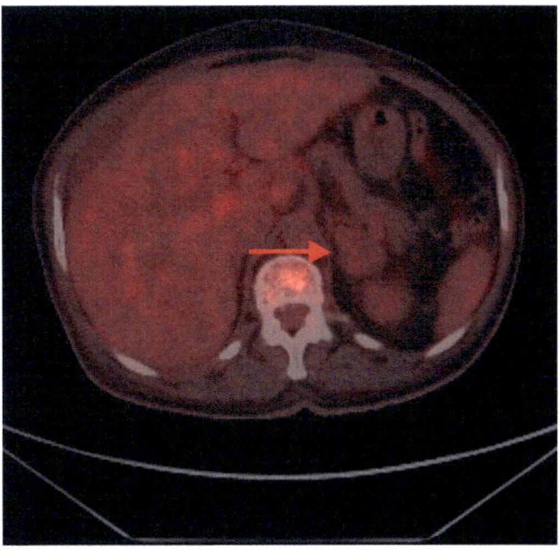

Fig. 11.32 PET/CT F18-FDG transversal slice of fused image, showing a left adrenal tumor mass, without pathologic uptake of FDG, in a patient with breast cancer, suggestive for left adrenal adenoma

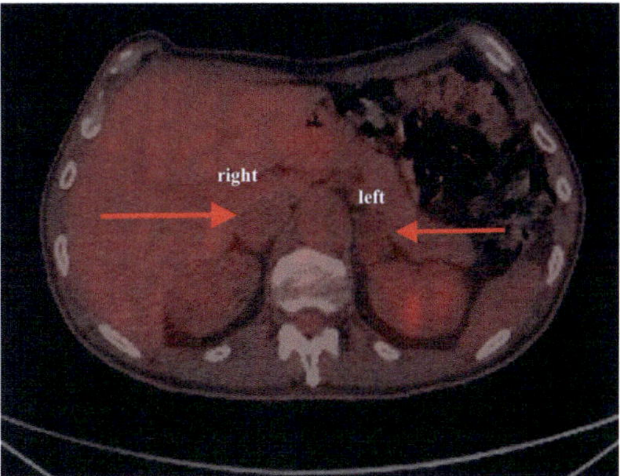

Fig. 11.33 PET/CT F18-FDG transversal slice of fused image, showing bilateral adrenal tumor masses, without pathologic uptake of FDG, in a patient with lung cancer, suggestive for bilateral adrenal adenomas

Conclusion:

The diagnosis was left adrenal adenoma, in a patient with lung cancer.

Similar clinical cases are presented in Figs. 11.32 and 11.33.

Key Points

- The PET/CT FDG examination is essential in the workup of lung nodule and lung cancer, being highly sensitive in this pathology.
- During its evolution, lung cancer frequently develops metastases in the adrenal glands; the differential diagnosis among the benign and malignant adrenal masses made by FDG PET/CT is able to change dramatically the treatment protocols.

Case 2: Adrenal Metastasis Discovered During F18-FDG PET/CT Examination for Other Primary Cancers

History:

A 67-year-old male, with the diagnosis of non-small cell lung adenocarcinoma operated 5 months before and with chemotherapy. He was examined in the follow-up.

Clinical examination:

The patient had no signs of respiratory dysfunction. The thorax examination revealed a postsurgery scar, without any palpable tumor mass or lymph nodes in the cervical and axillary area. Important weight loss of 7 kg/2 months, sweating, and tachycardia.

Examinations:

Thorax CT—tumor mass in upper left lung, enlarged multiple lymph nodes in the mediastinum; bilateral pleurisy.

Abdominal CT—tumor mass in the right adrenal gland, raising the suspicion of adrenal metastasis.

Findings:

The PET/CT F18-FDG revealed increased pathologic right adrenal uptake, suggestive for adrenal metastasis from lung cancer; intense, highly increased uptake of F18-FDG in a tumor mass of the left lung and in multiple lymph nodes of the mediastinum; bilateral pleurisy, left rib metastasis.

The patient was reevaluated, and the stage of the disease was upgraded (Fig. 11.34).

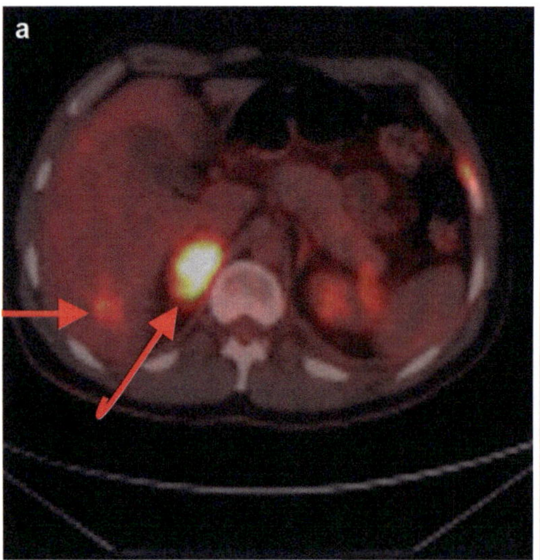

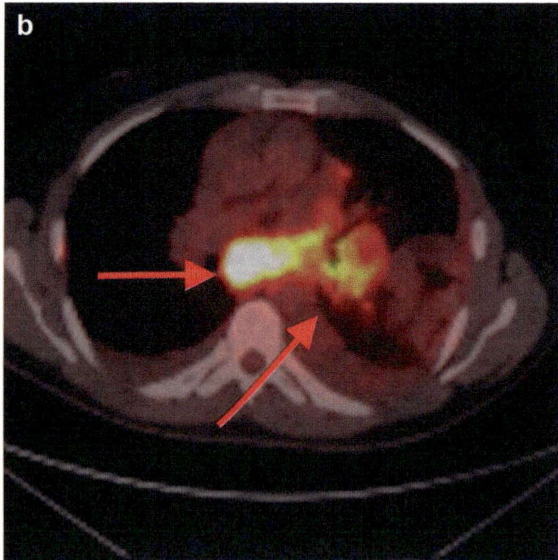

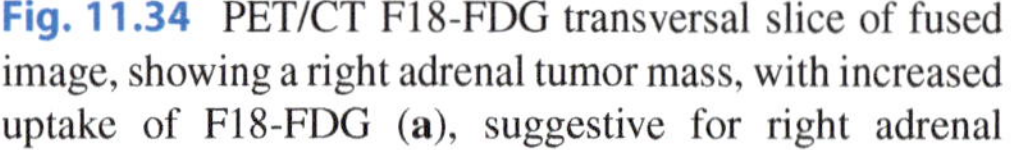

Fig. 11.34 PET/CT F18-FDG transversal slice of fused image, showing a right adrenal tumor mass, with increased uptake of F18-FDG (**a**), suggestive for right adrenal metastasis, in a patient with left lung cancer and left rib, mediastinum lymph nodes and liver metastases (**b**)

Conclusion:

The diagnosis was right adrenal metastasis, in a patient with lung cancer.

Key Points

- PET/CT F18-FDG examination is essential in the workup for lung nodule and lung cancer, being highly sensitive in this pathology.
- In more than 30% of cases with lung cancer, the strategy is changed after F18-FDG PET/CT.

Case 3: Adrenal Metastasis Discovered During F18-FDG PET/CT Examination for Other Primary Cancers

History:

A 51-year-old male, with the diagnosis of colon adenocarcinoma, newly diagnosed. He was examined in the initial staging.

Clinical examination:

The patient had mild abdominal pain, diarrhea, and palpable lymph nodes in the left axilla. Important weight loss of 5 kg/2 months.

Examinations:

Thorax CT—tumor mass in upper right lung, enlarged multiple lymph nodes in the left axilla;

Abdominal CT—tumor of the descending colon and tumor mass in the right adrenal gland, raising the suspicion of adrenal metastasis.

Findings:

The PET/CT F18-FDG revealed increased pathologic right adrenal uptake, suggestive for adrenal metastasis from colon cancer; intense, highly increased uptake of F18-FDG in a right lung metastasis and in multiple lymph nodes of the left axilla.

The patient was reevaluated, and the stage of the disease was upgraded (Fig. 11.35).

Conclusion:

The diagnosis was right adrenal metastasis, in a patient with colon cancer.

Similar case is presented in Fig. 11.36.

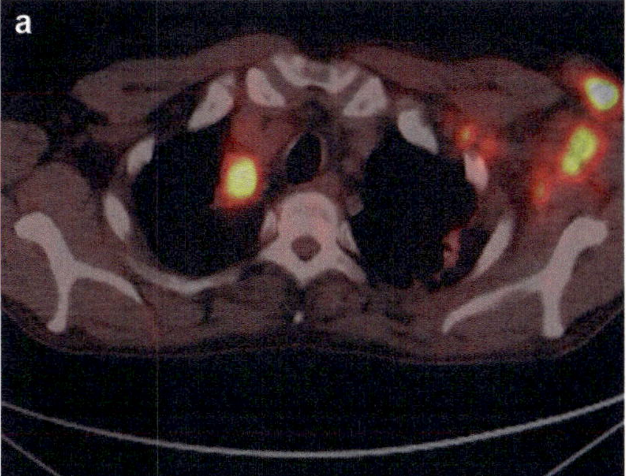

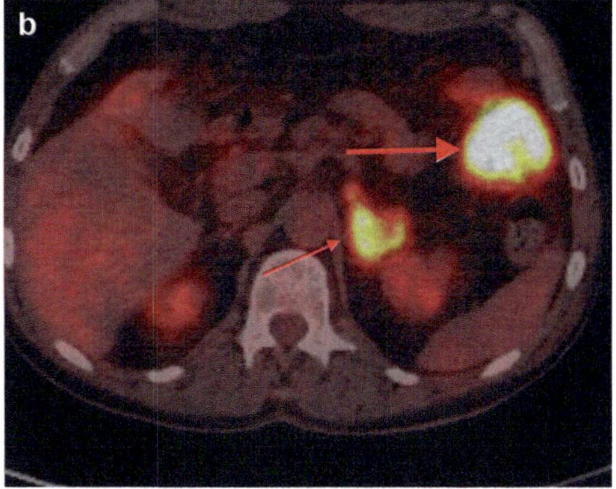

Fig. 11.35 PET/CT F18-FDG transversal slice of fused image, showing a left adrenal tumor mass, in a patient with colon cancer and right lung and left axillary lymph node metastases (**a**), with increased uptake of F18-FDG (**b**) in the left adrenal gland, suggestive for left adrenal metastasis

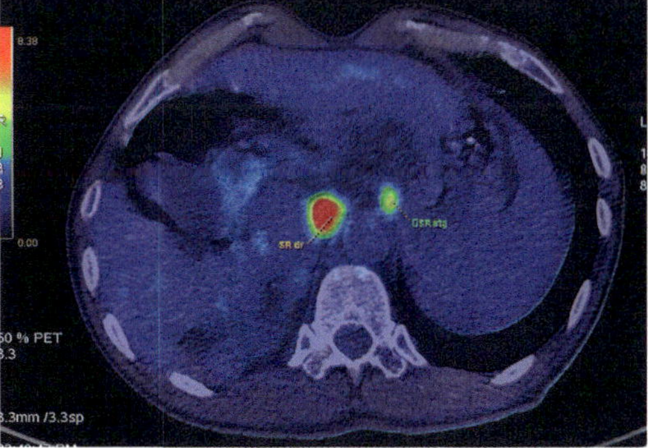

Fig. 11.36 PET/CT F18-FDG transversal slice of fused image, showing bilateral adrenal tumor masses, in a patient with non-Hodgkin lymphoma with increased uptake of F18-FDG in both glands

Key Points

- The PET/CT FDG examination is essential in the restaging of colon cancer, rarely being necessary ab initio.
- The key indication of PET/CT is the rising of tumor markers, with negative conventional structural imaging.
- The metastases in the adrenal glands from colon cancer are exceptionally rare but can occur, and we should be aware on this possibility.

Case 4: Adrenal Primary Malignant Tumor on F18-FDG PET/CT Examination

History:

A 47-year-old female, with the diagnosis of left adrenal carcinoma operated 2 years before. She was examined during the follow-up.

Clinical examination:

The patient had mild abdominal pain; weight loss of 8 kg/2 months, fatigue, and nausea.

Examinations:

Thorax CT—nothing to be mentioned..

Abdominal CT—tumor mass in the left adrenal area, raising the suspicion of adrenal recurrence.

Findings:

The PET/CT F18-FDG revealed increased pathologic left uptake in the left adrenal area, suggestive for adrenal recurrence of the tumor (Fig. 11.37).

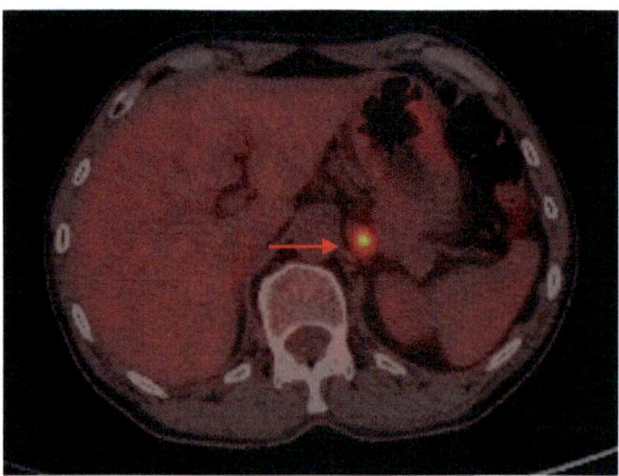

Fig. 11.37 PET/CT F18-FDG transversal slice of fused image, showing a left adrenal tumor mass, with increased uptake of F18-FDG suggestive for left adrenal tumor recurrence

Conclusion:

The diagnosis was right adrenal metastasis, in a patient with colon cancer.

Case 5: Adrenalitis During the Molecular Therapy of Malignant Melanoma on F18-FDG PET/CT Examination

History:

A 37-year-old woman presented with fatigue and headache after receiving three doses of ipilimumab, a monoclonal antibody against cytotoxic T-lymphocyte antigen 4, for the treatment of metastatic melanoma.

Clinical examination:

The patient had severe fatigue and nausea.

Examinations:

Thorax CT—nothing to be mentioned.

Abdominal CT—CT scans of the abdomen show the change in size of adrenal glands during treatment.

Findings:

The PET/CT F18-FDG revealed increased pathologic FDG uptake in both adrenal glands, suggestive for adrenal inflammation ipilimumab-related (Fig. 11.38).

Conclusion:

The diagnosis was adrenalitis ipilimumab-related.

Similar case in Fig. 11.39.

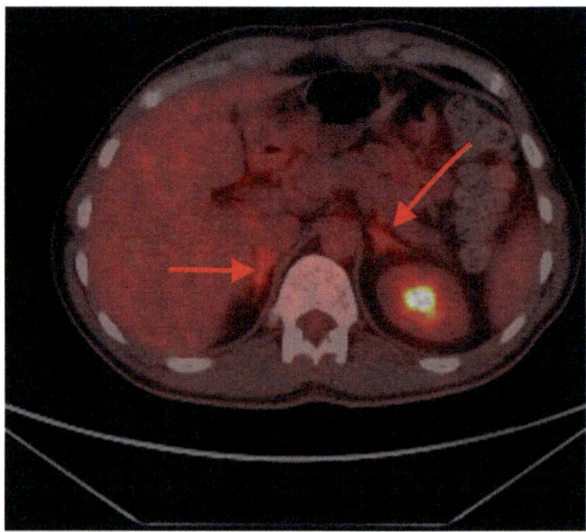

Fig. 11.38 PET/CT F18-FDG transversal slice of fused image, showing a bilateral adrenal increased uptake of F18-FDG suggestive for adrenalitis, in a patient with ipilimumab therapy for metastatic malignant melanoma

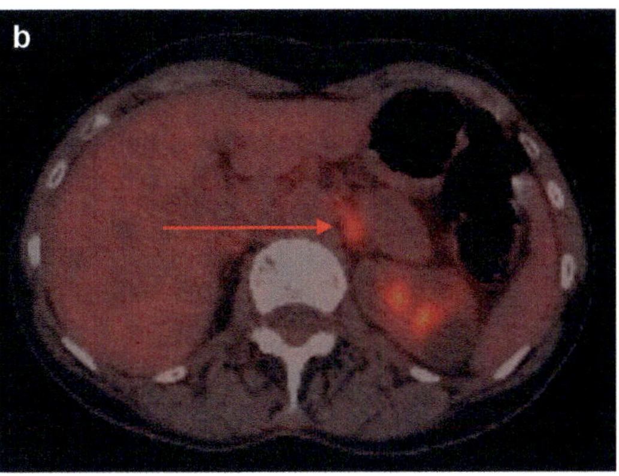

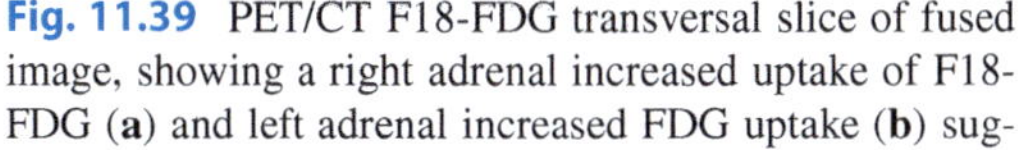

Fig. 11.39 PET/CT F18-FDG transversal slice of fused image, showing a right adrenal increased uptake of F18-FDG (**a**) and left adrenal increased FDG uptake (**b**) suggestive for ipilimumab-related adrenalitis, in a patient with metastatic malignant melanoma

11.9 PET/CT in Neuroendocrine Tumors (NETs)

NETs are rare neoplasms characterized by overexpression of somatostatin receptors (SSTRs). These SSTRs are G-protein-coupled transmembrane receptors and are internalized after binding to specific ligand; among these, SSTR2 and SSTR5 are predominantly overexpressed in NETs. Krenning et al. (1993) published, in a study with more than 1000 patients, that somatostatin receptor scintigraphy (SRS) is an important tool for imaging of NETs and has been shown to be superior as compared to other morphological imaging modalities, for the detection of both primary NET and their metastatic lesions.

Recently introduced PET/CT with Ga-68-labeled somatostatin analogues has shown better results than conventional SRS, based on the principle that Ga-68 SSTR binds to the somatostatin receptors overexpressed on NET cells. The "gold standard" of NET functional imaging, In-111-SSTR, or Tc-99m tektrotyd allows whole-body imaging with planar, SPECT, or SPECT/CT, but nowadays, the name becomes the "old standard," due to rapid development of PET/CT-SSTR, with better resolution and sensitivity.

Three major Ga-68 SSTRs are currently available for imaging, all having gallium-68 a positron emitter, DOTA (tetraazacyclododecane-tetraacetic acid), and another chain, as follows:

- Ga-68 DOTATOC: Ga-68 DOTA-Phe^{1}-Tyr^{3}-Octreotide-affinity for SSTR2 and SSTR5
- Ga-68 DOTANOC: Ga-68 DOTA-Nal^{3}-Octreotide-affinity for SSTR2, SSTR5,
- and SSTR3
- Ga-68 DOTATATE: Ga-68 DOTA-Thy^{3}-Thre^{8}-Octreotide (octreotate)-affinity for SSTR2 and SSTR5

Recent studies (Deppen et al. 2016) evaluated toxicity related to administration of Ga-68 DOTATATE, a tracer with high-affinity binding to subtype 2A, and compared with In-111 pentetreotide imaging. The authors showed that PET/CT changed management in 37% of patients. In-111 pentetreotide did not add value compared with Ga-68 DOTATATE in any patient. Given the superior performance for tumor detection, lower radiation dosimetry, and shorter completion time, their results conclusively demonstrate that Ga-68 DOTATATE PET/CT imaging is safe and should replace In-111 pentetreotide imaging, where available.

Despite different affinities, there is currently no evidence of a clinical impact of these differences in SSTR binding affinity, and therefore no preferential use of one compound over the others can be advised.

A comprehensive overview of Ga-68 SSTR PET/CT was published in 2014 (Sharma et al.), where the authors underlined the advantages of Ga-68 SSTR over SRS. Behind the economic reasons, the higher resolution, they mentioned that Ga-68 SSTR has about tenfold higher affinity for SSTRs as compared to SRS. Also, the Ga-68 DOTANOC has broad-spectrum affinity for SSTRs (SSTR2, SSTR3, and SSTR5) as compared to SRS (SSTR2 only) and provides the possibility of quantification of the tracer uptake in a given region of interest (SUV).

In gastroenteropancreatic NET (GEP-NET), Ga-68 SSTR has a sensitivity of 93% and specificity of 91% (Treglia, 2012), while other authors (Ambrosini 2012) showed specificity of 98%. The ESMO (2012) and European Neuroendocrine Tumor Society (ENETS) and the World Health Organization (WHO) recommend the use of either mitotic rate or Ki-67 labeling index, for GEP-NETs. Tumors with higher Ki-67 expression are associated with poorer prognosis. In this case, there is a well-defined place also for F18-FDG PET/CT. Since 1998, Adams et al. have showed a linear relationship between higher proliferative rate (Ki-67) and uptake of the F18-FDG. A cutoff value was established at Ki-67 > 10%.

In lung NET, the majority of them are typical carcinoids, with good prognosis, where the role of Ga-68 SSTR is a little controversial; in different studies, the results are equivocal and the number of patients very limited (Jindal et al. 2011); compared with F18-FDG (Kayani et al. 2009), Ga-68 SSTR was superior in the differential diagnosis of atypical/typical carcinoids.

Prasad et al. (2010) were the first to evaluate the role of Ga-68 SSTR PET/CT for metastatic unknown primary tumor. They demonstrated that PET/CT was able to localize the primary tumor in 59% of the patients.

In other NET the role of Ga-68 SSTR PET/CT is considered in direct relation to overexpression of SSTR (Sollini et al. 2014):

- Paraganglioma: the majority are SSTR2 and SSTR1
- Pheochromocytoma: predominantly SSTR2 and SSTR1
- Pituitary adenoma:
  - GH secreting: mostly SSTR2 and SSTR5
  - ACTH secreting: predominantly SSTR2 and SSTR5
  - TSH secreting: SSTR2, SSTR3, and SSTR5
  - PRL secreting: SSTR1 and SSTR5

In case of negative I-123 MIBG scan in patients with a high pretest probability of pheochromocytoma or paraganglioma, Ga-68 SSTR PET/CT should be considered as the next investigation. Additionally, PET/CT should be considered in the staging of patients in whom metastatic spread, particularly to the bone, is suspected.

The overexpression of SSTR has been reported in highest-grade gliomas, and it may be an interesting target for PRRT. Ga-68 SSTR PET/CT has been used to select patients for PRRT and to evaluate treatment response combined with other imaging modalities.

A summary of hybrid PET/CT imaging in NET is presented in Fig. 11.40.

EANM/SNMMI/ESMO Recommendations

1. DOTA PET imaging is imaging of choice in GEP-NET.
2. DOTA PET imaging is superior to MIBG in pheochromocytoma.
3. DOTA PET imaging is superior to octreotide in unknown primary NET.
4. FDG PET is indicated in grade 2/3 NET/NEC.
5. FDG PET is useful to predict prognosis.
6. DOTATOC PET is equal to DOTATATE PET.

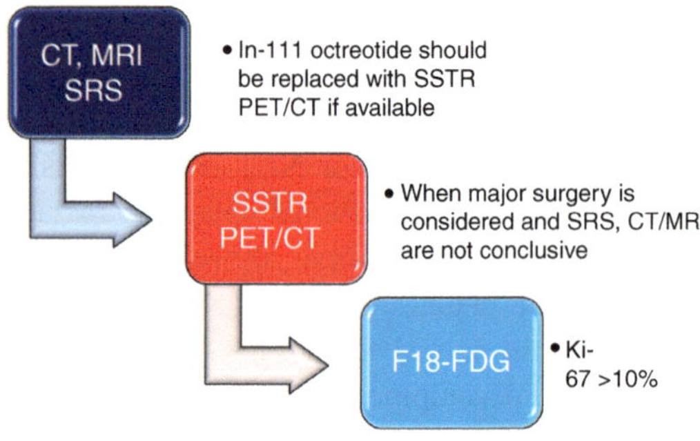

Fig. 11.40 Protocol of imaging in NET

Case 1: Well-Differentiated NET Grade 2 on F18-FDG PET/CT Examination

History:

A 67-year-old female, with the diagnosis of liver metastasis of well-differentiated NET and low-grade Ki-67 < 7%, diagnosed by liver biopsy, was referred for PET/CT FDG for the evaluation of the extent of the disease and for the diagnostic of the primary tumor.

Clinical examination:

The patient had mild abdominal pain, weight loss, jaundice, diarrhea, and nausea.

Examinations:

Thorax CT—nothing to be mentioned.

Abdominal contrast CT—tumor mass in the left liver lobe, raising the suspicion of metastasis.

Findings:

The PET/CT F18-FDG revealed *NO* increased pathologic uptake in the liver and failed to discover the primary NET (Fig. 11.41).

Conclusion:

The diagnosis was liver NET without pathologic FDG uptake.

Similar case is presented in Fig. 11.42; the NET located in the head of the pancreas does not express high aggressiveness and does not uptake FDG pathologically.

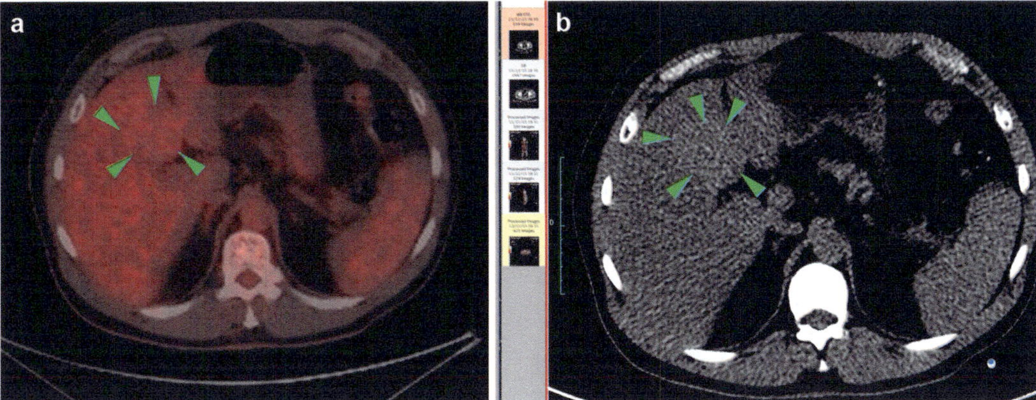

Fig. 11.41 PET/CT F18-FDG transversal slice of fused image PET/CT (**a**) and CT slice (**b**) showing normal FDG distribution; the exam failed to detect the primary tumor

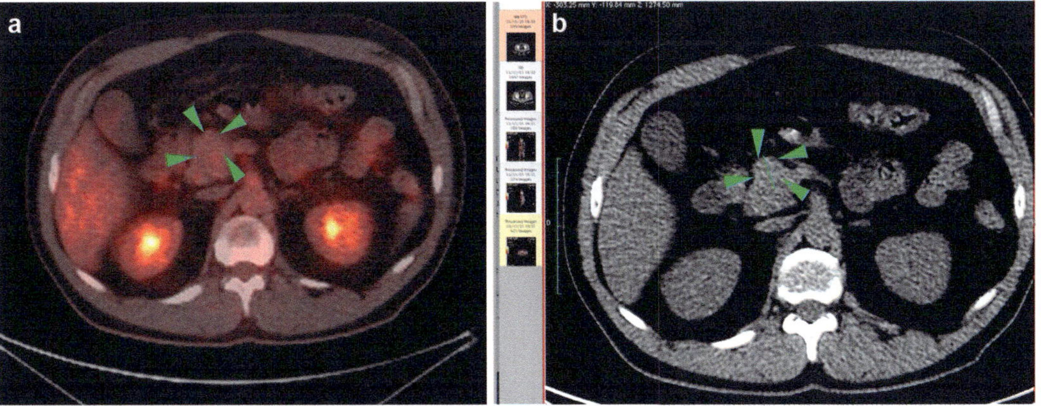

Fig. 11.42 PET/CT F18-FDG transversal slice of fused image PET/CT (**a**) and CT (**b**), showing normal FDG distribution; the NET located in the head of the pancreas has normal FDG distribution

Case 2: Ileum NEC (Neuroendocrine Carcinoma) with Liver Metastases on F18-FDG PET/CT Examination

History:

A 58-year-old female, with the diagnosis of liver metastasis of poorly differentiated NEC and G3 Ki-67 82%, diagnosed by liver biopsy, was referred for PET/CT FDG for the evaluation of the extent of the disease and for the diagnostic of the primary tumor.

Clinical examination:

The patient had severe abdominal pain; important weight loss, headache, and nausea.

*Examinations***:**

Thorax CT—nothing to be mentioned.

Abdominal contrast CT—multiple metastases in the liver.

*Findings***:**

The PET/CT F18-FDG revealed multiple tumor masses in the liver with increased pathologic uptake; also there was detection of primary NEC, in the ileum (Fig. 11.43).

*Conclusion***:**

The diagnosis was ileum NEC with multiple liver metastases.

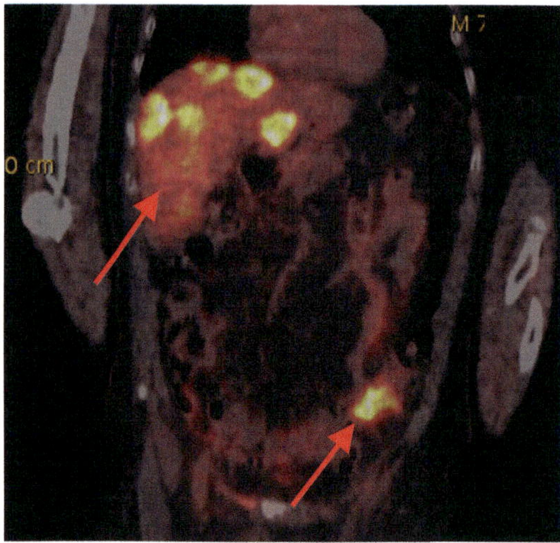

Fig. 11.43 PET/CT F18-FDG coronal slice of fused image PET/CT showing pathological increased FDG uptake in the ileum NEC (neuroendocrine carcinoma) and the liver metastases; the NEC was grade 3 and stage IV

Key Points

- F18-FDG is a marker of aggressiveness in NET, so the positive image plays a role in the prognosis and in therapy monitoring.

Case 3: Ileum NET on Ga-68 DOTATOC PET/CT Examination

History:

A 61-year-old female, with the diagnosis of ileum NET G2 and Ki 67–11%, was operated 1 year before; during the follow-up, Ga-68 DOTATOC PET/CT was performed for the evaluation of the remission.

Clinical examination:

The patient had no clinical signs and no positive imaging tests.

*Examinations***:**

Thorax CT—nothing to be mentioned.

Abdominal contrast CT—nothing pathologic to be mentioned; partial ileum resection.

*Findings***:**

The Ga-68 DOTATOC PET/CT revealed no pathologic uptake of the tracer, except a discrete hyperactivity in the left thyroid lobe (Fig. 11.44).

*Conclusion***:**

The diagnosis was ileum NET in complete remission; suspicion of thyroid nodule in the left lobe and possible medullary thyroid tumor. The patient was referred to an endocrinologist and had the following results:

Anti-Tg 20 kIU/L (N.V. <115 kIU/L)—normal.

TSH 2.1mIU/L (N.V. 0.4–4.5 mIU/L)—normal.

Calcitonin 139 pg/mL (N.V. < 13 pg/mL)—increased.

Thyroid ultrasound revealed—hypoechogenic nodule in the left thyroid lobe of 17/12 mm, with irregular margins that exacerbate intranodular vascularity.

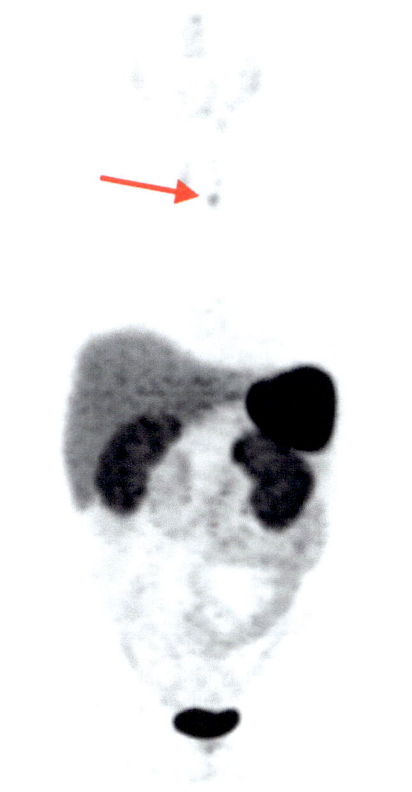

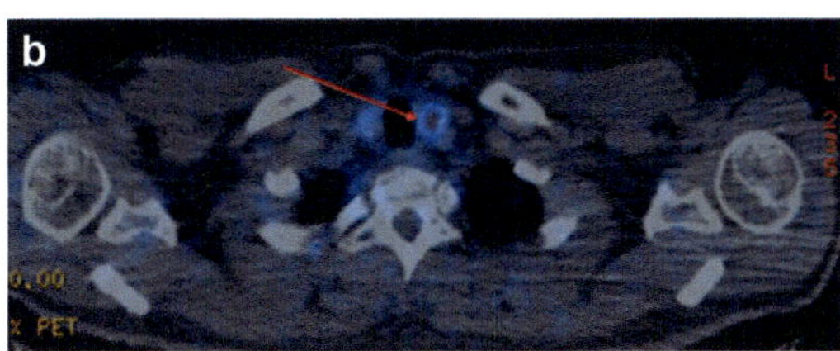

Fig. 11.44 Ga-68 DOTATOC PET/CT coronal slice of fused image PET/CT showing pathological increased uptake in the left thyroid lobe (**a**) and transversal slice (**b**); complete remission of ileum NET; the uptake was related to a medullary thyroid carcinoma

The patient refused the FNAB and genetic test being submitted to total thyroidectomy, with the histologic result of medullary thyroid carcinoma T1N0Mx.

11.10 PET/CT in Endocrine Receptor Imaging

Estrogen receptor imaging: F18-estradiol (FES)-PET/CT

Breast cancers in the majority of cases have low affinity for F18-FDG, so this imaging test is not routinely recommended for the diagnosis of primary tumor. If the aggressiveness of the tumor is high, FDG PET/CT turns rapidly in a positive test (Fig. 11.45).

A more personalized approach is knowing the receptor expression in different tumors, which is the key for targeted cancer therapy. Tumor receptor imaging aims to characterize the tumor biology, the therapeutic targets, and the pharmacodynamics of targeted treatments.

Breast cancer is already identified as one of the most suggestive examples. The metastases and the primary tumor sometimes express different cellular lines, so the treatments not always will act similarly in all sites of the tumor. The expression of estrogen receptors in the primary breast tumor and its metastases might be different, so the possibility of knowing this in a noninvasive manner would be of special importance and interest. Nowadays, it is possible to use such a protocol, considering estrogen receptor imaging, as is presented in Fig. 11.46.

Androgen receptor imaging: F18-dihydrotestosterone (FDHT)-PET/CT

In prostate cancer, like in breast cancer, F18-FDG normally is not indicated in front line, due to its well-differentiated pattern. Other PET tracers have been explored: F18-fluorocholine, F18-prostate-specific membrane antigen (PSMA), C-11 acetate-targeting lipogenesis, tracers radiolabeling bombesin and targeting gastrin-releasing peptide receptor (GRPR), and amino acid transport with anti-1-amino-3-F18-fluorocyclobutane-1-carboxylic acid (FACBC). Among these tracers is F18-fluoro-5α-dihydrotestosterone (FDHT), which was designated to target the androgen receptors. There are several drugs already

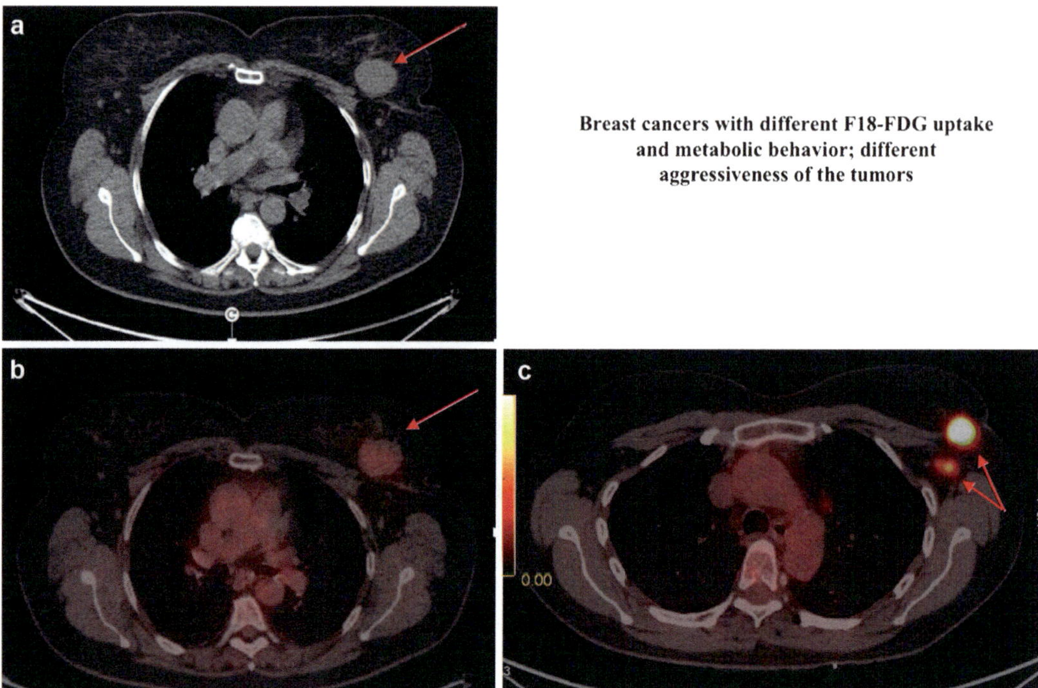

Fig. 11.45 F18-FDG PET/CT transversal slices of CT (**a**), fused image F18-FDG PET/CT (**b**) showing slight increased uptake in a tumor of the left breast; and transversal slice F18-FDG PET/CT (**c**) of a similar located tumor, but with completely different aggressiveness, with high FDG uptake and with an axillary lymph node metastasis

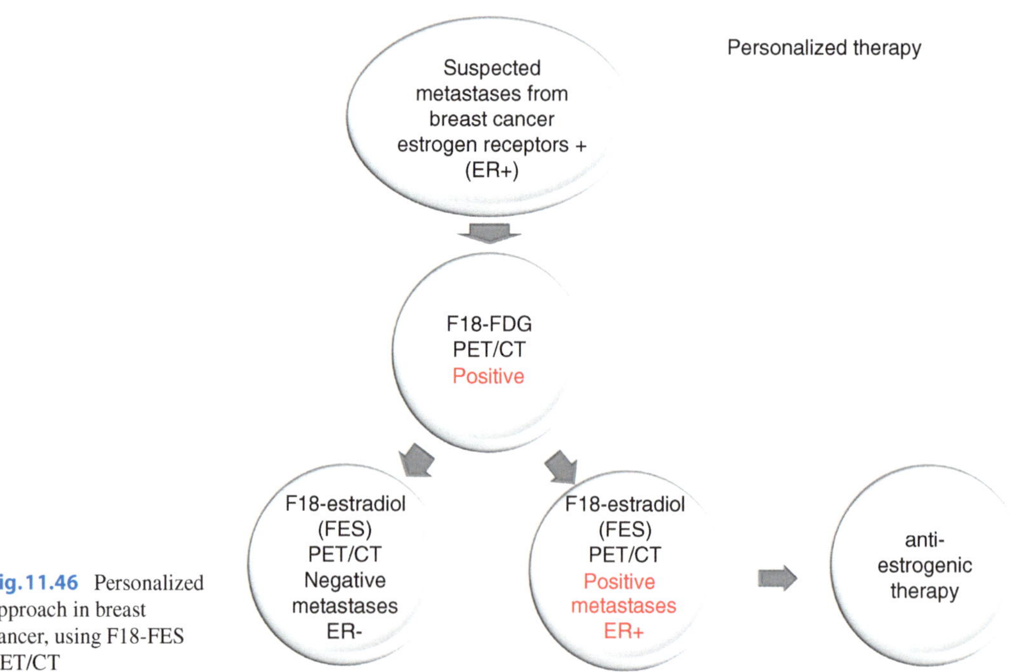

Fig. 11.46 Personalized approach in breast cancer, using F18-FES PET/CT

approved to be used in these cases, imaging being specific and systemic, unfortunately not yet largely available to common use.

11.11 PET/CT in Ovaries and Testis

Ovarian tumors: F18-FDG PET/CT

In premenopausal patients, normal endometrial uptake of F18-FDG changes cyclically, increasing during the ovulatory and menstrual phases. This physiologic expression in hybrid imaging should be known and mentioned in the report. It has a particular importance in case of already established diagnosis of cancer. Increased uptake in the endometrium adjacent to a cervical tumor does not necessarily reflect endometrial tumor invasion. Increased ovarian uptake in postmenopausal patients is associated with malignancy (Fig. 11.47), whereas increased ovarian uptake may be functional in premenopausal patients (Fig. 11.48). In case of pure cystic or benign enlarged ovary, the uptake is normal (Fig. 11.49). In women of reproductive age, the imaging should preferably be done within a week before or a few days after the menstrual flow phase to avoid any misinterpretation of pelvic F18-FDG PET image. Borderline ovarian tumors (BOTs) are more common in young women of

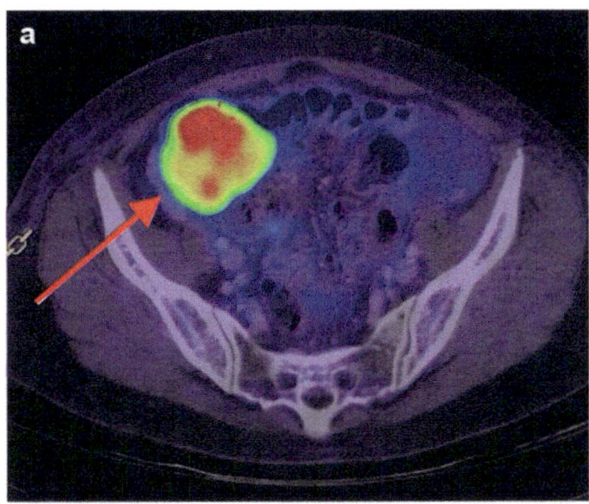

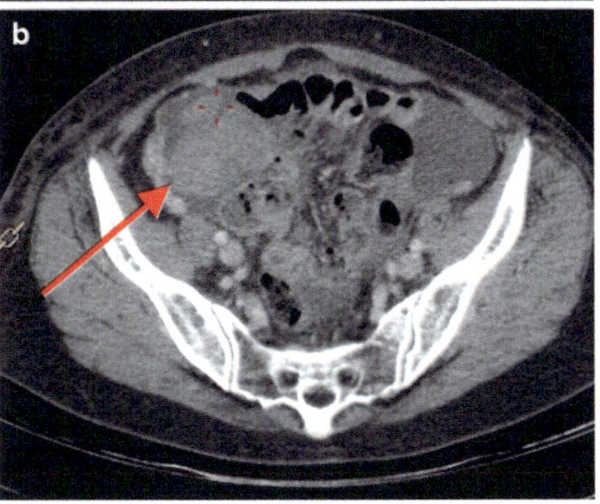

Fig. 11.47 F18-FDG PET/CT transversal slices of fused image F18-FDG PET/CT (**a**) and CT (**b**), showing increased uptake in a right ovarian tumor confirmed, ovarian adenocarcinoma

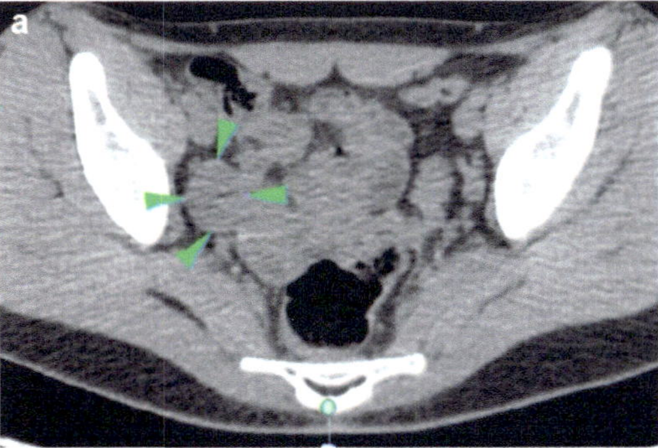

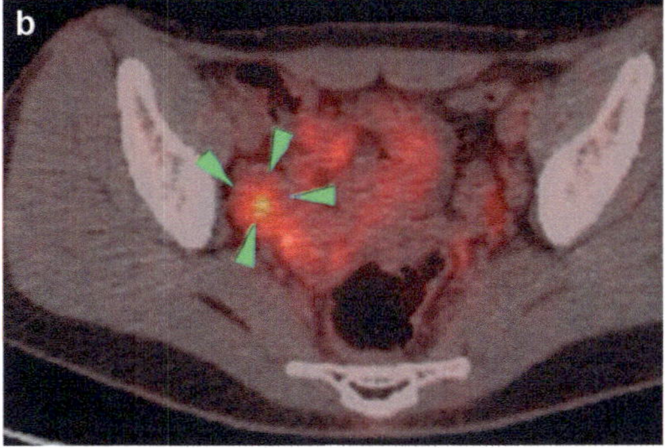

Fig. 11.48 F18-FDG PET/CT transversal slices of fused image F18-FDG PET/CT showing benign increased F18-FDG uptake in a right ovarian cyst during the menstrual phase

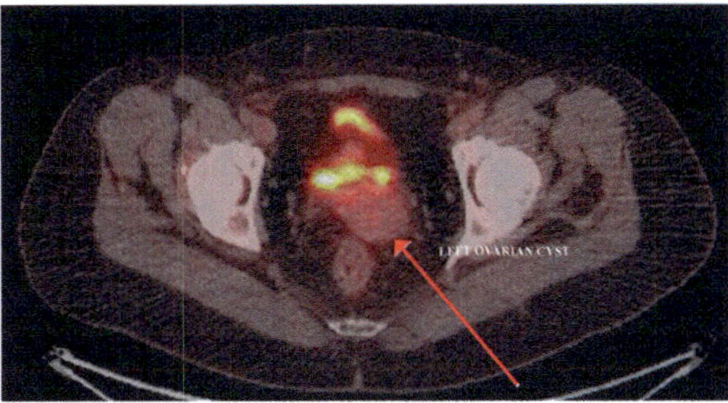

Fig. 11.49 F18-FDG PET/CT transversal slices of fused image F18-FDG PET/CT showing normal to low F18-FDG uptake in a left ovarian cyst (Piciu D, 2016)

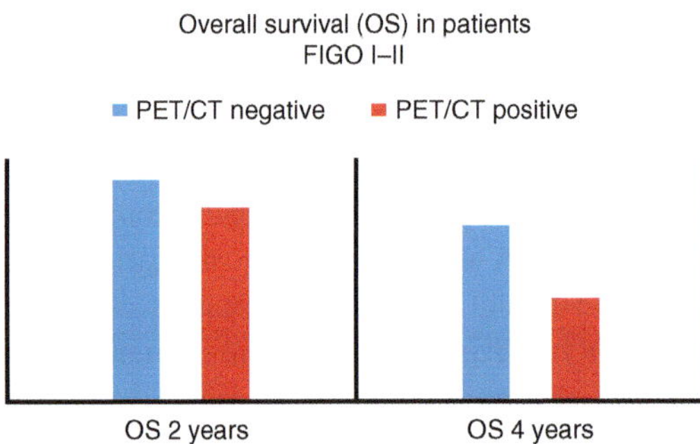

Fig. 11.50 The difference in overall survival (OS) rates at 2 and 4 years, between same FIGO group I and II, according to negative or positive F18-FDG PET/CT status (adapted from Caobelli F et al. 2016)

reproductive age and exhibit a better prognosis than malignant ovarian tumors (MOTs). F18-FDG PET/CT was used to differentiate BOTs from stage I MOTs (Kim et al. 2013). The author mentioned that SUV max was significantly lower in BOT group than in MOT stage I: 2.9 ± 1.5 vs 6.6 ± 2.9 (p = 0.0223).

The hybrid imaging PET/CT became an essential tool in monitoring the ovarian cancer disease. It has a prognostic value as was demonstrated by Caobelli et al. (2016). The authors mentioned that in same FIGO group I and II the patients with positive F18-FDG PET/CT have significant lower overall survival rates at 4 years than those with negative PET/CT (p = 0.003) (Fig. 11.50, adapted from Caobelli).

Testicular tumors: F18-FDG PET/CT

In male gonads, the topic where F18-FDG PET imaging has been used the most is the testicular tumors. PET with F18-FDG has no defined role in imaging of primary tumors where CT is the first-choice imaging modality. For assessing the success of chemotherapy in the presence of residual masses, especially in pure seminoma, F18-FDG PET has an important role. In nonseminomatous tumors, false-negative results are a common problem. F18-FDG PET performs best in predicting relapse in seminoma and in the evaluation of postchemotherapy residual mass in both seminoma and nonseminomatous germ cell tumors of the testis. After chemotherapy, for the assessment of a US-, CT-, or MR-visualized residual mass, F18-FDG PET/CT should be the test of choice, being a critical step in determining the subsequent management approach of these tumors (Figs. 11.51 and 11.52).

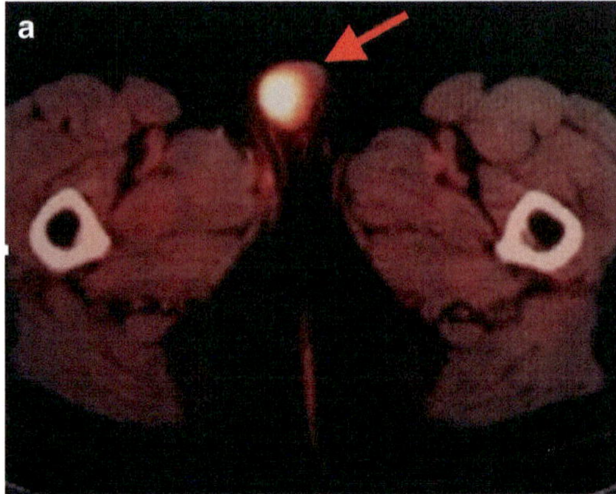

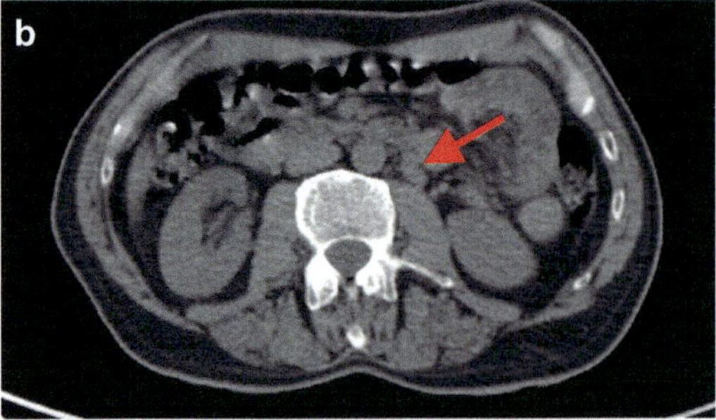

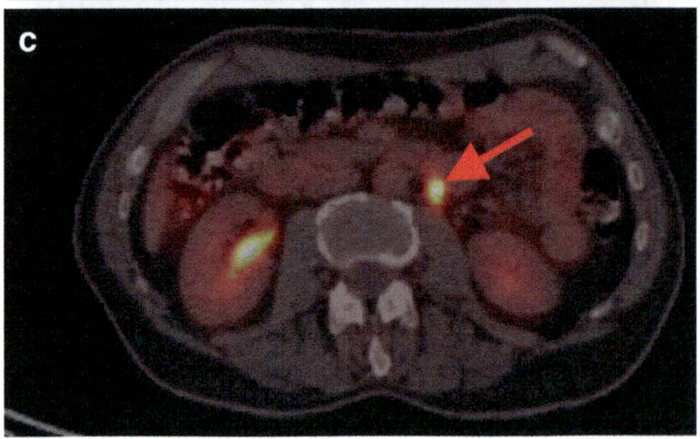

Fig. 11.51 F18-FDG PET/CT transversal slices (**a**) showing right testicular tumor with high F18-FDG uptake; PET/CT transversal slices of CT (**b**), fused image F18-FDG PET/CT (**c**) showing increased pathologic uptake in an abdominal lymph node mass in a case of operated seminoma postchemotherapy, suggesting persistent disease

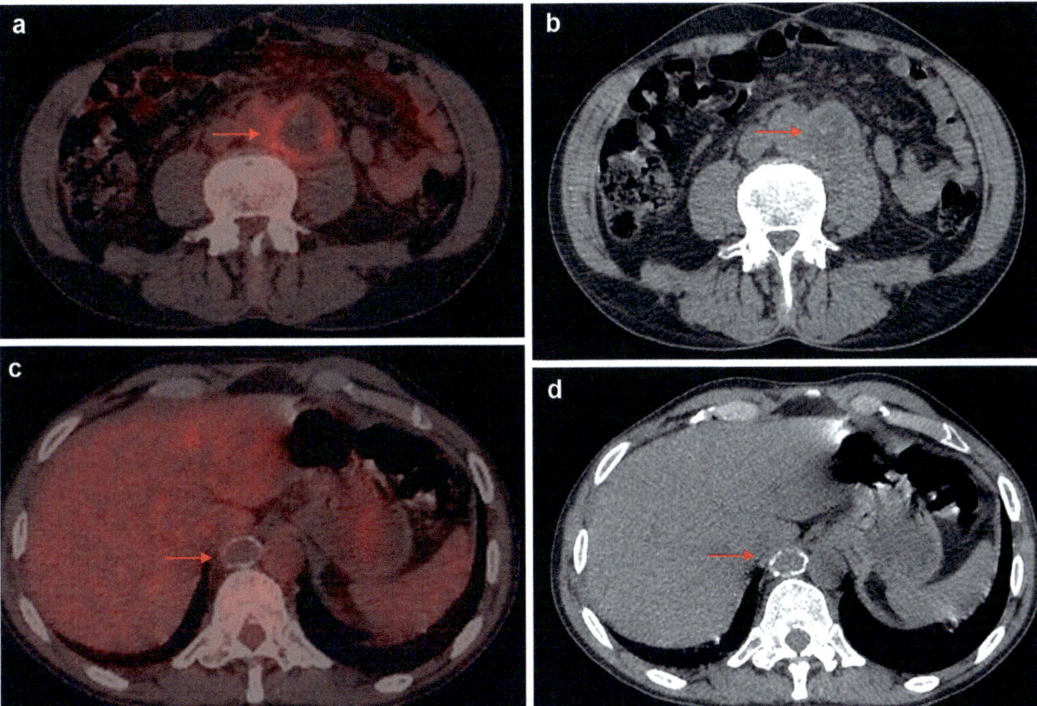

Fig. 11.52 F18-FDG PET/CT transversal slices of fused image F18-FDG PET/CT (**a** and **c**) and CT (**b** and **d**) showing abdominal residual masses in a case of seminoma postchemotherapy, with low uptake suggesting metabolic remission, despite the aspect of structural CT images

Further Reading

Adams S, Baum RP, Hertel A et al (1998) Metabolic (PET) and receptor (SPET) imaging of well- and less well-differentiated tumours: comparison with the expression of the Ki-67 antigen. Nucl Med Commun 19(7):641–647

Ambrosini V, Campana D, Nanni C et al (2012) Is Ga68-DOTA-NOC PET/CT indicated in patients with clinical, biochemical or radiological suspicion of neuroendocrine tumour? Eur J Nucl Med Mol Imaging 39(8):1278–1283

Ambrosini V, Campana D, Tomassetti P et al (2012) Ga68-labelled peptides for diagnosis of gastroenteropancreatic NET. Eur J Nucl Med Mol Imaging 39 Suppl 1: S52–S60

Ambrosini V, Nicolini S, Caroli P et al (2012) PET/CT imaging in different types of lung cancer: an overview. Eur J Radiol 81(5):988–1001.

Archier A, Heimburger C, Guerin C et al (2016) (18) F-DOPA PET/CT in the diagnosis and localization of persistent medullary thyroid carcinoma. Eur J Nucl Med Mol Imaging 43(6):1027–1033

Baras N, Dahm S, Haberland J et al (2017) Subsequent malignancies among long-term survivors of Hodgkin lymphoma and non-Hodgkin lymphoma: a pooled analysis of German cancer registry data (1990-2012). Br J Haematol. ;177(2):226–242 doi: 10.1111/bjh.14530. [Epub ahead of print]

Basu S, Rubello D. (2008) PET imaging in the management of tumors of testis and ovary: current thinking and future directions. Minerva Endocrinol 33(3):229–256.

Bertagna F, Bosio G, Biasiotto G et al (2009) A- F-18 FDG-PET/CT evaluation of patients with differentiated thyroid cancer with negative I-131 total body scan and high thyroglobulin level. Clin Nucl Med 34(11):756–761

Bertagna F, Treglia G, Piccardo A, Giubbini R (2012) Diagnostic and clinical significance of F-18-FDG-PET/CT thyroid incidentalomas J Clin Endocrinol Metab 97 (11): 3866–3875

Bogsrud TV, Karantanis D, Nathan MA et al (2007) The value of quantifying 18F-FDG uptake in thyroid nodules found incidentally on whole-body PET-CT. Nucl Med Commun 28:373–381

Caobelli F, Alongi P, Evangelista L et al (2016) Predictive value of (18) F-FDG PET/CT in restaging patients

affected by ovarian carcinoma: a multicentre study. Eur J Nucl Med Mol Imaging 43(3):404–413
Chang CA, Pattison DA, Tothill RW et al (2016) (68)Ga-DOTATATE and (18)F-FDG PET/CT in Paraganglioma and Pheochromocytoma: utility, patterns and heterogeneity Cancer Imaging;16(1):22
Chittiboina P, Montgomery BK, Millo C et al (2015) High-resolution (18)F-fluorodeoxyglucose positron emission tomography and magnetic resonance imaging for pituitary adenoma detection in Cushing disease. J Neurosurg 122(4):791–797
Chin BB, Patel P, Cohade C et al (2004) Recombinant human thyrotropin stimulation of fluoro-D-glucose positron emission tomography uptake in well-differentiated thyroid carcinoma. J Clin Endocrinol Metab 89:91–95
Choi JY, Lee KS, Kim HJ et al (2006) Focal thyroid lesions incidentally identified by integrated 18F-FDG PET/CT: clinical significance and improved characterization. J Nucl Med 47:609–615
Fahy FH. (2009) Dosimetry of pediatric PET/CT. J Nucl Med 50:1483–1491
Deppen SA, Liu E, Blume JD et al (2016) Safety and efficacy of 68Ga-DOTATATE PET/CT for diagnosis, staging, and treatment management of neuroendocrine tumors. J Nucl Med 57(5):708–714
Deppen SA, Blume J, Bobbey AJ et al (2016) 68Ga-DOTATATE compared with 111In-DTPA-Octreotide and conventional imaging for pulmonary and gastroenteropancreatic neuroendocrine tumors: a systematic review and meta-analysis. J Nucl Med 57(6):872–878
deGroot JW, Links TP, Jager PL (2004) Impact of 18F-fluoro-2-deoxy-D-glucose positron emission tomography (FDG-PET) in patients with biochemical evidence of recurrent or residual medullary thyroid cancer. Ann Surg Oncol 11:786–794
Giraudet AL, Taïeb D (2016) PET imaging for thyroid cancers: current status and future directions. Ann Endocrinol (Paris). doi:10.1016/j.ando.2016.10.002. pii:S0003-4266(16)31139-8 [Epub ahead of print]
Perros P et al. (2014) Guidelines for the management of thyroid cancer in adults. 3rd ed. Publication unit of the Royal College of Physicians. British Thyroid Association and Royal College of Physicians, London. Clin Endocrinol 81 (Suppl. 1), 1–122
Haugen BR, Alexander EK, Bible KC et al (2016) American Thyroid Association management guidelines for adult patients with thyroid nodules and differentiated thyroid cancer: The American Thyroid Association guidelines task force on thyroid nodules and differentiated thyroid cancer. Thyroid 26(1):1–133
Iagaru A, Kalinyak JE, McDougall IR (2007) F-18 FDG PET/CT in the management of thyroid cancer. Clin Nucl Med 32(9):690–695
Iagaru A, McDougall IR (2007) F-18 FDG PET/CT demonstration of an adrenal metastasis in a patient with anaplastic thyroid cancer. Clin Nucl Med 32(1):13–15
Jeong SY, Lee SW, Lee HJ et al (2010) Incidental pituitary uptake on whole-body 18F-FDG PET/CT: a multicentre study. Eur J Nucl Med Mol Imaging 37(12):2334–2343
Jindal T, Kumar A, Venkitaraman B et al (2011) Evaluation of the role of [18F] FDG-PET/CT and [68Ga] DOTATOC-PET/CT in differentiating typical and atypical pulmonary carcinoids. Cancer Imaging 15:70–75
Kayani I, Conry BG, Groves AA et al (2009) A comparison of 68Ga-DOTATATE and 18F-FDG PET/CT in pulmonary neuroendocrine tumors. J Nucl Med 50(12):1927–1932
Kang KW, Kim SK, Kang HS et al (2003) Prevalence and risk of cancer of focal thyroid incidentaloma identified by 18F-fluorodeoxyglucose positron emission tomography for metastasis evaluation and cancer screening in healthy subjects. J Clin Endocrinol Metab 88:4100–4104
Kim C, Chung H, Oh SW et al (2013). Differential diagnosis of borderline ovarian tumors from stage I malignant ovarian tumors using FDG PET/CT Nucl Med Mol Imag 47(2), 81–88.
Komninos J, Vlassopoulou V, Protopapa D (2004) Tumors metastatic to the pituitary gland: case report and literature review 89 (2): 574–580
Krenning EP, Kwekkeboom DJ, Bakker WH et al (1993) Somatostatin receptor scintigraphy with [111In-DTPA-D-Phe1]- and [123I-Tyr3]-octreotide: The Rotterdam experience with more than 1000 patients. Eur J Nucl Med 20:716–731.
Kroiss A, Putzer D, Uprimny C et al (2011) Functional imaging in phaeochromocytoma and neuroblastoma with 68Ga-DOTA-Tyr 3-octreotide positron emission tomography and 123I-metaiodobenzylguanidine. Eur J Nucl Med Mol Imaging 38(5):865–873
Maurice JB, Troke R, Win Z et al A comparison of the performance of Ga68-DOTATATE PET/CT and I123-MIBG SPECT in the diagnosis and follow-up of phaeochromocytoma and paraganglioma. Eur J Nucl Med Mol Imaging 2012;39:1266–1270.
Michaud L, Burgess A, Huchet V et al (2014) Is 18F-fluorocholine-positron emission tomography/computerized tomography a new imaging tool for detecting hyperfunctioning parathyroid glands in primary or secondary hyperparathyroidism? J Clin Endocrinol Metab 99(12):4531–4536
Michaud L, Balogova S, Burgess A et al (2015) A pilot comparison of 18F-fluorocholine PET/CT, ultrasonography and 123I/99mTc-sestaMIBI dual-phase dual-isotope scintigraphy in the preoperative localization of hyperfunctioning parathyroid glands in primary or secondary hyperparathyroidism: influence of thyroid anomalies Medicine 94(41):e1701
McDougall IR, Davidson J, Segall GM (2001) Positron emission tomography of the thyroid, with an emphasis on thyroid cancer. Nucl Med Commun 22(5): 485–492
Nahas Z, Goldenberg D, Fakhry C et al (2005) The role of positron emission tomography/computed tomography in the management of recurrent papillary thyroid carcinoma. Laryngoscope 115:237–243

National Comprehensive Cancer Network)(2016 National Comprehensive Cancer Network Clinical Practice Guidelines in Oncology. Thyroid carcinoma, vol 1. http://www.nccn.org/professionals/physician_gls/PDF/thyroid.pdf

Öberg K, Knigge U, Kwekkeboom D, Perren A, on behalf of the ESMO Guidelines Working Group (2012) Neuroendocrine gastro-entero-pancreatic tumors: ESMO Clinical Practice Guidelines for diagnosis, treatment and follow-up. Ann Oncol 23 (suppl_7): vii124-vii130

Palmedo H, Bucerius J, Joe A et al (2006) Integrated PET/CT in differentiated thyroid cancer: diagnostic accuracy and impact on patient management. J Nucl Med 47(4):616–624

Petrich T, Borner AR, Otto D et al (2002) Influence of rhTSH on [(18)F] fluorodeoxyglucose uptake by differentiated thyroid carcinoma. Eur J Nucl Med Mol Imaging 29(5):641–647

Piciu D (2016) Imagistica de fuziune PET/CT in oncologie. Editura Iuliu Hatieganu Cluj-Napoca

Piciu D, Irimie A, Duncea I et al (2010) Positron emission tomography – computer tomography fusion image, with 18-fluoro-2-deoxyD-glucose in the follow-up of patients with differentiated thyroid carcinoma. Acta Endocrinol (Buc) 6:15–26. doi:10.4183/aeb.2010.15

Piciu D, Pestean C, Barbus E et al (2016) Second malignancies in patients with differentiated thyroid carcinoma treated with low and medium activities of radioactive I-131. Clujul Med 89(3):384–389

Prasad V, Ambrosini V, Hommann M et al (2010) Detection of unknown primary neuroendocrine tumors (CUP-NET) using 68Ga-DOTANOC receptor PET-CT. Eur J Nucl Med Mol Imaging 37:67–77

Putzer D, Gabriel M, Kendler D et al (2010) Comparison of (68)Ga-DOTA-Tyr(3)-octreotide and (18)F-fluoro-L-dihydroxyphenylalanine positron emission tomography in neuroendocrine tumor patients. Q J Nucl Med Mol Imaging 54(1):68–75

Robbins RJ, Wan Q, Grewal RK et al (2006) Real-time prognosis for metastatic thyroid carcinoma based on FDG-PET scanning. J Clin Endocrinol Metab 91:498–505

Sandeep TC, Strachan MW, Reynolds RM et al (2006) Second primary cancers in thyroid cancer patients: a multinational record linkage study. J Clin Endocrinol Metab 91:1819–1825

Schluter B, Bohuslavizki KH, Beyer W et al (2001) Impact of FDG PET on patients with differentiated thyroid cancer who present with elevated thyroglobulin and negative 131- I scan. J Nucl Med 42(1):71–76

Seong Bae J, Chae BJ, Park CW et al (2009) Incidental thyroid lesions detected by FDG PET/CT: prevalence and risk of thyroid cancer. World J Surg Oncol 7(1):63–69

Singh I, Bikas A, Garcia CA et al (2017) (18)F-FDG-PET SUV as a prognostic marker of increasing size in thyroid cancer tumors. Endocr Pract 23(2):182–189

Sharma P, Singh H, Bal C, Kumar R (2014) PET/CT imaging of neuroendocrine tumors with (68)Gallium-labeled somatostatin analogues: an overview and single institutional experience from India. Indian J Nucl Med 29(1):2–12

Sollini M, Erba PA, Fraternali A et al (2014) PET and PET/CT with 68gallium-labeled somatostatin analogues in NonGEP-NETs tumors Scientific World J 13;194123

Soelberg KK, Bonnema SJ, Brix TH, Hegedüs L (2012) Risk of malignancy in thyroid incidentalomas detected by 18F-fluorodeoxyglucose positron emission tomography: a systematic review. Thyroid 22(9):918–925

Sundin A. Adrenal (2016) Molecular imaging Front Horm Res 45:70–79

The American Thyroid Association (ATA). Guidelines Taskforce on Thyroid Nodules and Differentiated Thyroid Cancer (2009) Revised American Thyroid Association Management Guidelines for patients with thyroid nodules and differentiated thyroid cancer. Thyroid 19(11):1195–1214

Treglia G, Castaldi P, Rindi G et al (2012) Diagnostic performance of Gallium-68 somatostatin receptor PET and PET/CT in patients with thoracic and gastroenteropancreatic neuroendocrine tumors: a meta-analysis. Endocrine 42:80–87.

Verkooijen RB, Smit JW, Romijn JA et al (2006) The incidence of second primary tumours in thyroid cancer patients is increased, but not related to treatment of thyroid cancer. Eur J Endocrinol 155:801–806

Index

D. Piciu, *Nuclear Endocrinology*, DOI 10.1007/978-3-319-56582-8

S

U

GPSR Compliance

The European Union's (EU) General Product Safety Regulation (GPSR) is a set of rules that requires consumer products to be safe and our obligations to ensure this.

If you have any concerns about our products, you can contact us on ProductSafety@springernature.com

In case Publisher is established outside the EU, the EU authorized representative is:

Springer Nature Customer Service Center GmbH
Europaplatz 3
69115 Heidelberg, Germany

Batch number: 10371063

Printed by Printforce, the Netherlands